CULTURAL AWARENESS
IN NURSING AND HEALTH CARE

CULTURAL AWARENESS IN NURSING AND HEALTH CARE

An Introductory Text

SECOND EDITION

Karen Holland SRN BSc(Hons) RNT MSc
Research Fellow, School of Nursing, University of Salford, Manchester, UK

Christine Hogg BSc(Econ) RGN RMN PgDE MSc PhD
Senior Lecturer, School of Nursing, University of Salford, Manchester, UK

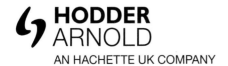

HODDER
ARNOLD

AN HACHETTE UK COMPANY

First published in Great Britain in 2001 by Arnold
This second edition published in 2010 by
Hodder Arnold, an imprint of Hodder Education, an Hachette UK company,
338 Euston Road, London NW1 3BH

http://www.hodderarnold.com

Hachette UK's policy is to use papers that are natural, renewable and recyclable products and made from wood grown in sustainable forests. The logging and manufacturing processes are expected to conform to the environmental regulations of the country of origin.

Whilst the advice and information in this book are believed to be true and accurate at the date of going to press, neither the authors nor the publisher can accept any legal responsibility or liability for any errors or omissions that may be made. In particular (but without limiting the generality of the preceding disclaimer) every effort has been made to check drug dosages; however it is still possible that errors have been missed. Furthermore, dosage schedules are constantly being revised and new side-effects recognized. For these reasons the reader is strongly urged to consult the drug companies' printed instructions before administering any of the drugs recommended in this book.

British Library Cataloguing in Publication Data
A catalogue record for this book is available from the British Library

Library of Congress Cataloging-in-Publication Data
A catalog record for this book is available from the Library of Congress

ISBN   978-0-340-97290-8
2 3 4 5 6 7 8 9 10

Commissioning Editor:	Naomi Wilkinson
Project Editor:	Joanna Silman
Production Controller:	Rachel Manguel
Cover Design:	Lynda King
Indexer:	Lisa Footitt

Cover image © Getty Images

Typeset in ITC Century Light 10pt by Transet Ltd., Coventry, England.
Printed in India

What do you think about this book? Or any other Hodder Arnold title?
Please visit our website: www.hodderarnold.com

This book is dedicated to my husband Terry and daughter Sera, for their continuing commitment to charitable work and voluntary services, supporting and helping those from all cultures to a better quality of life.

Karen Holland

This book is dedicated to my mum and dad, Ken and Sheila Hogg. Thanks for helping me see people differently.

Christine Hogg

Contents

Foreword viii

Preface ix

Acknowledgments xiii

1. Culture, race and ethnicity: exploring the concepts 1
2. Understanding the theory of health and illness beliefs 16
3. Working with health and illness beliefs in practice 32
4. Religious beliefs and cultural care 43
5. Cultural care: knowledge and skills for implementation in practice 58
6. Culture and mental health 78
7. Women and health care in a multicultural society 99
8. Men and health care in a multicultural society 116
9. Child and family centred care: a cultural perspective 131
10. Care of older people from black and minority ethnic groups 150
11. Caring for the health needs of migrants, refugees and asylum seekers 165
12. Death and bereavement: a cross-cultural perspective 185
13. Cultural diversity and professional practice 199

Appendices 213

References 223

Index 243

Foreword

In the 21st century, many countries have become multicultural in their overall population and local communities. This is partly a result of a global shift in where people choose to live in relation to families and work opportunities. It is also a direct result of natural and man-made disasters and wars, leading to displacement of people from their country of origin or homeland.

For health and social care this has had significant implications for those who seek to ensure equality of care delivery and access across all ages and cultures. In the United Kingdom there has been not only regional and local response to this need but a central government response, with the introduction of strategic direction by the NHS and implementation of guidance for its workforce to deliver culturally appropriate and non-discriminatory care. One such example is the publication of 'Religion or Belief: a practical guide for the NHS' (Department of Health, 2009), which offers a broad overview of possible responses to service user needs as well as a valued resource for nurses and other health care professionals.

'Cultural Awareness in Nursing and Health Care' focuses on more specific care issues, presenting an invaluable, timely resource. Each chapter offers discussion of key concepts related to culture, religion and health beliefs as they impact on individuals and communities, as well as taking into account issues such as gender and age. The authors have combined their long experience and expertise in teaching undergraduate and postgraduate students with their enthusiasm, passion and commitment to cross-cultural health care.

This text combines a pragmatic approach whilst addressing the needs of patients from a sensitive and humanistic perspective. The authors have made extensive use of current evidence throughout the book and the inclusion of two new chapters on men's health and migrants, refugees and asylum seekers, is reflective of key areas of care that have been previously less well supported. Case studies provide realistic guidelines for good practice and sensitive topics are dealt with in a responsive way, ensuring that the reader reflects on their own beliefs and practices, as well as understanding how others may act. Reflection on practice is important for all healthcare professionals, as is understanding the evidence base to decision making, in order to provide competent and appropriate care.

Although the book is aimed at a nursing readership in the main, it is of relevance to other health workers, given that the care of any patient in the NHS today is dependent on an integrated and multidisciplinary approach. I recommend this book to individual healthcare practitioners, to service managers and to educationalists and to all who care for and support people from multicultural backgrounds.

Professor Sir Ara Darzi KBE

Preface

Given that many societies are multicultural in nature, all healthcare professionals working in hospital and community settings now require a different set of skills and knowledge to be able to ensure both quality and equality of health care provision.

The first edition of this book was published in 2001. The idea for writing a book about cultural care and nursing arose from frustration with the lack of UK texts and material that we could use for our teaching. It was also apparent that, despite the recognition in statute (United Kingdom Central Council for Nursing, Midwifery and Health Visiting, 1989), and by professional bodies and others at the time, that cultural care delivery was seen as an essential part of the nurse's role, but that there was no clear direction being given on how to ensure that nurses became more knowledgeable and aware of the different cultural needs of patients and clients. Compared to the USA, where Madeline Leininger and others had made an impact in this area, it appeared that we had a long way to go in order to achieve similar recognition of the importance of cultural care and cultural competence. The impact that prejudice and racist behaviour had on the teacher and student in the classroom and in clinical practice was also a major factor in our decision to undertake writing a book that would acknowledge the importance of meeting the cultural needs of the patients as well as those of healthcare staff.

During discussions with students and colleagues who wished to enhance their knowledge and practice of caring for individuals from multicultural backgrounds, it became apparent that what was required was a book that would allow them to explore the theoretical concepts through their own clinical and educational experiences. Implementing cultural care also requires both knowledge and skills to deliver it in a sensitive way. Consequently, we decided to combine the theoretical ('know-that') knowledge (Polanyi, 1962; Kuhn, 1970) required with a case-study/problem-solving approach. The reader could then explore concepts as they were encountered or applied to practice ('know-how') knowledge (Polanyi, 1962; Kuhn, 1970), and reflect upon those experiences in order to enhance their own skills.

Since the publication of the first edition there have only been a small number of books published by UK authors on subjects related to cultural awareness, competence and ethnicity as they relate to nursing and health care. Examples are Burnard and Gill (2008), Culley (2001), and Papadopoulos (2006). In the US there have been new editions of books referenced in some of our chapters, for example Andrews & Boyle (2008), but not many new titles. In journals, however, there has been an increase in the number of articles which have focused on various aspects of culture in nursing and health care in UK and other countries; for example Nayaranasamy (2003) and Nyatanga (2008) from the UK, and DeSouza (2008) from New Zealand. However in comparison to other topics in nursing education, the issue of students learning how to meet the needs of patients and clients from different cultural groups is not well represented.

The Nursing and Midwifery Council (NMC) in the UK make it clear that student nurses on qualifying should 'practice in a fair and anti-discriminatory way, acknowledging the differences in beliefs and cultural practices of individuals or groups' (NMC 2004, p27). This competency statement relates specifically to professional and ethical practice but it is implicit in the other competencies that student nurses must achieve: that acknowledging and understanding cultural beliefs and practices is essential in order to deliver culturally appropriate care.

This new edition covers a wide range of topics which we have explored with students and practitioners. We have tested the case studies and reflective exercises and many have been used as 'triggers' in some of our problem-based learning activities with pre- and post-registration nursing students. We have made every attempt to avoid stereotyping of people and groups in society in the case studies but for teaching and learning purposes, it may be inevitable that a level of generalization occurs in order for students to fully appreciate the various issues which could arise in care situations.

Much of the material is also relevant to any healthcare practitioner who wishes to ensure that the care they deliver to patients is culturally appropriate and sensitive to individual needs. We have also experienced its value to colleagues working as hospital chaplains, who have found the material helpful in understanding the way in which cultural and religious beliefs impact on actual nursing care and also in supporting their training of staff in aspects of their 'spiritual role and how to support different cultures during illness or bereavement .

Following peer review of the first edition and from our own experience of the needs of these groups we have added two new chapters - one on the health care of refugees and asylum seekers and the other on men's health.

In **Chapter 1** we explore the concepts of culture, race and ethnicity as they apply to health care and nursing. The terms are often confused in their interpretation by both healthcare professionals and the public in general. However, an understanding of their use is essential if a holistic approach to care is being promoted. This chapter is an essential prerequisite to reading and understanding the issues addressed in the rest of the book.

Chapter 2 explores the different health and illness beliefs of individuals and cultures, in an attempt to understand how people behave when they are ill, and why.

Holistic nursing care relies on an agreed understanding of the patient's illness experience. **Chapter 3** explores the way in which the health and illness beliefs of the patient affect the way in which care is planned and delivered.

Caring for individuals who are sick requires an insight into the way in which they cope with their illness. Many rely on their spiritual and religious beliefs and, because of the nature of the work involved, so do the nurses and carers themselves. **Chapter 4** examines the way in which care is affected by the religious beliefs and practices of patients and their carers.

Implementing care that is both culturally appropriate and culturally competent relies on a common understanding of the knowledge and skills required. **Chapter 5** explores the knowledge and skills needed to undertake this care, and demonstrates through examples how a framework for assessment can be utilised.

Mental health problems are common within all cultures and societies. **Chapter 6** explores both the development of transcultural psychiatry and the skills required for caring for individuals with mental health problems from different cultural backgrounds.

The role of women in society may vary according to the value that their own culture places on them. In addition, their religion and culture may influence how they cope with both general health problems and those that are specific to women. **Chapter 7** examines how nurses can ensure that the care they give takes into account the personal needs and beliefs of women from different cultures as well as being responsive to their role within those cultures. **Chapter 8** explores how culture and ethnicity impacts on how men approach health and well-being generally, and how their cultural beliefs and values can then impact on any illness experience.

A family-centred approach to care will require an understanding of the nature of the family within different cultures. In addition, the experience of children within these cultures necessitates sensitive care by nurses in practice. **Chapter 9** explores the importance of understanding the cultural background of children and their families in order to ensure that care is culturally sensitive.

Ageing is a universal experience, but each culture and society values older people differently. In a world where there is a growing population of older people, there is a great need for nurses to appreciate and understand their cultural backgrounds. **Chapter 10** explores the way in which different cultures view care for the older person.

Chapter 11 focuses on health care for refugees and asylum seekers, who needs have become an integral part of health care in a number of communities across the United Kingdom .

Death is an inevitable part of human existence and, for the nurse, an understanding of how societies cope with death and the grieving of others is an essential part of their role, given the fact that for many patients this is the way in which their illness ends. **Chapter 12** explores the way in which different cultures manage the death experience, and the knowledge and skills required of nurses to manage this within different health care settings.

For nurses and other health care professionals to deliver care that is both culturally sensitive and competent, a major shift is needed in how the healthcare professions value culturally sensitive and competent care of patients as well as the cultural and religious needs of staff. **Chapter 13** explores the professional practice issues that exist in a culturally diverse society, including racial inequalities in the nursing profession.

In the **Appendices** we have retained the summary of religious beliefs and practices as they impact on individual care. They are not intended to be viewed as a 'recipe book', but as drawing together many of the issues identified throughout the text.

We recognise that, in taking a broader multicultural and not multiracial standpoint, we could be accused of not reflecting the importance of race in any meaningful way. However, our book makes reference to race as an important concept within care, as we recognise its importance as a key component of the nurse–patient relationship as well as patient-patient and nurse-nurse relationships . We also acknowledge that the way in which literature uses the phrases 'black and minority ethnic' and 'white' to define cultural groups could in fact indirectly exclude individuals in society who normally consider themselves to be 'white' but who are also members of a minority ethnic group (e.g. members of the Polish or gypsy traveller community).

In order to ensure continuity and clarity of terminology, the word patient is used in the majority of the text. However, the word client is used in relation to mental health care, consistent with the literature in this area. For convenience, where the pronoun is necessary we have used 'she' to refer to the nurse, but this is not to disregard the fact that many nurses are men, as discussed in Chapter 8.

Each chapter concludes with a list of further reading which will enhance the reader's understanding of the issues discussed, as well as a list of relevant web-sites for additional resources. Throughout the book we have endeavored to ensure that the text is referenced to supporting literature, reflecting our recognition and belief that practice needs to be evidence-based. However, this has not always been possible due to the dearth of material in nursing literature that reflects the issues we have chosen to discuss, in particular research studies related to nursing practice and cultural issues. The whole text is a reflection of our own ideas, values and interpretations of events, and not those of the publishers. We have made every attempt to ensure that these have been represented and dealt with sensitively.

Karen Holland
Christine Hogg

Acknowledgements

As with the 1st Edition we wish to offer our thanks to a number of people who have given us their support throughout the writing of this book.

We begin however by thanking all those who have both read and purchased copies of our first book and for all the helpful feedback we have received over the past 9 years since its publication. This has been gratefully received and used to update the book as much as possible. We are aware that many of those who have read chapters applicable to their work have been enabled to change their practice as a result. This has made us believe that another edition was necessary in order to enhance, whenever possible, the evidence-base for their practice.

At Hodder Arnold we wish to thank Naomi Wilkinson (Commissioning Editor) for commissioning this second edition and for her support for the new chapters, Joanna Silman (Project Editor) for her unstinting support and encouragement throughout the whole of the writing and publishing process as well as helping us decide on the most appropriate cover colour for the book! We would also like to thank Andy Anderson for his copyediting skills and spotting those 'deliberate mistakes'! And finally Clare Patterson for her attention to detail and patience with us through the proofreading stage of the final manuscript. This has truly been a team effort.

On a personal level we would like to thank the following individuals , some of whom are student nurses at the University of Salford , who have contributed to our understanding of all things 'cultural ' and for their advice as to the content of the book: Aysha Badat , Catherine Green , Jenny Hodgkiss, Peggy Mulongo, James Murray, Nicola Rushton., Pam Sherlock.

We would like to thank our colleagues in the School of Nursing & Midwifery at The University of Salford who have always supported us in our cultural endeavours and by using the book and its content in their own teaching. In particular Elizabeth Collier, Angela Darvill and Moira McLoughlin who have provided endless hours of enthusiasm, and space for reflection.

Finally we wish to thank our families who continue to give us their support in various ways during the writing period, and for ensuring that many of Maslow's hierarchy of needs are met!

1 Culture, race and ethnicity: exploring the concepts

Karen Holland

INTRODUCTION

This chapter aims to explore and discuss the concepts of culture, race and ethnicity. This will enable the reader to gain an understanding of their individual meaning as well as their application and interpretation within nursing and healthcare practice. Reading this chapter will also inform and underpin all the other chapters in the book.

This chapter will focus on the following issues:
• cultural care in context;
• the meaning of culture;
• the meaning of race;
• the meaning of ethnicity;
• culture, race and ethnicity in nursing and health care.

CULTURAL CARE IN CONTEXT

Nurses have been advised in the past that the needs of different cultural groups were not being catered for (Chevannes, 1997; Le Var, 1998), and that there was a need to ensure that healthcare practitioners are suitably prepared to cater to these needs (Gerrish *et al.*, 1996b). However, there has been very little guidance offered by the statutory and professional bodies on how to make these recommendations a reality within healthcare practice and nurse education. The publication of the English National Board research report (Iganski *et al.*, 1998b) on the recruitment of minority ethnic groups into nursing, midwifery and health visiting was another example of the evidence clearly indicating a need for a national policy. The Department of Health began this cultural change in health care by ensuring that National Health Service (NHS) Trusts adhered to Patients' Charter standards with regard to privacy, dignity and religious and cultural beliefs (Department of Health, 1992) and in 2009 published guidance for NHS organizations on how to manage the issue of belief and religion in order 'to implement and comply with the requirements of legislation on religion or belief enacted recently', and also provides general practical guidance around the issues that fall out of that for the NHS (Department of Health, 2009).

However, despite the increase in information and research concerned with ensuring that the culture and religious beliefs of patients and clients are considered in health care and nursing, there remains a distinct lack of evidence on what is available to help us to achieve this. The United

Kingdom Central Council for Nursing, Midwifery and Health Visiting (UKCC) 1992 Code of Professional Practice set out for nurses, midwives and health visitors how they were expected to relate to the general public in the course of their work. It stated the need to:

> **Recognize and respect the uniqueness and dignity of each patient and client and respond to their need for care, irrespective of their ethnic origin, religious beliefs, personal attributes, the nature of their health problems or any other factor[.]**

(UKCC, 1992)

The updated Nursing and Midwifery Council (NMC) professional code (*The Code – Standards of Conduct, Performance and Ethics for Nurses and Midwives*, 2008) no longer makes this an explicit issue as in 1992 but an implied one, where ensuring that the specific needs of individuals is met is an accepted part of ensuring that nurses 'make the care of people your first concern, treating them as individuals and respecting their dignity'. For example, it states that as nurses we 'must not discriminate in any way against those in your care'.

The Australian Code of Professional Conduct (2008), however, has retained a more explicit statement: 'Nurses respect the dignity, culture, ethnicity, values and beliefs of people receiving care and treatment, and of their colleagues' and offers four explanatory statements as to how this is visualized (see Box 1.1).

Box 1.1 Conduct Statement 4: Nurses respect the dignity, culture, ethnicity, values and beliefs of people receiving care and treatment, and of their colleagues.

Explanation

1. In planning and providing effective nursing care, nurses uphold the standards of culturally informed and competent care. This includes according due respect and consideration to the cultural knowledge, values, beliefs, personal wishes and decisions of the persons being cared for as well as those of their partners, family members and other members of their nominated social network. Nurses acknowledge the changing nature of families and recognize families can be constituted in a variety of ways.

2. Nurses promote and protect the interests of people receiving treatment and care. This includes taking appropriate action to ensure that the safety and quality of their care is not compromised because of harmful prejudicial attitudes about race, culture, ethnicity, gender, sexuality, age, religion, spirituality, political, social or health status, lifestyle or other human factors.

3. Nurses refrain from expressing racist, sexist, homophobic, ageist and other prejudicial and discriminatory attitudes and behaviours toward colleagues, co-workers, persons in their care and their partners, family and friends. Nurses take appropriate action when observing any such prejudicial and discriminatory attitudes and behaviours, whether by staff, people receiving treatment and care or visitors, in nursing and related areas of health and aged care.

4. In making professional judgements in relation to a person's interests and rights, nurses do not contravene the law or breach the human rights of any person, including those deemed stateless such as refugees, asylum seekers and detainees.

From *Code of Professional Conduct for Nurses in Australia* (2008)

From this we can see very clearly what those involved in the education of student nurses would be able to promote in the undergraduate curricula and this incorporates a clear statement in Point 4 around the vulnerable group that we have now included in Chapter 11. A major report published in New South Wales, Australia, was a National Review of Nursing Education, with one element focusing specifically on multicultural nursing education (Eisenbruch, 2001). The conclusion from the review was that, at least in Australia, 'nursing has embedded within it a notion of multiculturalism which is both new and old'. In the UK this is not as clear, and Lauder *et al.* (2008) in their report on the evaluation of pre-registration nursing and midwifery programmes in Scotland, found that there was generally an exposure to cultural issues rather than any development of competency and, again, this was variable across the education providers. This raised the issue of how students were both prepared for, and experienced meeting the needs of, a multicultural community.

Reflective exercise

Consider your own learning experiences either as a student nurse or a healthcare professional and, focusing on one encounter with someone from a different culture from yours, decide what you would have liked to know about their culture which would have helped you to manage their care differently.

The outcomes of research studies (Iganski *et al.*, 1998b; Beavan, 2006) and Department of Health initiatives focusing on meeting the needs of diverse communities in the UK are essential to supporting the implementation of professional recommendations, but there is first a need for a common understanding and appreciation of the issues to be addressed. One of the important factors influencing decisions about the needs of multicultural groups is that there is a shared understanding of different cultural backgrounds. This involves understanding the use of language and terminology related to care. In the literature, three terms are frequently used in discussion about cultural care practices, namely culture, race and ethnicity. An understanding of the meaning of these terms in relation to health care is the focus of this chapter.

However, Baxter (1997) cautions us about using the terms 'culture' and 'multicultural', in that such usage ignores issues of race and 'does not provide an adequate explanation of how racial discrimination arises or how it can be addressed'. While this is acknowledged, we have observed when teaching that if the broad cultural issues are explored first and students are clear about the background of different cultural groups (e.g. in terms of lifestyle and beliefs), then the subsequent teaching and discussion of issues related to race and racism become easier and less confrontational because the student has a clear and safe framework within which to explore his or her own views and experiences. Each chapter in this book will give both student and teacher the opportunity to begin this reflective learning process in order, hopefully, to bring about change in their own beliefs and practice, and in addition to begin to influence that change in others.

THE MEANING OF CULTURE

The terms culture, race and ethnicity are often confused in their interpretation by healthcare professionals and the public in general. In order to determine what is meant by culture, let us examine the following definitions:

> Culture is ... a complex whole, which includes knowledge, beliefs, art, morals, law, custom, and any other capabilities and habits acquired by man as a member of society.
>
> *(Tylor, 1871, cited in Leininger, 1978b, p. 491)*

> Culture is the learned and transmitted knowledge about a particular culture with its values, beliefs, rules of behaviour and lifestyle practices that guides a designated group in their thinking and actions in patterned ways.
>
> *(Leininger, 1978b, p. 491)*

> Culture is ... a set of guidelines (both explicit and implicit) ... that an individual inherits as a member of a particular society and that tell them how to view the world and learn how to experience it emotionally, and how to behave in it in relation to other people, to supernatural forces and gods and to the natural environment. It also provides them with a way of transmitting these guidelines to the next generation – by the use of symbols, language, art and ritual. To some extent, culture can be seen as an inherited "lens" through which the individual perceives and understands the world that he inhabits and learns how to live within it.
>
> *(Helman, 2007, p. 2)*

There appears to be agreement in these definitions that culture is an inherited or learned set of guidelines through which we come to know how to live in our own social group or within society. Henley and Schott (1999, p. 3) point out that culture is 'not genetically inherited', nor is it 'fixed or static', but in fact 'changes in response to new situations and pressures'. Andrews and Boyle (1995) viewed culture as having the following four main characteristics.

> 1. It is learned from birth through the process of language acquisition and socialization. From society's viewpoint, socialization is the way culture is transmitted and the individual is fitted into the group's organized way of life.

> 2. It is shared by all members of the same cultural group: in fact, it is the sharing of cultural beliefs and patterns that binds people together under one identity as a group (even though this is not always a conscious process).

> 3. It is an adaptation to specific activities related to environmental and technical factors and to the availability of natural resources.

> 4. It is a dynamic, ever-changing process.
>
> *(Andrews and Boyle, 1995, p.10)*

Different cultures have established values and norms that govern how individuals communicate with one another and how they behave towards each other. All societies have 'norms' that guide the ways in which individuals do this, and they can be either rewarded or punished as they conform to, or deviate from, the established norm. Our culture therefore determines the pattern in which we undertake both roles and responsibilities related to family, friends and the workplace.

For example, nurses have their own professional and social culture and student nurses learn through gaining experience in different types of practice placements and establishing what knowledge and skills are essential in order to 'survive' in that culture. So, student nurses have to know how to behave when in uniform and what is expected of them when they are working on a ward. Holland (1993) found that there were aspects of nurses' culture, such as the order in which they carried out their work, which had remained unchanged since Florence Nightingale's day. She also found that there were many rituals that were important in ensuring that everyone, including the patients, knew what to do in hospitals. One of the most important rituals was that of the handover report, when information was communicated by nurses about the patients and their care. Other researchers have also found rituals associated with nursing culture (Kaminski, 2006; Street, 1992; Wolf, 1988), including the handover (Strange, 1996).

De Santis (1994) believes that when patients and nurses meet one another, there is in fact a meeting of three cultures:

1. the nurse's own professional culture, with its beliefs, values and practices;
2. the patient's culture, based on the patient's life experiences of health and illness and their personal values, beliefs and practices;
3. the culture of the setting in which they meet (e.g. hospital, community or family setting).

If we can understand that these cultures exist when we are communicating with patients, this will enable us to begin to understand some of the actual and potential problems that may arise when assessing, planning and implementing care. One other culture that De Santis (1994) does not account for, and which can have a substantial effect on the nurse–patient relationship, is that of the nurse. For example, if the nurse is a Muslim and is caring for a Muslim patient (male or female) there may well be an occasion for conflict where body care or personal preference is concerned. In some situations, the student nurse may be asked to interpret for the patient as he or she speaks that particular language. However, this is not always viewed positively by students, especially if they are asked frequently to undertake this role:

> I didn't mind doing this [interpreting] for patients, as it saved time and helped them straight away – and I can speak four different languages, which, of course, was even more useful. But I found I was being asked to do it on other wards as well and it was not helping me to make sure I met my learning objectives on my ward.

> *(Adult nurse student, Year 1 Diploma course)*

Consider the following Case Study, which explains this meeting of cultures as explained by De Santis (1994) further.

Mr Mohamed Kalhid Quereshi, a 68-year-old Muslim man, is admitted to a large district general hospital after having been seen by the consultant in the diabetic clinic of the outpatients department. He has been admitted with glycosuria (sugar in the urine).

The first 'culture' he meets is that of the hospital (organizational culture). His previous experience of hospitals will determine his behaviour and his understanding of all that is taking place. If it is his first visit, he is immediately faced (like anyone coming into hospital) with the dilemma of where he has to go. The signs on the doors and walls will not necessarily be familiar. If it is a hospital that acknowledges the needs of a multicultural society, the signs will at least be in different languages, but it would be incorrect to assume that he can actually read these.

Walking through the hospital, this patient will encounter many different individuals in different uniforms of different colours. On reaching the outpatients department, again there will be an array of signs for different departments (e.g. Orthopaedic, ENT, CT Scan, Diabetic Clinic). To those who work in the hospital, these signs will be familiar as they have been learned and they are part of the hospital culture. However, to Mr Quereshi, even in his own language their meaning may not be readily understood unless he is familiar with the cultural language of the hospital. At this stage he may begin to experience what Herberg (1995) has termed 'culture shock'. This is similar to what happens when one travels to a different country and for the first few days everything is very strange or alien. People are also uncertain how to behave in such new environments (Burnard and Gill, 2008).

The second culture Mr Quereshi may encounter is that of the nurse (nursing culture), who may ask him for 'his sample' and who may, if she does not receive a response, hand him a container and ask him to go to the toilet and 'bring the sample back'. Here the nurse is assuming that the patient understands the terminology and the language used by healthcare professionals and which is specific to them. New student nurses may experience a similar situation to Mr Quereshi when, for example, listening to a handover report for the first time, with phrases such as 'nil by mouth', 'in situ', 'doing the obs', 'he's crashed' and 'she's not p.u.'d yet' being commonplace.

The patient's own cultural and individual beliefs (patient culture) about their body and how it works may also be completely different from those of the healthcare professionals. Mr Quereshi may believe that his diabetes has nothing to do with passing urine, and he may therefore wonder why he has to give this sample to the nurse. He may find that the toilet does not have adequate washing facilities for his personal needs, further increasing his anxiety and concern.

To be able to understand and manage these cultural encounters effectively, the nurse and other healthcare professionals must have the appropriate knowledge and skills. In order to determine your own needs in relation to ensuring culturally appropriate care, consider the issues with regard to Mr Quereshi's encounters with health care.

Imagine that Mr Quereshi is a patient on your ward. You are to be his named nurse and have to undertake an assessment of his needs on admission to hospital.

1. What will you need to know about his admission to hospital from the outpatients department?
2. How will you ensure that he understands the role of the nurse and other healthcare workers who will be caring for him?
3. What knowledge of his culture will you need in order to ensure that the assessment of his needs is culturally appropriate?

Your responses may have considered the following issues with regard to the three cultures identified by De Santis (1994).

Organizational culture

Organizations such as NHS Trusts have equal opportunity policies which ensure that all patients, regardless of culture, are afforded equal care. For example, any information that is given to Mr Quereshi about his admission to hospital should be provided in his own language as well as in English.

In addition to written information, many hospitals employ the services of trained interpreters or link workers who offer a very valuable service to both health service staff and non-English-speaking clients. In 1994, the Royal College of Nursing (RCN) published a learning unit on meeting the needs of black and minority ethnic clients. Although this unit is no longer available on the RCN site, the key issues remain relevant and are supported by more recent evidence (Bradby, 2001). It focused on three roles, namely interpreters, health advocates and link workers, and it highlighted the problems associated with untrained interpreters, who were very often members of staff, the patient's immediate family or relatives. These problems were listed as:

- *Inaccurate translation* – because of inability to translate important ideas and words;
- *Bias and distortion* – caused by inability to put aside personal bias;
- *No confidentiality* – the importance of confidentiality may not be recognized, and this may inhibit clients from being open in interview;
- *Not understanding their role* – untrained interpreters may answer questions from staff without putting them to the clients, and may only relay part of the information to the client;
- *No explanation of cultural differences* – untrained interpreters may not be sensitive to differences in culture, values and expectations, and this limits their effectiveness;
- *Personal unsuitability* – people brought in to interpret on an *ad hoc* basis may be the wrong sex or much older or younger than the client. Their backgrounds may be very different and they may even belong to a group which is antagonistic towards the client's own group.

Royal College of Nursing, 1994, p.5

The trained interpreter would have clear role parameters to work with, but would not necessarily be viewed as part of the health team. Health advocates, on the other hand, are employed to provide a service that will ensure equality for non-English-speaking patients, and they 'are on the side of clients rather than that of the health professionals' (Royal College of Nursing, 1994). Link workers are specially trained interpreters and health advocates, and they have become important members of healthcare teams in hospital and community services (Tribe and Raval, 2002). They have different skills and are 'trained to observe a strict code of professional ethics' (Royal College of Nursing, 1994). Many of them speak a number of languages and dialects, and work with the healthcare team to ensure effective communication (see Chapter 6 for a further discussion of the role of interpreters and intercultural communications). Mr Quereshi may or may not require the services of a link worker to ensure that his admission to hospital takes into account his cultural needs as well as his health needs.

Reflective exercise

As a student nurse have you ever been asked to interpret for a patient while in clinical practice?

1. If yes, reflect on the experience and consider how it affected your learning experience and the person you were interpreting for.
2. If no, consider how effective communication would be achieved without an interpreter being available for a patient unable to speak English.

Nursing culture

As Mr Quereshi will usually be cared for by female nurses, he may find receiving care an embarrassing and uncomfortable experience. Being aware of his specific beliefs and needs as they relate to his Muslim culture will help nurses to interact with him in a sensitive manner. The way in which he relates to the nurses may also be influenced by his views about women and nursing. The role and status of nurses in some societies may be lower than those in the UK because of the links to beliefs about 'dirt and pollution' (Jervis, 2001). Lawler (1991) and Somjee (1991) cited the example of Indian nurses, where the touching of excreta is linked to low status and low caste in Indian society. Nurses need to ensure that patients of all cultures understand their role in order to avoid misunderstanding. Being cared for by nurses from his own culture would not necessarily help Mr Quereshi, even though communication on cultural needs would be an asset. This is because the relationship between men and women in Muslim culture is very restrictive and to be cared for intimately by a Muslim female nurse might be more embarrassing than being cared for by a non-Muslim nurse. Iganski *et al.* (1998b) identified the low status of nursing as a career in some cultures and the role of the nurse in care in an interview with a senior administrator responsible for student recruitment, who stated that:

> We are in an area of all different cultures ... but we are having problems with the parents and the grandparents of the Sikhs and Muslims and that, because it's not seen to be a thing to nurse people – you know, touch bodies and things like that – we're hoping that in another

generation, if you like, that would have gone out of the window. It is getting better because the children that are born in this country actually grow up with a different idea from the parents or the grandparents, so it's getting better, but it's got a long way to go yet.

(Senior Administrator; Iganski et al., 1998b, p. 37)

Patient culture

Mr Quereshi is a Muslim man and, in order to ensure that his care is appropriate, the nurse must have an awareness of his specific cultural needs. For example, diet will be an important aspect of care, given that he has glycosuria (sugar in the urine) and may be diabetic. Any medicine he may be prescribed should be alcohol-free, and 'capsules should not contain gelatine' (Community Practice, 1993, p. 333). If he requires insulin, the human form would be prescribed, because pork is a prohibited food (Pennachio 2005). A devout Muslim would need to be able to pray five times a day while in hospital. This is essential to well-being, although illness does allow exemptions. If it was the time of Ramadhan, he would be required to fast in the hours between dawn and sunset. This may cause personal conflict because of the treatment for his diabetes. If he is a very devout Muslim, he may refuse to take anything at all into his body – 'through the mouth, the nose, by injection or suppository between dawn and sunset' (Henley, 1982). The Holy Qur'an (Holy Koran) allows for flexibility, and if Muslims cannot fast at all 'they are permitted in the Qur'an to perform another virtuous act such as providing food for the poor' (Henley, 1982).

> ### Key points
>
> 1. Culture is an inherited or learned set of guidelines which social groups use to live in wider society.
> 2. Different cultures have their own values and beliefs about health and health care.
> 3. Nurses have a different role and status according to how individual societies view their work and their gender.

THE MEANING OF RACE

There appears from the literature to be general agreement with regard to the definition of race. For example, Fernando (1991) defines race as 'a classification of people on the basis of physical appearance ... with skin colour the most popular physical characteristic'.

Country of origin is also frequently used with this concept of race (e.g. African–Caribbean). However, race has not just been expressed in this way. Jones (1994) reminds us that in the past it was 'a way of dividing humankind which also denoted inferiority and superiority, which was linked to patterns of subordination and domination'. She cites colour as being a very important determinant in this classification, with 'black' people being defined as inferior and more primitive whereas 'white' people were viewed as superior. However, Cashmore (1988) points out that the main issue is not what 'race' is, but how the term is used. He states that nearly all social scientists, for example, use the term to define social groups according to their physical or bodily attributes, which are then linked to their social behaviour.

Because race has become such a crucial concept in health care generally, it is important to examine how theorists view it. This will also help us to understand why and how people adopt such different views about living in a multicultural society both generally and locally. Jones (1994) believes that there are two distinct theories of race, namely consensus (functionalist) theories and conflict theories. Consensus theories suggest that following an initial disruption of society by large numbers of immigrants, 'social consensus will be restored through resocialisation and integration' (Jones, 1994, p. 298). It is believed that any new social group, with its individual customs, will become no different from the rest of society, and that it is they who have the 'problem' not the majority culture. They become 'indistinguishable from the majority and integrate through mixing with the host society' (Jones, 1994), while not losing their cultural norms and values altogether. Another theory is one in which there is a more liberal view and acceptance of 'subcultures, norms and values, which are different but equal' (Jones, 1994). In communities that adopt this view, there may be a more open acceptance of other cultures (e.g. in regular multicultural religious services).

In contrast, conflict theories view race relationships as part of an ongoing struggle between the dominant and subordinate groups in society. This creates racial conflict where they experience racism, which, according to Dobson (1991), is 'a mixed form of prejudice (attitude) and discrimination (behaviour) directed at ethnic groups other than one's own'. This occurs at two different levels: 'individual and institutional' (Dobson 1991).

An example of institutional racism can be seen in the recruitment of African–Caribbean women to enrolled nurse and pupil nurse training because the entry qualifications for SRN training were geared to UK education criteria and values (Jones, 1994; Culley and Mayor 2001). This experience is discussed in more detail in Chapter 11.

Fernando (1991) stresses that in any 'racist' society the identification of individuals according to their race and ethnicity is not to be undertaken lightly, and he points out that they both carry 'racial' connotations. He stresses that simply renaming a racial group as 'ethnic' does not get rid of the racial persecution of that particular group.

Reflective exercise

1. Examine your own views with regard to how different cultural groups should live alongside one another.
2. How could these views affect your caring for people in both community and hospital settings?

To help you to explore your own views on this issue, consider the following scenario:

> During attendance at a Summer School, a student is asked to share a room with a colleague who is Asian. Her reply is: 'I'm not racist but ... I don't think that's a good idea. I'd rather share with an English colleague just in case there are any problems with food or something, like she may want to pray on her own.'

The statement 'I'm not racist but' indicates that the student cannot be considered non-racist. The additional comment that she would prefer to share with an English colleague also indicates a view of culture and race that excludes members of minority ethnic communities as not being English – yet they may have been born in England. These types of comments could be viewed as harmful if they intrude into the nurse–patient relationship. Nurses who hold such views could let them influence the way in which they deliver care. For example, if Mr Quereshi rang the nurse call-bell, the response could be that 'I'm not racist but … you go and answer that; he doesn't make any effort to understand me so why should I go? You're better with him than I am'. These are examples to help you to explore your views, and they are adapted from real situations.

Reflective exercise

Consider other situations where you have heard the phrase ' I'm not racist but …' and reflect on how you felt when you heard this. What, given your reading of this chapter, do you believe was the cause of the speaker's statement? What was the outcome?

Key points

1. The nurse has a responsibility to ensure that patients 'come to no harm' while in their care. This includes protecting them from racist behaviour by other patients and healthcare colleagues.
2. Racism can occur at both individual and organizational levels.
3. Racial discrimination and prejudice can prevent the implementation of equal opportunities policies.

THE MEANING OF ETHNICITY

Jones (1994) states that the term ethnicity:

> …refers to cultural practices and attitudes that characterise a given group of people and distinguish it from other groups. The population group feels itself and is seen to be different by virtue of language, ancestry, religion, common interests and other shared cultural practices such as dietary habits or style of dress. Ethnic differences, in other words, are wholly learned – they are the result of socialisation and acculturation – not genetic inheritance.

> *(Jones, 1994, p. 292)*

However, it is important to remember that in belonging to an ethnic group, each individual within that group must still be acknowledged. In addition, using the term 'ethnic' to describe differences between cultures has often led to discrimination and prejudice owing to differences in customs, dress and language. Baxter (1997) defines an ethnic group as:

> a group of people who have certain background characteristics such as language, culture and religion in common; these provide the group with a distinct identity, as seen by themselves and others. Although the term also covers white people (ethnic majorities) and includes such groups as Greeks, Poles, Italians, Welsh and Irish, it is often used inaccurately to describe black or ethnic minority groups in Britain.

> *(Baxter, 1997, p. xvii)*

From these two definitions we can see that belonging to an ethnic group will affect the way in which we communicate both verbally and visually with others. They also show that we all belong to an ethnic group. However, the problem with using the terms 'race' and 'ethnicity' to differentiate between social groups is highlighted in a report published by the British Medical Association (BMA) in 1995 on the need for multicultural education for doctors and other healthcare professionals. The report considered that ethnicity has replaced 'race' as a health research definition but that it is 'a fluid variable; its meaning can change over time and the borderlines between groups are not clearly demarcated' (British Medical Association, 1995).

This is unlike race, which is related to physical attributes (Cashmore, 1988). The report concludes that this makes it very difficult to create an effective system for differentiating between groups in order to determine specific health needs. There are problems with any such classification system. A system that is based on racial categories fails to take into account the many individual and cultural differences between groups, and one that is based on ethnicity may not address specific issues about 'discrimination and equal opportunities' (British Medical Association, 1995). From April 1995 it has been a mandatory requirement by the Department of Health that ethnic monitoring of inpatients takes place (Karmi, 1996). Previously this was undertaken mainly for 'employment practices' but it has now become increasingly important for monitoring health services (Department of Health, 2005). Karmi (1996) believed that:

> ...if properly implemented, ethnic monitoring can provide valuable information on the epidemiology of disease in ethnic groups. It can also reveal inequalities of access. The information can be used to make changes, which should go towards improving the service and ensuring that it is sensitive, equitable and appropriate.

> *(Karmi, 1996, p. 10)*

However, as noted previously, there are limitations to any classification system, and if it is not used properly (i.e. collecting the data without any consequent change), then it could be viewed suspiciously as collecting 'race data for clandestine use' (Karmi, 1996). The Department of Health in the UK published a practical guide to ethnic monitoring in the NHS and Social Care, which includes an outline of why ethnic monitoring is important in ensuring equality of health and social care provision to all cultural groups (Department of Health, 2007).

During the assessment process on admission to hospital, nurses may be required to collect data on ethnic origin, and it is important that they explain to patients the rationale for this in terms of healthcare planning.

CULTURE, RACE AND ETHNICITY IN NURSING AND HEALTH CARE

In order to establish an understanding of these concepts as they apply to healthcare practice, consider the following Case Study.

Mrs Dorothy Jones is a 60-year-old woman from Jamaica who moved to the UK in 1952 with her parents. She has worked as a nursing auxiliary for the past 30 years in a large teaching hospital and has been married to Ernest for 40 years. They have four children and 10 grandchildren who, apart from one daughter who is a ward sister at the hospital, have all made their home in Jamaica. For the past four years Dorothy's diabetes has been gradually getting worse, and she has now developed two large ulcerated areas on both legs. This has necessitated long periods off work, and she is becoming increasingly house-bound. The district nurse, Sister Jan Rowan, visits Dorothy daily and has experienced some difficulty in trying to encourage her to lose weight. Dorothy is reluctant to do so, as she says she is happy with her body and her shape. Jan has recently completed a short course on cultural awareness and is trying to understand Dorothy's health and illness beliefs in order to help her. Unfortunately, Dorothy does not have a good relationship with her general practitioner (GP), Mr Vijaykumar Patel, a Hindu man. She feels that he has not been very helpful with her pain relief, and she has no faith in the medication he does prescribe. Dorothy and her husband would like to retire to Jamaica, as she feels that this is where she 'belongs', but her health problems are making it less likely to happen. She feels that her only link to her home is the Pentecostal church, which she is now also finding increasingly difficult to attend.

1. How are culture, race and ethnicity reflected in this Case Study?
2. Has Mrs Jones become integrated into UK society?
3. What are the specific ethnic differences between Mrs Jones, Sister Rowan and Dr Patel?
4. What needs to happen in this healthcare scenario to enable Mrs Jones to improve her health?
5. Reflect on your personal experiences of caring for patients in similar situations and identify personal objectives for future learning needs.

Some key points that you could explore in your reflections could include:
- Mrs Jones' 'cultural' roots in Jamaica and her need to return there to live with her family;
- the use of the term African–Caribbean (or Afro-Caribbean) which Karmi (1996, p. 44) defines as being a term used to 'describe people of African origin, who came to Britain from the Caribbean Islands, notably Jamaica, Trinidad, Tobago, Grenada, Dominca, Barbados, St Lucia and the British Virgin Islands'.
- her health and illness beliefs with regard to her body and body image (see Chapter 3);
- the three different cultures of Mrs Jones (patient), Sister Rowan (healthcare profession – nursing) and Dr Patel (healthcare profession – medicine);
- Dr Patel and Sister Rowan's own cultural and religious beliefs as well as their professional ones;

continued

Case study

- the need for Mrs Jones to improve her health by losing weight;
- an altered diet would also improve the diabetes and healing of the leg ulcers;
- Mrs Jones' personal beliefs may not help the district nurse to implement a mutually agreed plan;
- Mrs Jones' poor relationship with her GP – a man from another culture and healthcare profession – is also contributing to her non-compliance with care/treatment which would help her to realize her long-term goal of 'going home' to Jamaica.

Pierce and Armstrong (1996) believe that:

> … diabetes is a particular problem for African–Caribbean people living in the UK, for two reasons. The first is that rates of diabetes are very high in this population … reflecting the high prevalence of the disease in the Caribbean … and is according to Alleyne *et al.* (1989) a leading cause of death in Jamaica … The second reason why diabetes is a particular problem is the importance of patients' beliefs about diabetes and their effect on health-related behaviours.

(Pierce and Armstrong, 1996, p. 91)

In the Case Study above, Mrs Jones would have to make radical changes to her lifestyle in order to manage her diabetes with any degree of success (Brown *et al.*, 2007). However, as Pierce and Armstrong (1996) have highlighted, the cultural beliefs of African–Caribbean people about their diet and body shape (e.g. the relative merits of African–Caribbean food versus English food and the concept of 'ideal' body size) can make it very difficult for health professionals to recommend changes with which Mrs Jones would agree (see Chapter 3 for further information on food and diabetes in African–Caribbean culture).

CONCLUSION

As the above Case Study illustrates, it is essential to understand all three cultures in a nurse–patient encounter in order to ensure culturally safe and appropriate care. It is important to recognize that the nurse's own culture can influence the nurse–patient relationship. The responsibility for ensuring that nurses have the knowledge and skills to do this should lie with both them and their employers.

CHAPTER SUMMARY

1. Any understanding of the terms culture, race and ethnicity is essential if culturally safe and appropriate care is to be ensured.
2. In every nurse–patient relationship there is a meeting of three cultures, namely those of the organization, the patient and the nurse.
3. Racism, discrimination and prejudice continue to prevent the implementation of care that is culturally safe and appropriate.

FURTHER READING

Bhopal R S (2007) *Ethnicity, race and health in multicultural societies: Foundations for better epidemiology, public health, and health care.* Oxford University Press, Oxford.
This book discusses race and ethnicity as seen internationally as well as practical examples of the key concepts in a health context.

Kelleher D and Hillier S (eds) (1996) *Researching cultural differences in health.* Routledge, London.
This book is a collection of research studies focusing on the management of illness by minority ethnic groups. These include studies related to diabetes, hypertension and mental illness.

Culley L and Dyson S (2001) *Ethnicity and nursing practice.* Palgrave, Basingstoke.
This book introduces theories of race, ethnicity and racism and explores how an understanding of these can help nurses and other healthcare professionals meet the needs of minority ethnic communities.

WEBSITES

http://anthro.palomar.edu/culture/culture_2.htm
A website which discusses through exercises and examples the nature of human culture and its characteristics and the methods used by anthropologists to study it.

http://openlearn.open.ac.uk/mod/resource/view.php?id=166547
This website links to an Open University Learning Unit example 'Diversity and Difference in Communication', which includes a section on interpreters.

http://www.practicebasedlearning.org/resources/diversity/ethnicity.htm
This website hosts a number of links and resources in relation to ethnicity and culture. The outcome of a Higher Education Academy funded project on inter-professional practice based learning.

http://www.maryseacole.com/maryseacole/melting/validated.asp
This website hosts a number of resources developed as an outcome of a project called Multi-Ethnic Learning and Teaching in Nursing, including a number of other websites and resources.

http://visiblenurse.com/nurseculture6.html
This website focuses on aspects of Kaminski's study of nursing culture and access to her whole study.

http://www.dhsspsni.gov.uk/eq-raceeqhealth
This website hosts a good practice guide to racial equality in health and social care by the Northern Ireland Department of Health, Social Services and Public Safety.

http://www.dh.gov.uk/en/Publicationsandstatistics/Publications/ PublicationsPolicyAndGuidance/Browsable/DH_4116927
This link leads directly to the publication 'A Practical Guide to Ethnic Monitoring in the NHS and Social Care'.

2 Understanding the theory of health and illness beliefs

Christine Hogg

INTRODUCTION

Views and beliefs about health and ill health are reflected in different cultures. Health and illness are experienced as individuals, but we behave according to the norms and values that shape us.

> **This chapter focuses on the following issues:**
>
> - health beliefs;
> - the importance of understanding health beliefs in nursing practice;
> - the three systems of health beliefs, namely biomedicine, personalistic and naturalistic systems;
> - the sectors of health care, namely the popular sector, the folk sector and professional medicine.

HEALTH BELIEFS

In modern or Western medicine, the term 'health beliefs' generally describes beliefs and practices that are held or maintained by others (i.e. individuals from other cultures). The health beliefs and practices of some people may therefore conflict with those from the indigenous or majority group. Conflicting ideas can result in both nurses and patients feeling frustrated and failing to understand each other. Ultimately, this may cause the patient to abandon or ignore healthcare services. Culture and tradition influence everyone's beliefs about health and illness. Jones (1994) suggests that health is subject to widely variable individual, social and cultural interpretations produced by the interplay of individual perceptions and social influences; she believes that 'all of us, whether we are professional healthworkers or lay people, create and recreate meanings of health and illness through our lived experience' (Jones, 1994, p. 2).

The concept of health is broad and complex and has a wide range of meanings. People's perceptions of health may change over their lifespan. Older people may view health in terms of functioning and coping (e.g. can I get to the shops this week?), whereas young people may view health in terms of their level of fitness and energy.

Thus, health is not simply a well-functioning physical state, but rather it is a complex dynamic interplay of forces that is dependent on many variables, not least social, psychological, spiritual and emotional factors. Health beliefs are also ideas and conceptualizations about health and illness that are derived from the prevailing world-view. Often they relate closely to the world in which we live, where we live and the dominant social and economic environment. They are extremely complex and, like the notion of 'culture', they may change and evolve over time.

Health beliefs are activities undertaken by people in order to protect, maintain or promote health. Health maintenance practices are those guidelines and actions that are specific to each cultural group. These actions help people to stay well. Spector (2010) notes that in the United States black populations stress the need for diets that include three meals a day and in particular a 'hot breakfast'. Laxatives are also considered to keep the system 'running' or 'open'. Kaunonen and Koivula (2006) note that Finnish people place great value in the role of the sauna in maintaining health. Saunas are said to alleviate physical and mental stress, pain and tension, and promote good sleep. Parry *et al.* (2004) noted in interviews with Gypsy Traveller women that they placed great importance in keeping a clean home as a matter of pride and because cleanliness and hygiene was considered very important for health as a precaution against infection. Another woman noted that 'if this place wasn't clean I'd be depressed'. Indeed, in some Traveller sites bathrooms, toilets and laundry facilities may be kept separate from the main living areas as people may fear contamination.

A study by Prior *et al.* (2000) investigated the health beliefs of Cantonese-speaking communities in England and found that happiness was thought to be a central part of leading a healthy life: one respondent noted 'If you are happy (kuaile), have a happy family, have no heavy pressure, then you will be in good health'. Happiness was important to the extent that unhealthy behaviours were seen to be acceptable if they led to inner contentment. For example, if smoking made you happy then it was acceptable to smoke.

However, beliefs may also cause people to neglect or jeopardize their health status. An example of how health beliefs can change over time is the practice of sunbathing. In Victorian Britain, tanned or bronzed skin was considered unfashionable and a sign of working outdoors and therefore belonging to the agricultural or lower classes. Women especially would shield their faces with a parasol, as fair skins were fashionable – a porcelain skin was much sought after. However, in the UK today a sun-tan is generally associated with health ('looking good' and 'feeling healthy'). Sun-tans are a status symbol that signals affluence (i.e. the freedom to holiday abroad). Individuals may spend the whole of their annual holiday cultivating a sun-tan and, on returning home, are eager to show off their brown skin to their friends and relatives. They are often met with cries of 'don't you look well!'. Although medical advice warns against sun-tans, as they are associated with a high incidence of skin cancer, they continue to be associated with health and well-being. This example demonstrates that attitudes and beliefs are often socially constructed and change over time.

The importance of understanding health beliefs in nursing practice

Spector (2010) argues that, as nurses, we enter the profession with ideas about health and illness that are unique and which have been shaped by our ethnic and cultural background. Spector (2010) encourages nurses to explore their cultural heritage by considering their own beliefs and practices that may have been passed on through female members of the family (for example, through mothers and grandmothers). Nurses then bring these beliefs to the health arena, wards, community settings and therapeutic encounters in which they are engaged and these can influence nursing practice in the prevention and treatment of illness. However, these beliefs may change as nurses integrate with their professional groups and absorb the beliefs, values and attitudes of the culture of nursing. An example of this is nursing language. Nursing has its own language – a set of phrases, idioms and terms that may be alien to others (for example, 'doing the obs', 'off duty', 'doing the cares', 'doing the backs' and 'handovers').

This culture of nursing, with its rites of passage, language, codes of behaviour and expectations, may be evident at many levels. However, it is often hidden and, as nurses, we may regard these distinct practices as the norm. Unless we are aware of this, a gap may develop between the provider of health care (e.g. the nurse) and the recipient (e.g. the patient or client).

However, if the provider becomes more sensitive to the issues surrounding health care, then more comprehensive and holistic care will be delivered (see Chapter 1 for a discussion of nursing culture). As nurses it is impossible for us to become experts on every cultural or ethnic group. Indeed, it is argued that becoming an 'expert' leads to stereotyping and making generalizations about people. Henley and Schott (1999) emphasize that not everyone in a particular culture may have the same attitudes and assumptions about illness and health:

> ... there may be more similarities between the health beliefs or practices of different ethnic groups at the same socio-economic level than there are within the same ethnic group at different socio-economic levels
>
> *(Henley and Schott, 1999, p. 25)*

The health services in the UK are based on models of health and disease that are part of the UK culture and way of life. In many respects these customs and practices are taken for granted or we treat them as the norm. They are almost woven into the fabric of our healthcare system. It is only when we distance ourselves or view them through someone else's eyes that these practices may seem strange or illogical. An example in the UK is the custom of calling a surgical consultant by the title of Mr, Mrs or Miss, whereas a medical consultant will always be referred to as Dr.

Key points

1. Health beliefs are individual, but they are also influenced by the culture that envelops us.
2. Understanding health beliefs is fundamental to nursing practice if we are to care for people holistically.
3. Nurses bring their own health beliefs into the profession, but they are also influenced by the culture of nursing.

HEALTH BELIEF SYSTEMS

Health beliefs can be broadly divided into three categories or systems, namely biomedicine, personalistic systems and naturalism.

Health beliefs based on biomedicine

Biomedicine is also referred to as Western medicine, modern medicine or allopathic medicine. The term Western medicine is perhaps most appropriate because it was developed in, and is the dominant health system of, North America and Europe. Biomedicine came to dominate Western thinking about health and illness after about 1800, and as such it is a relative newcomer.

In general, biomedicine is regarded as the superior system of healthcare delivery in the world. It is a system that has been exported all over the world in the same way that Christianity was exported to the developing world (Thorne, 1993). According to biomedicine, illness and disease are caused by abnormalities in the structure and function of the body organs and systems. In the biomedical or scientific system, physical and biochemical processes are studied and manipulated. Biomedicine draws from the natural sciences such as chemistry and physics, which rely on the patterns of cause and effect to explain illness. For example, bacteria entering the body (cause) will result in an infection (effect). Diseases are therefore caused by pathogens (bacteria and viruses) entering the body, or by biochemical changes taking place in the body owing to conditions or events (e.g. wear and tear, accidents, nutritional deficiencies, the ageing process, injury, stress, environmental factors, cigarette smoke or alcohol). Biomedicine views the body or the mind as a complex machine in which all of the parts function together to ensure health. If malfunctioning occurs, the clinician intervenes to limit damage and to help to resume normal functioning.

The diagnostic process in biomedicine requires the identification of the pathogen or process responsible for causing particular abnormalities. This usually involves physically examining the patient, and then removing or destroying the entity that is causing the disease. If cure is not possible, treatment may involve repairing or controlling the affected body systems. Biomedicine may be regarded as an attacking force, and militaristic terminology such as 'battling cancer', 'fighting disease' or 'winning the war against germs' is commonly used. Practitioners in biomedicine are highly educated and respected specialists. They are scientists who practise in settings that resemble laboratories and other scientific institutions. The law upholds their position and authority and they have the right to treat patients, to prescribe powerful medicines and to withhold treatment if they believe this is necessary. They also have the right to detain patients in hospital if, for example, it is believed that they are suffering from a mental illness or are a danger to other people. Practitioners are expected to remain objective and analytical, drawing from their powers of observation and specialist knowledge. In general, they concentrate solely on treating the diseased or injured part of the body (e.g. the broken leg). Biomedicine views the mind and body as two separate entities.

In biomedicine, health is acquired by illness prevention activities such as restoration through exercise, medication and other means. In maintaining health it is assumed that individuals are responsible for their own bodies and that they have freedom to determine or choose their own lifestyle (Jackson, 1993; Helman, 2007).

Health beliefs based on personalistic systems

Personalistic health belief systems may also be known as magico-religious systems. In such systems, illness is caused by the active intervention of a sensate agent, possibly a supernatural force. In personalistic systems there are three main causes of illness:

- supernatural forces (e.g. a god or deity);
- non-human (e.g. ghosts, ancestors or evil spirits);
- human (e.g. witches or sorcerers).

People may believe that God and supernatural forces control the world and that human beings are at the mercy of natural forces. According to this view, the sick person is therefore a victim and may be the object of aggression or punishment, with or without justification (Jackson, 1993).

The cause of ill health is therefore not organic malfunctioning but rather forces beyond the individual's control. For example, ill health may be interpreted as a breach of good behaviour (e.g. not saying prayers at the traditional times).

In smaller-scale societies, where interpersonal conflict is more frequent, it is common to blame other people for one's ill health. The practice of witchcraft, which is particularly common in Africa and the Caribbean, is associated with malevolent or mystical powers to harm others. Witches are often 'different' from other people, either in the way they behave or in their appearance. They are an easy target for ascribing blame or misfortune, particularly when an unexplained or untreatable illness occurs, as they are then seen as the causative agents. Their powers to cause misfortunes may be either inherited or acquired by gaining membership of a particular group. Witchcraft beliefs were common in Europe in the Middle Ages and there are still echoes of these beliefs in the UK today (e.g. traditions such as Hallowe'en and images in children's fairy stories such as Hansel and Gretel).

The practice of sorcery is also common in some non-Western societies. Sorcery is the ability or power to manipulate or alter supernatural events with magical knowledge and ritual. It is a powerful force and may be used consciously among family and friends. The practice of 'Voodoo' or 'Hoodoo' is found in African and African-American cultures. Sorcery may be used to manipulate social relationships (e.g. dealing with envy or jealousy, or a partner who is straying) or it may be used to deal with ill health. The terms 'fixing' or 'hexing' are used to describe the process of sorcery. Spector (2010) has described some of the practices used in black American communities (e.g. the use of powerful oils and powders to bring luck or ward off evil).

The notion of the 'evil eye' as a cause of illness or distress is found in Europe, the Middle East, North Africa and Central and South America. The evil eye relates to the malevolent power of the look or glance of a jealous person. The glance may cause ill health or damage in the recipient of the look. The person accused of the evil eye may be totally unaware of the act, and may be a stranger or an outsider in a community; for example, a tourist or traveller may be believed to be an offender (Helman, 2007).

In Nigeria, the Yoruba people have developed a complex belief system in which a person is perceived to be at the centre of a web of personal and spiritual relationships. The Yoruba believe that a person's health is influenced by ancestors, their god, the spirits and the plants and animals in the environment (Mares *et al.*, 1985).

In personalistic systems, the patient or the victim must identify the agent behind the act and then render it harmless, as well as lift the spell. The 'curers' within this system have supernatural powers and use magical practices (e.g. trances) to detect the cause of the disease or illness. The curer will be anxious to find the cause of the disease rather than just cure it. He or she may use special powers or curing rituals, and later the victim may consult another 'lesser' curer such as a herbalist.

In this system, preventing illness involves the maintenance of good social relationships with friends and family, paying respect to ancestors through prayers and devotions and avoiding all conflict. Individuals may also wear special clothing or jewellery, or be embraced by spells to protect themselves and their families. Supernatural forces may also be responsible for other non-physical misfortunes such as crop failures, earthquakes and floods, and they may be blamed for petty misfortunes, lost articles or minor injuries.

In personalistic health belief systems, individuals are generally more conscious and mindful of the power and presence of spiritual forces. The shaman or spiritual curer is found in many cultures, and is similar to the 'clairvoyants' or 'mediums' of Western cultures. The shaman has special powers whereby they allow themselves to become possessed by certain spirits until they are able to master or neutralize them. The shaman's powers are healing in that they are able to alleviate guilt, anxieties, fears and conflicts and eradicate them. The shaman is also a part of the community, so they usually hold the shared beliefs of that community (Lipsedge, 1990).

Personalistic health belief systems are more likely to be found in rural communities or in remote communities that have little contact with the rest of the world. For example, such systems are found in remote Australian Aboriginal communities where levels of literacy are low and people have strong ties to their ancestors and their land (Jackson, 1993). However, elements of the personalistic system may be found in the UK.

Case study

Mrs Bibi was referred to the community psychiatric nurse by her GP and health visitor, who were very concerned about her low mood, insomnia and complaints of pains in her legs following the birth of her fourth child 6 weeks ago. Her husband said that he had heard Mrs Bibi talking to herself at night. Mrs Bibi moved to England 9 years ago. In England she felt very isolated and found it difficult to learn the language, mainly owing to time limits and the demands of bringing up four children. She began to express feelings of unease and anxiety about the house in which they lived. Her husband explained that the previous owners had been Hindus and Mrs Bibi felt that since they had moved in the 'Jinns' had taken possession of the house. They described the Jinns as bad spirits that caused trouble around the house. The couple revealed that they blamed Mrs Bibi's poor health on the Jinns. She felt that the Jinns were making her life miserable and making her feel like a bad mother. The couple decided to contact the Imam at their local Mosque. After visiting the house he decided that they were justified in their interpretation of the situation. The Imam returned to the house and performed a ceremony to drive out the Jinns. Mrs Bibi soon began to feel better. She described feeling more in control and having more patience with the children; her sleep had also improved. She had no further contact with the community psychiatric nurse.

Mrs Bibi, a Muslim, clearly felt that her illness was caused by malevolent spirits or Jinns. In the Islamic world, the Jinns (or ginns) are malevolent spirits that cause ill health. In a biomedical framework Mrs Bibi might have been diagnosed as suffering from postnatal depression or puerperal psychosis and treated with antidepressant medication. Instead, her beliefs (and those of the people around her) were understood – in the context of her life and her health beliefs – to be the cause of her distress. The appropriate treatment involved removing the cause of her distress by consulting the Imam who performed the relevant ceremony.

In contrast to biomedicine, the personalistic system does not have a strong scientific basis. It is characterized by a strong sense of connection to the spiritual world, and by strong beliefs based on traditions and values that are passed on from one generation to the next. Personalistic belief systems may also have connections to religion, but they are not religious in origin. These beliefs are powerful and deeply held, and people might not always be dissuaded from practising their health beliefs by the arguments for biomedicine.

Health beliefs in naturalistic systems

Unlike biomedicine, which is a relative newcomer, naturalism (also known as holism) has a long tradition and originates in the ancient civilizations of Greece, India and China. Naturalistic systems explain illness in personal and systemic terms. Health is seen as the balance of elements (e.g. heat and cold) in the body. Human life is only one aspect of nature and is part of the natural cosmos. Any disturbance and imbalance causes illness and disease or misfortune. Unlike personalistic beliefs, naturalistic approaches to health are widely believed and form the basis of traditional health practices in many Asian countries, including China, Japan, Singapore, Taiwan and Korea. They are also found in South America, the Philippines, Iran and Pakistan.

According to naturalistic systems, illness is caused by either excessive heat or cold entering the body and causing an imbalance. Sometimes this involves actual temperatures (e.g. standing in a cold room or in a cold wind). Everyday objects are also often ascribed hot or cold properties. Thus foods, medicines, physical conditions (e.g. childbirth) and emotional conditions may be given hot and cold properties.

Health in traditional Chinese medicine

In Chinese medicine, for example, the normal functioning of the body is perceived as a balance between two opposite energies – yin and yang. Traditional Chinese medicine is a well-organized and highly respected system of medical knowledge based on observations and trials on the human body. The fundamental premise of Chinese medicine is the principle of maintaining balance and harmony in the body. The key concepts include yin, yang and chi. The Chinese regard the human body, the natural surroundings, the social relationships that pervade society and the supernatural world as elements that are linked and regulated by the adequate management of opposites and similarities.

Chi is force or energy that irrigates the human system, and health results in sufficient and adequately distributed energy. The strength and flow of chi depends on the correct balance of yin and yang – two opposing forces. Yin is regarded as a cold, dark, watery (female) force, while yang is a hot, fiery (male) energy. The relationship and interaction between yin and yang produce changes in the body, and illness and disease occur when there is a deficiency of an energy or energy disequilibrium.

The role of the traditional practitioner is to restore the balance of these vital forces so that the patient is able to overcome their illness. Illness is diagnosed by questioning the patient about the complaint, observing their general appearance and taking their pulse. The practitioner may then prescribe a variety of cures to restore the balance. Various practices may be used, such as acupuncture, foods, herbs, exercise, dietary restrictions and enema poultices, all of which are aimed at restoring the balance between hot and cold. In contrast to Western medicine, there are few invasive procedures. Practitioners are highly respected in Chinese cultures. Sometimes coins may be used on the skin to treat headaches and other minor ailments (Jones, 1994; Schott and Henley, 1996; Gervais and Jovchelovitch, 1998).

In Chinese culture, food plays an integral role in the restoration of health. For example, an individual who experiences too much anger over a long period of time may expose the body to excessive heat and risks becoming ill with a 'hot' disease. In this case, prescribing the appropriate cold food may restore the balance between yin and yang. Cold (yin) foods may vary between cultures, but they are generally bland foods such as boiled and steamed foods, including vegetables and fruits. However, hot (yang) foods include spicy foods or those containing high levels of animal protein. Hot and cold foods may vary within communities and between families (Mares *et al.*, 1985).

Gervais and Jovchelovitch (1998, p. 38) note the use of other food in illness, and quote an interviewee as follows: 'For flu, some people they drink a lot of ginger. They bang the ginger and they get the juice of the ginger, the drink of the root flowing out'. Another interviewee cited other cures for rheumatism and arthritis: 'You have to buy the piece of snake and put it in alcohol. ... It's good medicine to treat the joints. I mean the snake contains some medicine'.

Pillsbury (1978) discussed traditional postnatal customs in China. After childbirth it is believed that women are vulnerable to illness because the body has become depleted of heat. In many traditional cultures it is stipulated that women should be confined to the home for 1 month. During this time a woman is said to be 'sitting out' the month, and she is expected to observe a set of extremely restricted prescriptions and codes of behaviour. Many of these rules are based on the balance of yin and yang. For example, the woman may be forbidden to wash her hair during the month (because water is believed to cause wind to enter the body, which may lead to asthma later in life). She is also forbidden to go outside during the month, as this may cause the gods to look down and catch sight of her. She is forbidden cold or raw foods (e.g. Chinese cabbage, leafy green vegetables and most fruits), but she is encouraged to eat chicken (which is a hot food and may 'create fire' which helps to restore balance). She must also avoid exposure to the wind or a breeze, as cold air may open up the joints and lead to rheumatism later in life.

The findings of this research are also highlighted in the study by Gervais and Jovchelovitch (1998). One man who was interviewed said: 'We believe [women] lose a lot of blood [during delivery], they lose a lot of yang already so they have to bring it back to the neutral'. In the same study, fried and baked foods as well as ginger and ginseng were taken during the postnatal month. People also recognized the importance of sitting at home and waiting for the balance to be restored.

Pillsbury (1978) notes:

> My observations of interpersonal reactions in Chinese households during the month give the impression that far more attention is lavished upon the mother relative to the newborn infant than in the United States. This extra attention their families and social networks show them while they are doing the month seems in fact to preclude Chinese women from experiencing postpartum depression as understood and taken for granted by Americans.
>
> *(Pillsbury, 1978, p. 20)*

Ayurvedic medicine

Ayurvedic medicine, practised mainly on the Indian subcontinent, is a traditional Hindu system of medicine which is over 2000 years old. Health is again viewed as a state of balance and disease as a state of disharmony, and treatment is concerned with finding internal remedies to restore harmony. The term 'Ayurvedic' is derived from 'Ayur', meaning life and longevity, and 'veda', meaning science. The universe is believed to be composed of five elements or bhutas, namely earth, air, fire, ether and wind. These are the five basic constituents of all life, and they also make up the three dosas (or humours) in the body. The dosas or doshas are the person's qualities, or humours, and they vary according to the time of life or the season:

- vata – wind, linked to dryness and old age;
- pitta – bile, linked to water, the rainy season and middle age;
- kapha – phlegm, linked to the earth, springtime and the growing season.

The body is said to be composed of seven tissues, the dhatus, which need to balance in order to ensure good health. Tensions are created by the changing seasons, the lifespan and habits that may cause ill health. Health is maintained by ensuring a balance between the humours. Notions of heat and cold in the diet also exist in Ayurvedic medicine and diet may be used as therapy. Unbalanced diets may cause disease (Helman, 2007; Jones, 1994; Schott and Henley, 1996).

The role of medicine is to control the dosas and restore the humours of the body to balance. Ayurvedic medicine is very popular in India, where there are Ayurvedic universities where Hakims (the practitioners of Ayurvedic medicine) are trained. Ayurvedic medicine is funded by the Indian government and coexists with Western scientific medicine, which was imposed during the British colonial period (Healey and Aslam, 1990).

Key points

1. There are three broad health belief systems, namely biomedicine, personalistic (or magico-religious) and naturalistic (or holistic systems).
2. Biomedicine is the most dominant form of health belief system in the developed world.
3. Other forms of health beliefs are powerful and prominent in many cultures.

SECTORS OF HEALTH CARE

When people become ill or need medical help they may have several options open to them, depending on where they live, who they are and the prevailing healthcare practices in that culture. Healthcare systems always exist in context – they cannot be isolated from the prevailing social, religious, political and economic organizations that surround them and indeed shape and influence them.

Kleinman (1986) suggests that in any complex society there are three sectors of health care that often coexist. Each sector has its own way of understanding and treating health problems, deciding who the appropriate person to treat the problem is and how the patient and the healer should behave towards each other. These three sectors of health care are the popular, folk and professional sectors and will be used to explore how patients access health care and healthcare advice.

The popular sector

This sector may also be called the lay sector, and it is usually the first port of call when people are ill. It does not usually involve financial transactions. For example, people may choose to self-medicate or to consult relatives, friends or neighbours. There is often heavy reliance on family members, especially on women. In a study of Gypsy Travelling communities, Parry *et al.* (2004) note that many people placed great trust in family carers and the lay referral system. Close family was seen as important in a 'hostile world where sometimes people may be met with hostile reactions from health workers':

> in a second, you can tell by their attitude, they don't look you in the eye, it's just sort of 'what's the problem'... they do palm you off the minute they find out you are Travellers.

(Parry et al. 2004, p. 70)

Lay referral systems are also important as many people lack confidence in dealing with bureaucracy and in particular with 'form filling' – 'If you don't read and write it's difficult to get information' (Parry *et al.* 2004).

In many cultures, however, mothers and grandmothers are often the first point of consultation, as a friend so vividly pointed out to me:

> When I had my first baby, I was really lucky as I had my sister and my mum living close by. It was great because if there was anything wrong with Danny, I would just get on the phone straight away and they would come round to see us. It's easier and quicker than ringing the doctor or health visitor – and you know that they're not going to think you are just another neurotic mother. Now I have three of my own – they're a bit older so I help my younger sister, giving a bit of advice here and a few tips there etc. It's nice to be able to pass on your experience.

In this case the main credentials or qualifications for giving advice are past experiences, which are regarded as effective and worthwhile, and are 'passed on' through families. When people become ill they often treat themselves (e.g. using traditional medicines or foods that have been passed on as cures). I asked some friends and relatives how they treat a common cold and the replies varied widely (see Box 2.1).

Box 2.1 Health beliefs and the common cold

'I go to bed with a hot-water bottle and drink lots of lemonade'
'Oh, I just try to carry on as normal – after all, a cold is just a cold'
'I drink lots of honey and lemon – my grandma always said it is soothing'
'I like to take Lemsips (aspirin and citric acid). I like the taste and it makes me feel a bit brighter'
'Vitamin C is very good for colds. It helps fight them off'
'I go to the doctor's for some antibiotics in case it goes to my chest'
'I just take Panadol and water – the water helps to rehydrate me and the Panadol gets my temperature down'
'I take whisky, water, lemon and honey, all boiled together'

In a society that places great value on biomedicine, we might have expected to see some uniform standard practices based on sound medical evidence. Health beliefs and practices vary even within the biomedical framework and, interestingly, in this 'straw poll' only one person considered consulting a doctor. The only common feature was the reliance on vitamin C, which took the form of lemons or lemonade. Vitamin C therefore seems to take on medicinal properties.

Other practices that may be considered effective or useful are those that help the individual to stay well or ward off ill health. These may include wearing lucky charms or medals, saying prayers or adopting the correct behaviours. Spector (1996) emphasizes that these health protectors may take many forms. For example, charms such as amulets are worn on a string around the neck, wrist or waist to protect the wearer from the evil eye. The mano milagroso is worn by people of Mexican origin for luck and the prevention of evil. In Muslim communities, a fragment of the Qur'an may be worn on the body. In Catholic countries, small medals of favourite saints may be pinned to clothing to protect the individual from adversity. In other countries, garlic is thought to protect health, and for this reason may be found hanging in some people's homes.

I asked a group of student nurses to give examples of health beliefs that they knew and had grown up with; the resulting list is shown in Box 2.2.

Box 2.2 Health beliefs of student nurses at the University of Salford

An apple a day keeps the doctor away

Eat the crusts on bread – it makes your hair curly

Eating lots of fish makes you intelligent – 'good brain food'

Sitting on a cold wall gives you haemorrhoids

Coughs and sneezes spread diseases

Eating lots of raw jelly makes your nails strong

Drink Guinness when you're pregnant – it's rich in iron

Don't go to bed with your hair wet or you'll get pneumonia

If you suffer heartburn in pregnancy, your baby will have lots of hair

Bananas are good for digestion

Bananas and hot milk are very good for insomnia

Feed a cold and starve a fever

Wear a thick vest or liberty bodice in winter – it stops chills on the kidneys

Garlic thins the blood

Colicky babies should be given treacle – it settles the stomach

Fresh air for babies – strengthens the lungs

Keep your feet warm – this stops colds and chills

Carrots make you see in the dark

Masturbation makes you blind/mad

Cheese gives you nightmares (avoid at bedtime)

Avoid sexual intercourse when you're pregnant – it may damage your baby's head

During pregnancy, boys are carried at the back and girls are carried at the front

Avoid swimming/sexual intercourse/washing your hair when you are menstruating

Laughter is the best medicine

When a person has shingles (herpes zoster), if the lines meet in the middle they may die

Ways to induce labour in pregnancy:

    Castor oil

    Sexual intercourse

    An enema

    A hot curry

    Walking with one foot on the pavement and one food on the road

    A bumpy car drive

Reflective exercise

1. Which of the statements in Box 2.2 do you agree with, and why?
2. Which statements are based on scientific theory?
3. Which of them do you reject as untrue, false or an 'old wives' tale'?
4. Think of other beliefs that you grew up with and share them with colleagues.

Individuals that may be consulted in the popular sector include women with several children, friends, neighbours, paramedics, nurses, people that have had the same illness, doctors' receptionists, and the spouses or partners of doctors. As nurses, we may often be regarded as a source of knowledge among our family, peers or even the community. Popular help may even extend to anyone who regularly deals or interacts with the public (e.g. the police). A local hairdresser told me the following:

> I have just started a certificate in counselling. The reason I'm doing it is because it occurred to me some time ago that I spend much of my working life listening to people's problems. I thought, 'Well, I might as well try to do it properly', so I'm learning how to help people at night school. I just think of it as another skill. To me it's just as important to some people as the perm they have or the right cut.

Another important and popular source of non-professional help is self-help groups, where people may share advice, seek or give support (a factor involved in healing) or help novices and newcomers. Self-help groups and voluntary organizations value their members' experience rather than their professional expertise. They value mutual help, and often seek to destigmatize and demystify the health problem.

Key points

1. In the popular sector, help is non-professional.
2. The popular sector values experience and mutuality.
3. In the popular sector self-help and self-medication is important.

The folk sector

The folk sector is often a feature of developing countries or non-Western societies. It may take an intermediate position between the popular and professional sectors. The practitioners or healers in the folk sector are usually based in the community, and are well known and valued by the local people. Consequently, they may share the same values and beliefs as the local community and so are in an ideal position to adopt a holistic approach to the person being treated. For example, they may be able to advise on all aspects of the individual's life or their family position. Although this position is more formalized than in the popular sector, there is little training, and education may be acquired through an apprenticeship. People may also become healers as a result of special gifts or signs that are bestowed upon them. They may receive the 'gift' of healing from a 'divine' source (e.g. in a vision), or they may gain their skills from their family (usually through the mother). In Ireland, for example, the seventh son of the seventh son is believed to have special powers.

There are many different types of folk healer, (e.g. clairvoyants, spiritual healers, shamans). Treatment in the folk sector may include the use of special herbs and medicines. Parry *et al.* (2004) in a study of Gypsy Travellers in the UK found that some people spoke of their belief in 'curing people' or specific religious healers in the community. Seeking the help of curing people may be combined with going to pilgrimage sites such as Lourdes in France or Knock in Ireland.

Spector (2009) describes the healing practices of Native American healers. She notes that they are wise in the ways of the land and of nature. They know well the interrelationships of human beings, the Earth and the universe. Herbs are regarded as spiritual helpers and are prescribed and used in treatments. For example the Hopi Indians use sunflower to treat spider bites and the stem of a yucca plant to treat constipation.

Divination is a ritual that is found world-wide. It aims to uncover the supernatural causes of illness by the use of supernatural powers. Among Navaho Indians, motions of the hands are used in conjunction with sand-sprinkling to guide the healer to the cause of illness. Songs and chants may also accompany the ritual. Star-gazers pray to the stars, asking for the cause of illness, and listening may be used to guide the healer to the cause of illness (the sound heard guides the healer). Spector (2009) argues that many of these effects are psychological, and that the chanting and hand motions may bring calmness and a sense of being cared for. These healing gifts are not inherited or learned, they are received as a gift. The rituals follow a complex pattern and are cherished within the community.

The folk sector plays an extremely important role in helping people to maintain their psychological health, but unfortunately practitioners are often dismissed as 'quacks' or charlatans by professional health workers. However, it must be acknowledged that there are unscrupulous operators who masquerade as 'healers', and they need to be distinguished from those who have genuine healing powers.

There are several advantages to healing by traditional practitioners that are often overlooked. Spector (2009) emphasizes that the healer in folk medicine may maintain an informal friendly relationship with the patient and may place great emphasis on building and maintaining a good rapport with the individual and their family. Thus, in folk medicine, people may feel that they have a greater degree of control with regard to the treatment that they are expected to follow. Patients may also find that they are given more time and consideration. Their background and social circumstances are understood, so they are not regarded as impersonal malfunctioning units, but as individuals in their own social context.

Key points

1. Folk medicine lies in an intermediate position between lay and professional medicine.
2. Folk medicine healers may have a central role to play in the spiritual and social welfare of the client.
3. Folk medicine healers employ ritualistic and complex methods of treatment.

Professional medicine

This system of health care is generally regarded as the most highly organized and developed approach. Professions, by definition, have their own collective system of management, education and codes of conduct. They are usually self-regulating and have their own powers and policies. They also have their own knowledge base and highly developed skills. Professional medical practitioners may include not only doctors but also the paramedical professionals (e.g. nurses, physiotherapists).

However, the medical profession has its own group with a powerful hierarchy and a set of prescribed rules and codes of conduct. The medical profession is prestigious and respected in Western society, and members of the profession are financially well rewarded. In the UK, members of the medical profession are categorized within complex hierarchies of knowledge and power, such as professors, lecturers, consultants, registrars and house officers. They also work in very specialized and highly defined areas of practice related mainly to the nature of patients' problems (e.g. cardiac care, gastroenterology, rheumatology).

When a patient consults a doctor, he or she will use problem-solving skills to determine the cause or individual nature of a specific problem that the patient is experiencing. In the past, patients were often treated away from home in specialist centres, and their problems were considered in isolation, away from their families or communities. However, there has been an increased focus on primary and community care (Department of Health, 2008) whereby patients not only have more say about the nature of professional medicine received but also work together with the medical profession, enabling the patients to take more control over their health.

Doctors are highly trained, with scientific and intellectual skills that are used to diagnose illness (as opposed to spiritual or intuitive processes). They may use technical instruments or make a diagnosis by using quantifiable measurements based on the physiological details of the patient (e.g. blood pressure). In general, the families of patients being treated in hospital are only allowed to visit at designated times, although this does vary from region to region. Hospitals and health centres have their own rules and codes of behaviour, and these largely reflect cultures and prevailing ideologies in society.

CONCLUSION

In this chapter I have described the three categories of health belief systems, namely biomedicine, personalistic and holistic systems, and the ways in which healthcare delivery is organized. These distinct classifications are useful, but in practice they are rarely mutually exclusive. They represent different ways of viewing the world and values about health. In the UK, for example, biomedicine dominates health practice, yet complementary therapies and alternative healers are becoming increasingly popular. There are many nurses and doctors who have skills in therapies such as massage or aromatherapy. The growing popularity of alternative or complementary therapies in the UK may simply be because of the increased availability of, and publicity about, these practices, as well as some dissatisfaction with biomedicine. This dissatisfaction may have arisen in response to reductionist approaches to health and illness, prompting people to seek more holistic approaches. For example, holism rejects the notion of the mind–body split, and instead recognizes the relationship between individuals and their environment.

Jackson (1993) argues that in alternative or complementary therapies the individual is viewed as an active central participant in health care, as opposed to the passive recipient of biomedicine. There is a growing body of thought that acknowledges the concept of holism as being central to successful health care, and nursing itself has embraced the fundamental principles of holism, ensuring that care is individualized as well as holistic.

CHAPTER SUMMARY

1. Health beliefs are universal and central to the way in which health care is practised and delivered.
2. The three main health belief systems, namely biomedicine, personalism and holism, are rarely mutually exclusive.
3. Biomedicine – the dominant health belief system in the developed world – is becoming increasingly influenced by other belief systems, particularly holism.

FURTHER READING

Armstrong E (2002) Scorpions, snakes and qi gong in Chinese medicine. *Practice Nursing* **13**, 361–3.
This article explores Chinese medicine and in particular the concept of yin and yang. It is informative and interesting.

Brewer J and A, Bonalumi N (1995) Cultural diversity in the Emergency Department: health care beliefs and practices among the Pennsylvania Amish. *Journal of Emergency Nursing* **21**, 494–7.
This article discusses the health care practices of the Amish, an ethnic group in Pennsylvania in the USA. The article is a sensitive and illuminating consideration of a cultural group and the authors demonstrate how seemingly 'traditional' healthcare beliefs and practices may be approached with a 'modern' perspective.

Bury M and Gabe J (2003) *Sociology of health and illness: a reader.* Routledge, London.
This book offers a wide range of papers focusing on health beliefs and knowledge and related themes.

Ohnuki-Tierney E (1993) *Illness and culture in contemporary Japan. An anthropological view.* Cambridge University Press, New York.
This work gives a fascinating insight into a description of Japanese health care.

WEBSITES

http://ethnomed.org/

This website is an excellent site for information on many cultures, their beliefs and customs, including patient education information and access to other related websites. There are also video clips in different languages. It has a US focus but useful knowledge for any reader.

http://www.intute.ac.uk

This is an excellent portal to access different websites world wide on a wide range of topics such as beliefs and cultures.

http://openlearn.open.ac.uk/course/view.php?id=3371&topic=all

This is the web-link to the Open University Learning Space site for the *issues in complementary and alternative medicine* unit, which looks at a range of issues including different health belief models.

3 Working with health and illness beliefs in practice

Christine Hogg

INTRODUCTION

In Chapter 2, I examined the major divisions in health beliefs and the way that health care is delivered depending on the prevailing cultural beliefs about health and illness. At the end of that chapter I stressed that the boundaries of health practices are often blurred. Indeed, Helman (2007) argues that the larger and more complex the society, the more therapeutic options are available.

Helman (2007) states that:

> Modern urbanized societies, whether Western or non-Western, are more likely, therefore to exhibit health care pluralism. ... Though these therapeutic modes coexist, they are often based on entirely different premises, and may even originate in different cultures, such as Western medicine in China, or Chinese acupuncture in the modern Western world. To the ill person, however, the origin of these treatments is less important than their efficacy in relieving suffering.
>
> *(Helman, 2007, p. 81)*

This chapter will focus on the following issues:

- pluralism in health care;
- magico-religious beliefs in health care practices in the UK;
- caring for people with different health beliefs;
- eliciting health beliefs and working with them in practice.

PLURALISM IN HEALTH CARE

In health care, pluralism means the use of two or more different types of health care. These may be used concurrently or alternatively. In the UK there is a growing awareness of complementary or alternative medicines. For example, a mother whose child has a skin condition such as eczema may use homeopathic remedies at one time and switch to a conventional remedy, such as steroid cream, at another. Another example is a man with depression, who may be prescribed antidepressants by his GP, but may also use massage concurrently if he believes that stress is the root cause of his depression. In the UK, Muslims may consult the hakim before, after or instead of the GP, and in Hindu communities the Vaid may provide health care. Some people, for example, may use two systems. They may practise one system and consult their GP (professional), but ignore the advice given and instead follow the advice of someone else (e.g. a relative or friend). Many people use alternative practitioners as well as or instead of conventional practitioners.

Gervais and Jovchelovitch (1998) found that the Chinese people they interviewed tried to integrate the two systems of health beliefs (i.e. traditional Chinese and Western medicine). One participant said:

> I think most of us look at traditional Chinese medicine and Western medicine as coexisting quite nicely. I think that on the whole most of us would try anything as long as it works. You'll find that sometimes [the Chinese] go to both. They see the Western medical doctor and then toddle off to a herbalist to get the herbs, and then they'll use the two together. They wouldn't see the conflict.

> *(Gervais and Jovchelovitch, 1998, p. 51)*

Many individuals in this study believed that Western medicine was beneficial because it offered 'quick-fix' solutions, but that Chinese medicine tackles the root of the problem. Chinese medicines, tonics and herbs are used to maintain good health, whereas biomedicine is used to deal with serious diseases. In this study it has been clearly demonstrated that Chinese people integrate different systems of knowledge and combine health resources. Their approaches to health care were flexible and did not rely solely on one method at the expense of another.

Thorne (1993) has criticized Western medicine and its dominance and claims to superiority over other approaches to the treatment of health and illness. Non-biomedical systems are generally described as 'non-rational, superstitious and non-objective' and therefore inferior. Thorne also highlights the contradiction in our society:

> As a society, we abuse our physical selves in search of psychosocial well-being, we pay for expert medical advice we have no intention of following, and we express considerable anxiety about the extent to which crime, environmental destruction and social injustice influence the 'health' of nations.

> *(Thorne, 1993, p. 1934)*

Thorne (1993) highlights the fact that although Western medicine is purported to be superior, in reality the indigenous population often ignores it. This point can be demonstrated by the low uptake of health promotion relating to smoking. Although there are clear scientifically proven links between smoking and heart disease, a significant number of people continue to smoke. Interestingly, some people rationalize their smoking by claiming that they enjoy it or that it is a stress reliever. We have probably all heard the refrain 'if I don't die of this, I might die of something else' or 'I could get run over by a bus tomorrow'. These views about health are fatalistic – they assume that it is in someone else's hands. Another criticism that Thorne (1993) levels at biomedicine is the low priority given to maintaining good relationships. In Chinese mental health, for example, great emphasis is placed on health as a communal activity – it is the responsibility of everyone. Thus health may be restored by, for example, discovering and rectifying the source of animosity towards the patient. This is in contrast to Western biomedicine and can be seen in the following observation of a nurse working on an acute medical ward:

> I often wonder about the way we sort out people's problems on the wards, we just send them back to the same conditions that caused the illness in the first place. I mean it's OK for me to say to such and such a body, ' yes, you can go back home now and think that's that'. One lady was in here last month after being harassed by her neighbour's son. It caused her an acute asthma attack and yet as soon as she got better, we just sent her straight back home. Nobody thought about actually tackling her real problems – the fact that she can't even leave her house without getting abused in the street, must cause her to feel hemmed in and under a lot of pressure, yet we ignore that and just congratulate her when her peak flows are up.

A study by Parry *et al.* (2004) of Gypsies (Roma) and Travellers found that great emphasis was placed on self reliance, stoicism and tolerance of chronic ill health. There was a belief that you have to be 'tough' and not 'give in'. However, this notion was also linked to general mistrust of the people in 'outside' society, that is, settled people or 'Gorgios' as they are know in many Gypsy dialects.

Travellers' beliefs and attitudes led to great pride in taking control and self determination. There was also a fear of being weak or lazy and they expressed the need to keep going for the sake of their children's well-being. This may stop Traveller families from seeking the help and support that they need. Fatalism was expressed as 'if God borned you down to have a short life, you had a short life and if he borned you to have a long life, you'd have a long life – nothing you can do to alter it.' (Parry *et al.*, 2004). However these fatalistic attitudes to illness and a deep-rooted fear of cancer may lead to people avoiding screening as medical treatment is seen as unlikely to make any difference.

There is also evidence that the way in which illness is perceived in the biomedical system still relies on non-scientific rationale. Helman's work (2007) describes a set of beliefs about colds, chills and fevers that are commonly held by residents in a London suburb. The results of his research clearly demonstrate that in the UK, people's health beliefs are still enmeshed in humoural theories about health and illness, as opposed to biomedicine.

Helman's (1994) research revealed that people believe that 'colds' and 'chills' are caused by the penetration of the natural environment across the boundaries of the skin into the human body, with damp or wet conditions being believed to cause cold or wet conditions in the body, such as a 'runny nose' or a 'cold in the head'. Cold or dry environments caused cold or dry conditions such as a feeling of cold, shivering and muscular aches. The cold forces were found mainly in the upper part of the body, such as the head, and had the ability to move around the body so, for example, a head cold could 'go to the chest'. Chills occurred mainly in the lower part of the body (e.g. a bladder chill or a chill on the kidneys). These conditions were mainly caused by the individuals putting themselves at risk by careless behaviour (e.g. walking barefoot on a cold floor). Another example was 'washing your hair when you don't feel well' or 'sitting in a draught after a hot bath'. Colds and chills are therefore the individual's own responsibility caused, as one man explained, 'by doing something abnormal'.

Folk remedies for colds emphasized the return to a normal temperature and balance by treating cold with heat (e.g. hot drinks, hot food, rest in a warm bed) and generally comforting one's body (e.g. by feeding oneself – hence the phrase 'feed a cold').

In contrast, fevers were believed to be caused by invisible entities called 'bugs', germs or viruses. They penetrated orifices and caused a raised temperature as well as other symptoms. These 'germs' were considered to be amoral agents, like 'insects' that travel through the air. They were also endowed with personalities of their own. One person stated that 'I've got that germ, doctor, you know – the one that gives you the diarrhoea, and makes you bring up'. Once a germ enters the body and causes a fever, it can move to attack several parts of the body simultaneously: 'It's gone to my lungs' or 'I can feel it in my stomach'. The victims of fevers are blameless and are able to mobilize the sympathy and help of friends and relatives. Remedies and cures for fevers are aimed at restoring the temperature to normal and washing out the germ or starving it of any nourishment – hence the phrase 'starve a fever'.

Other remedies may include 'sweating' – that is, 'sweating it out of your system'. Germs cannot be seen but are 'invisible malign spirits' that have a combat status (hence the need to 'fight it off'). Remedies used may include many types of potions and mixtures, none of which have a scientific basis. Helman's (1994) research is familiar to anyone raised in the UK or European culture. The echoes of these beliefs are used by nurses in hospitals. When having a baby in hospital, I remember being told very firmly by a midwife (as I strolled around barefoot in the summer months): 'Put your slippers on! You'll catch your death of cold!'

Some practices and customs that are inherent to the UK healthcare system are based on health beliefs that are neither scientific nor rational. An example of this is the extent to which superstition (or magico-religion) still plays a part in our practices. Examples that are encountered on wards include the sayings and beliefs listed in Box 3.1.

Box 3.1 Superstitious beliefs encountered in nursing practice

'Deaths always come in threes'
'Bed number 13 is unlucky'
'Never put red and white flowers together in a vase' (because the colours symbolize death and are therefore unlucky)
'A full moon means there are more people with mental illness around'
'Whenever there's a death on the ward, open a window so that the soul can fly out'

Reflective exercise

1. Which of the above beliefs are you familiar with?
2. Do you know of any others?
3. How superstitious are you? List the superstitions you follow (e.g. touching wood, reading your horoscope).

SUPERSTITIOUS BELIEFS IN HEALTHCARE PRACTICE

In nursing practice, there are many health beliefs that are illogical or which are based on false or unscientific premises and assumptions. A mental health nurse recounted the following story:

> There was one ward where I had a placement, where the staff and patients never ate from the same plates or drank from the same cups. When I questioned this, a staff nurse said 'Oh that's because we don't want to catch anything from the patients'. I said, laughingly, do you mean like schizophrenia and manic depression, and to my astonishment she said 'Yes'. I couldn't believe it, in this day and age! It was like something out of the dark ages.

Thorne (1993) made the following observation:

> In my opinion, nurses committed to a more global orientation must fix their gaze beyond cultural sensitivity and begin to appreciate the way in which the western biomedical tradition has influenced all aspects of their practice and of the organizational structures within which that practice occurs.

> *(Thorne, 1993, p. 1939)*

Western medicine is a relative newcomer in terms of healthcare delivery and practice, but by the same token it is a system that has made huge advances in terms of life expectancy and treating illness and disease. In developing countries, Western medicine has provided people with protection against fatal diseases such as malaria, and its value cannot be underestimated. However, it is important to note that, although biomedicine is the dominant belief system in the UK, there are still echoes of superstition or magico-religious beliefs in everyday practice.

Key points

1. Pluralism is an important and significant factor in health care that pervades most healthcare systems.
2. People may use alternative or complementary systems concurrently with conventional systems.
3. Western or modern medicine incorporates other facets of health belief systems, such as magico-religious beliefs.

CARING FOR PEOPLE WITH DIFFERENT HEALTH BELIEFS

One of the greatest challenges in healthcare practice is to care for people with different health beliefs from one's own:

> Each of us tends to trust the system we have grown up with. We assume that practitioners in this system know what they are doing, and [we] often mistrust those who do things differently.

> *(Henley and Schott, 1999, p. 24)*

Let us consider some of the issues through one health problem.

The case of diabetes

The way that people understand health and illness issues in other cultures is demonstrated by the differing views of diabetes mellitus (DM).

A study by Hjelm *et al.* (1999) of Swedish people and Yugoslavian migrants with diabetes found that the Yugoslavian migrants discussed their adverse experiences as migrants when explaining the causes of their diabetes. They also retained some of their former traditions such as taking natural drops and foods that they believed might make them feel better, such as puréed carrots. They were also less inclined towards self care and seemed to behave in a more passive role when dealing with their diabetes. In a study in the UK, Meetoo and Meetoo (2005) also discovered that people from South Asian communities found that taking alternative medicines for DM was considered appropriate as they were thought to have fewer side effects. In a further study Hjelm *et al.* (2003) interviewing Arabic-speaking communities explained the causes of DM as being through the will of Allah or God.

A study by Lewis (2007) of British Indian patients in West London found that some had beliefs about the way that the vascular system of the body works. Hindus, for example, had concepts of channels (nadis) along which a 'mystical vital force' (prana) flows. They also believed that DM could be caused by the jealousy of other people who may curse you. Other causes may be being the victim of unprovoked malice or doing something wrong in a past life.

The following Case Study explores the complexities and challenges of caring for someone whose health beliefs may be in conflict with one's own.

Case study

Gloria is a 72-year-old woman who emigrated to the UK from the West Indies in 1952. She lives alone, her husband died 8 years ago, and she has a daughter and two sons living in the neighbourhood. She has been diagnosed with diabetes mellitus and the district nurses are baffled by her reluctance to follow their dietary advice. Gloria says that she gets bored with eating vegetables all day and every day.

Pierce and Armstrong's (1996) research examined the attitudes of African-Caribbean people towards diabetes. Using focus groups, they identified a variety of beliefs about the causes of diabetes and the appropriate care and treatment for the condition. For example, some people clearly associated diabetes with sugar. However, sugar had different properties for different people. One woman believed that her diabetes was 'part of the ovaries breaking down and being unable to handle sugar', and another believed that depression had contributed to her diabetes.

Other individuals in the study blamed their illnesses on English food, and one woman reported that she knew of someone who had returned to the West Indies and found that their diabetes had cleared up. There was also a belief that 'starchy foods were bad'. Foods that grow underground (e.g. yams and potatoes) were believed to be very starchy, whereas those that grow above ground (e.g. bananas and plantain) were not. Pierce and Armstrong (1996) stated that :

continued

Case study

> In the West Indies, a lot of starchy foods were eaten, but the hot sun and general heat ensured that these foods were 'burned up'. Perspiration then got rid of the food. Thus it was failure to perspire sufficiently in the UK that made starchy foods into a potentially dangerous factor.
>
> *(Pierce and Armstrong, 1996, p. 96)*

This research may provide some insight into Gloria's reluctance to follow dietary advice. It may be that Gloria is avoiding starchy foods, preferring instead to eat a diet of vegetables in the belief that she should avoid carbohydrates.

What action could the nurse who is caring for Gloria take in this situation?

In this situation, the nurse may find it useful to ask Gloria about her day-to-day life and her understanding of diabetes and the effects that it has on her body. It may also be useful to elicit her attitudes and feelings about the diabetes, and how she perceived the condition prior to diagnosis. For example, the nurse could ask her the following questions.

- What do you know and understand about diabetes?
- Do you know anyone else who is diabetic?
- What do your family think about diabetes?
- What has caused you to have diabetes, and how does it affect you?

ELICITING HEALTH BELIEFS

At the beginning of this chapter we stressed that healthcare professionals are socialized into one culture, and then resocialized into a provider culture. Subsequently, they come into contact with people who have chosen to retain and maintain their beliefs and practices with regard to health and illness. Differences in beliefs may result in conflicts with regard to care and treatment, as well as apathy and withdrawal from care that may be manifested, for example, by broken appointments or failure to comply with prescribed medication. As already discussed, nurses themselves incorporate a set of beliefs, values and customs as soon as they enter the arena of nursing. The culture of nursing has a language of its own, and it is all too common to hear a patient say 'I don't understand what the nurses and doctors are saying – they use all sorts of technical language and abbreviations'. This problem is compounded when there are also linguistic differences between the nurse and the patient (see Chapter 1).

The financial cost of mismanaging care is very high. If patients miss appointments, valuable slots on waiting lists are wasted. However, the human costs are perhaps even higher. For example, people who do not seek help or access care may be risking their health and ultimately their lives.

Mares *et al.* (1985) suggest the following practical ways to find out about people's beliefs and practices.

- Avoid trying to change the traditional practices of people because they do not fit in with the expectations of the health service institutions.

- Any proposal for practical action should be made as far as possible with representatives of the community. It is pertinent to find out what changes, if any, members of the community might like to see.
- It may be useful to undertake a detailed exploration of the health beliefs and practices of the people you are working with in relation to your area of practice.

They also suggest the following useful tips.

- Find out about the health beliefs and practices of people in your area by reading the available literature and information. It may be useful to compare this with what people in the local community tell you.
- Establish the use of traditional healers and, if possible, meet them and discuss their approaches to care.
- Establish which illnesses are significant in the community and what people are most concerned about. Find out about people's beliefs in the causes of illness and effective prevention and cures.
- Find out which symptoms are regarded as serious. Make sure that your colleagues know and are aware of the differences; be aware that people may need reassurance about symptoms that health staff do not consider to be serious.
- Give guidelines on symptoms that should be seen by a doctor.
- Try to build up a picture of the normal chain of referral within the community.
- Explain your role carefully and describe your relationship with other members of staff who may be involved in terms that patients can understand.
- Involve local people in education programmes, especially key members of the community (e.g. elderly people who are highly respected).

Health beliefs or traditional values may be at odds with one's own values. As one midwifery lecturer wrote:

> When I worked in the East End we put a lot of time and energy into trying to persuade Bengali women to put their babies on their tummies to sleep, but to no avail. They persisted in lying them on their backs. The Back to Sleep campaign made nonsense of our advice. I wonder how much else that we think is sacrosanct will also turn out to be wrong.
>
> *(Schott and Henley, 1996, p. 125)*

People are unlikely to change their beliefs and practices if they feel under pressure or if they consider that their views are under threat or will be ridiculed. Attempts to try to change people's beliefs are almost always counter-productive. Instead, it may be useful to involve clients in making decisions about their care in a way that does not make them feel threatened or stupid. This may result in greater compliance and cooperation.

Jackson (1993) suggests that the following questions should be asked in order to elicit information about the client's health beliefs.

- What do you think caused your problem?
- Why do you think it started when it did?
- What do you think your sickness does to you?
- How does it work?
- How severe is your sickness?
- Will it have a short or long course?
- What kind of treatment should you receive?
- What are the most important results you hope to receive from this treatment?
- What are the chief problems your sickness has caused you?
- What do you fear most about your sickness?

It is important to remember to establish rapport with the patient and to ask these questions with sensitivity and care. After eliciting this information, Jackson (1993) advocates taking the following steps in order to negotiate a care plan.

1. *Explain the relevant points of biomedicine in simple and direct terms.* This might involve explaining the cause, signs and symptoms and likely treatment for this particular illness. Although the information may seem alien to the patient, it may in fact be of value to him or her. It may be necessary to use interpreters at this stage.
2. *Openly compare the client's belief system with biomedicine.* Point out the discrepancies, but give the client opportunities to ask questions and clarify terms, and to raise objections.

Jackson comments that 'familiarity with the client's culture can be helpful to this process because it may give the practitioner clues about possible problems' (Jackson, 1993, p. 41).

If the client refuses the proposed plan of care, the nurse may find it useful to invite them to think of a solution to the problem. Any suggestions may then be discussed together until a plan that meets the needs of both parties can be agreed upon.

Jackson (1993) also emphasizes that, where possible, practitioners should seek to preserve helpful or non-harmful beliefs and practices, given that these often prove to be useful when studied by Western medicine. Some practices may be neutral in their effects but seem irrational to the outsider (e.g. the use of hot or cold foods in postnatal care). However, we need to remind ourselves that our own beliefs and practices are not always logical or scientific, and they may not always 'make sense' to someone from outside our own culture.

However, there may be conflict if health beliefs are considered to be positively harmful or dangerous. It may then seem urgent to change them immediately in order to protect the patient. However, some cultural practices may be ingrained in people's lifestyles, and may perhaps be part of a strict religious or moral code. They may be difficult to challenge without causing individuals to feel affronted or alienated. People may fear that changing their beliefs or complying with biomedicine may result in punishment (from God or their family, religious groups or peers). These are very difficult ethical dilemmas that are beyond the scope of this chapter (although it may be useful to refer to Chapter 4). However, the nurse has a duty to allow the patient to express their beliefs and ideas about care, and to negotiate and explain his or her perspective in a manner that is non-threatening and respects the other person's belief system as being both valid and meaningful.

Key points

1. People's health beliefs may have a direct impact on their behaviour and the way in which they respond to illness.
2. Nurses need to be aware of these factors and to take particular care when eliciting beliefs about health.
3. The patient needs to be understood in the context of his or her own life and personal circumstances.

CONCLUSION

Kleinman (1986) argues that medical systems do not just deliver health care. They are part of society and, as such, they reflect the wider social and cultural systems. Biomedicine is therefore merely a product of our UK culture – as is the National Health Service (NHS) that is the vehicle for UK health beliefs. In this chapter I have argued that, although in principle health beliefs can be divided into three distinct areas, in practice these distinctions are false and the three areas often overlap. In Chinese cultures, for example, the concept of holism is central to health beliefs yet people may be deeply superstitious and may worship and pray to their ancestors. In the UK healthcare system we live within a plurality of health belief systems. Ostensibly we adhere to, or align ourselves with, the biomedical model, but many nurses are superstitious at heart and may believe and employ practices that are neither scientific nor logical. However, it is important not to negate or ridicule these practices, but to place them within a social and cultural context and to recognize that they are a part of the culture of the healthcare system in the UK. They are not superior to other systems but need to be acknowledged as belonging to the UK notion of health. Thorne (1993) makes the following argument:

> Thus the nature of healing and the social expectations upon healers reflect a range of options which are better understood in the context of the culture than in contrast to one another. In each case there is considerable logic to the system, although the logic reveals considerable variation in the starting point. The prevalence of both the naturalistic and personalistic traditions in most cultures challenges us to examine our own healing practices for their own non-naturalistic elements.
>
> *(Thorne, 1993, p. 1938)*

CHAPTER SUMMARY

1. Pluralism is the use of concurrent approaches to health care.
2. Health beliefs that differ from one's own require careful and sensitive elicitation.
3. The exploration of health beliefs needs to be undertaken within the person's life and social context.

FURTHER READING

Brown K, Avis M and Hubbard M (2007) Health beliefs of African–Caribbean people with type 2 diabetes: a qualitative study. *British Journal of General Practice* **57**, 461–9.
This paper explores the accounts of the way in which African–Caribbean people living in Nottingham experience and manage their diabetes.

Fadiman A (1997) *The spirit catches you and you fall down.* Noonday Press, New York.
This work describes the dilemmas that face a child of a refugee's family from Laos who suffers from epilepsy in an American hospital. It vividly portrays the culture clash, and provides an interesting account of health beliefs that are at odds with biomedicine.

Fedorowicz Z and Walczyk T D (2007) A Trisomial concept of sociocultural and religious factors in healthcare decison-making and service provision in the Muslim Arab world.
In: Papadopoulos I (ed.) *Transcultural health and social care development of culturally competent practioners.* Churchill Livingstone, Edinburgh, 265–81.
This chapter (Chapter 16) gives an interesting and informative account of Islamic medicine and healthcare issues.

Helman C G (2007) *Culture, health and illness*, 5th edn. Hodder Arnold, London.
This book explores all aspects of cultural beliefs and practices and is also an excellent resource for other chapters in this book. Chapter 4, Caring and curing: the sectors of health care (pp. 81–121), is particularly relevant to this chapter.

Loewenthal K (2006) *Religion, culture and mental health.* Cambridge University Press, Cambridge.
This book explores a range of issues linking religion and cultural beliefs with mental health issues.

4 Religious beliefs and cultural care

Karen Holland

INTRODUCTION

Nurses care for individuals who have different religious beliefs and backgrounds, and Neuberger (1994) believes that: 'The first requirement for anyone caring for a patient and wishing to recognise his spiritual and cultural needs is to know something of the basic beliefs of the religion concerned' (Neuberger, 1994, p. 8).

This chapter provides an introduction to some of the main religions practised in the UK and the ways in which these influence healthcare practice. Four religions form the focus of this chapter, namely Jehovah's Witnesses, Christian faiths (see also Appendix 1), Islam (see also Appendix 4) and Hinduism (see also Appendix 3). These were chosen to reflect the impact of major belief systems on aspects of daily living and health care. Other religions and associated practices are introduced throughout the book, and a brief summary of Buddhism, Judaism and Sikhism can also be found in the Appendices.

This chapter will focus on the following issues:

- religion and spirituality;
- religions and healthcare practice:
  - Jehovah's Witnesses;
  - Christian faiths;
  - Islam;
  - Hinduism.

RELIGION AND SPIRITUALITY

The Department of Health in the UK has long recognized the need to ensure that religious and cultural beliefs of patients and their families are met by both staff and the wider organization (Department of Health, 1996). This is also important for their carers and members of community and hospital healthcare teams. The Department of Health (1996) stated that 'You can expect the NHS to respect your privacy, dignity and religious and cultural beliefs at all times and in all places' and a National Association of Health Authorities and Trusts (NAHAT) report (1996) offered the following guidance to NHS Trusts in their responsibilities to meet this standard:

- Adopt a holistic approach to the delivery of health care.

- Recognize that 'spiritual' does not necessarily mean 'religious'.

- Treat people as individuals and do not make assumptions about their spiritual needs because they come from a particular social or ethnic group.

- Accept that not all religions are based on the same criteria.

- Enable people in hospital to have access to those who are most likely to be able to help them to meet their spiritual needs.

- Provide a platform for all sections of the community to meet their spiritual needs in hospital.

(National Association of Health Authorities and Trusts, 1996, p. 5)

As a result of this commitment, NHS Trusts ensured that they had guidance in place to assist staff in meeting patients' needs through providing guidance on various religions and cultures and how this affected their care needs (see websites section for examples). The Department of Health in the UK have now published a new guide for the NHS entitled *Religion or Belief* (Department of Health, 2009) which offers not only guidance on how religion and belief should be considered in care but also offers some examples from practice and links to other resources. An example of this is information on how religious beliefs influence end-of-life care (see Chapter 12).

When people are ill we know, for example, that the way they feel about themselves or their attitude to life can affect their progress. This can be either positive or negative. Consider the following statement made by a woman with breast cancer:

> I relied on God mentally a lot. I was afraid and scared so I wanted someone to rely on. I begged him that I was repentant about the bad things that I had done, so wouldn't he please let me live. I believe that God is eternal and omnipotent, so he has enough power to take care of me. I sometimes get tired of him and sometimes not. But now he is a big help to me.

(Kyung-Rim, 1999, p. 91)

Reflective exercise

Consider how you would have reacted if a patient had said this to you, and then asked 'What do you think?'.

There is no right or wrong answer to this question. As nurses, we are expected to be able to communicate and reassure our patients, but sometimes this is difficult, especially if we have not come to understand our own beliefs about such life-threatening situations. However, not all religions are based on such beliefs in God, and it is important for nurses to have some understanding of the basic principles that underpin other religious and spiritual beliefs.

RELIGIONS AND HEALTHCARE PRACTICE

Jehovah's Witnesses

According to the BBC website (2009 – see end of chapter) there are reportedly 'about 6.9 million active Witnesses in 235 countries in the world (2007), including 1 million in the USA and 130,000 in the UK'.

Jehovah's Witnesses believe in both the Old and New Testaments of the Bible, and they regard Jesus Christ as the Son of God (Jehovah). However, they believe that the cross is a 'pagan symbol and shun its use' (Schott and Henley, 1996), they do not regard Sunday as a holy day, and they do not celebrate Christmas or Easter. Jehovah's Witnesses refer to each other as 'brothers' and 'sisters', and each congregation is led by a group of men known as Elders. They also believe in trying to reach the community with their religious messages, in much the same way that Jesus did. They have their own publication, called *The Watch Tower*, which they give to people during their household visits. Their religious beliefs about blood and blood products are of major significance in terms of health care. They are not allowed to eat blood or blood products, neither are they able to receive blood transfusions, as they believe that a human being must not have his or her life prolonged with another creature's blood (Schott and Henley, 1996).

The influence of Jehovah's Witnesses' beliefs on healthcare practice

Jehovah's Witnesses will normally accept all forms of medical treatment with the exception of infusion with blood and blood products. Most Witnesses carry cards which state this clearly and hospitals also have forms which Witnesses are required to sign refusing blood and blood products. This includes:

> **Whole blood, red cells, white cells, platelets and plasma. Blood fractions such as Factor 8, anti-D and globulins are considered to be substantially different from whole blood and from the constituents that nourish and sustain the body. These are therefore not strictly prohibited and it is up to individual Witnesses to decide whether to accept these products.**
>
> *(Schott and Henley, 1996, p. 326)*

Autotransfusion (transfusion of one's own blood) can be used, but only if the blood has not been stored and it is used immediately. It is acceptable for a patient to have a blood test provided that no blood is retained. A major ethical dilemma for many nurses and healthcare practitioners occurs when a parent refuses a blood transfusion for their child, and in some extreme cases the decision has been overruled by a court order. The Jehovah Witness Hospital Liaison Committee will offer help and advice on all matters related to the health of Witnesses (Henley and Schott, 1999).

Consider the following Case Study of Mr Alias.

Case study

Mr Alias, a 40-year-old man, is admitted to the intensive-care unit following a road traffic incident. He is diagnosed as having lacerations to his liver and abdominal injuries. The doctor orders that he is to go to the operating-theatre for surgery. The patient informs the nurses that he is a Jehovah's Witness and agrees to the surgery, but will not allow them to give him any blood transfusions. (Adapted from Carson, 1989.)

1. What are the implications for nurses of a patient refusing a blood transfusion?
2. How would the nurse ensure that the Nursing and Midwifery Council (NMC) Code of standards of conduct, performance and ethics for nurses and midwives (2008) was adhered to, and ensure that the patient's own spiritual and religious needs were met?

Points to consider

1. All events involving the nurse and the patient need to be documented as fully as possible in the patient's nursing notes.
2. Information that is given to the patient about alternatives to blood products must be recorded.
3. The patient's family may require additional support; they may or may not be Jehovah's Witnesses themselves.
4. If Mr Alias dies during surgery, the nurses and doctors may wish to discuss their own feelings and beliefs with someone, especially with regard to the religious beliefs of the patient. Such an incident can cause much stress among staff.

Jehovah's Witnesses are also not allowed to undergo termination of pregnancy or sterilization, as these interventions are interpreted as taking life and interfering with nature; euthanasia is, therefore, also not supported. There are no special practices related to death other than prayer and Jehovah's Witnesses can be either cremated or buried after death.

Christian faiths

Most people in the UK who are practising Christians belong to the Church of England (the Anglican Church), the Roman Catholic Church or the Free Churches (e.g. Methodist, Baptist or Pentecostal churches). The holy book of Christians is the Bible, and the Christian holy day is Sunday. Other important times of the year are listed in Box 4.1.

Box 4.1 Important days in the Christian calendar

Christmas Day (celebrates the birth of Jesus Christ)
Ash Wednesday (first day of Lent)
Lent (a 6-week period during which some people fast or abstain from certain foods as penance)
Good Friday (in remembrance of the torture and death of Jesus Christ on the cross)
Easter Sunday (celebrates Jesus rising from the dead)
Ascension (celebrates Jesus rising physically into heaven)
Pentecost (celebrating the descent of the Holy Spirit on the disciples)

In conjunction with these holy days there are special religious 'rites' which involve either the individual or the whole community. Some of these are particularly important for patients who are ill either at home or in hospital. In normal circumstances only an authorized person may carry out the associated rites which are also known as sacraments. Christian rites are listed in Box 4.2.

Box 4.2 Christian rites

Individual rites – baptism, confirmation and marriage
Community rites – communion and mass; penance and confession; anointing
Baptism – when a person is admitted to the Christian community
Confirmation – a personal commitment and acceptance by the individual (of the Christian community)
Marriage – the personal commitment of two individuals to family life
Communion/mass – 'feeding' of the community and spiritual communion with God (usually in a church or other consecrated area)
Penance – a formal acceptance of blame for some past wrongdoing, which requires the individual to strive for a better way of life
Confession – acknowledgement to a priest of some past wrongdoing and a request for forgiveness to enable the individual to begin to live in a better way
Anointing – a spiritual strengthening by a nominated chaplain or priest at times of stress, sickness or death

---

Prayer is very important to most practising Christians, especially during periods of stress and crisis (e.g. dying). They may wish to be provided with a Bible if they are admitted to hospital without their own copy. Roman Catholic patients may have rosary beads with them, or may wish to have religious pictures pinned to their bedclothes. Some Christians may also wear religious jewellery, such as a cross or medallions of saints (e.g. St Christopher). These must not be removed unless it is absolutely essential, and even then only with the patient's permission (as is the case for all cultures who wear jewellery of religious significance).

Reflective exercise

Find out what services and facilities are available for Christians in:
1. Your local hospital.
2. The community around your local health centre.

You will probably find that services and facilities vary according to the social and cultural groups to be found in the local population. Most hospitals have an area identified for multi-denominational worship, and many have a Christian chapel. In large district general and teaching hospitals there are hospital chaplaincies that employ either part-time or full-time chaplains. A local priest may also have special responsibility for the religious and spiritual care of Roman Catholics in hospital. In the community there will be church and chapel buildings, but as the population has changed with regard to its beliefs and culture, these may no longer be used for Christian worship. This has resulted in many of these buildings being converted for other uses (e.g. restaurants, private housing).

Effects of Christian beliefs on healthcare practice

Blanche and Parkes (1997) provide an insight into how Christian beliefs become evident during periods of crisis, and readers of this book may recall similar stories. Consider the following example of George Jones, aged 73 years, who was having a heart attack and, with his wife Phyllis and his neighbour, was waiting for the ambulance to take him to hospital.

Case study

Phyllis was an Anglican; she believed in God and went to the local Church of England regularly. She had learned her religion from her parents and saw the Godhead very much as a Holy Family. She loved Jesus, whom she knew to be the Son of God and regarded him as a personal friend. She particularly enjoyed the pictures of Mary and the baby Jesus which reminded her of her relationship with her own children. She had confidence that when her turn came, Jesus would find a place for George and her in heaven. She sometimes worried about his refusal to go to Church. George thought religion was nonsense but he explained to his friends that this did not mean that he was an atheist. He went to weddings and funerals, and he reprimanded his grandchildren when they swore. George survived in hospital for less than a day. (From Blanche and Parkes, 1997, p. 131.)

How do you think Phyllis (with her Christian beliefs) would cope with George's death?

Points to consider

1. Phyllis could gain great comfort from her beliefs and her church, but she might also feel that her God had let her down. This is particularly often the case in situations that involve a sudden bereavement or watching someone in severe pain.
2. After her husband's sudden death Phyllis might wish to spend some time on her own or in the hospital chapel. The hospital chaplain may already have been to see her husband in order to offer to pray with them both.

All practising Christians in hospital should be offered the support of the hospital chaplains, and many will want to continue with their normal Christian rites at this time. For example, on Good Friday or Ash Wednesday, Catholics do not eat meat or drink alcohol. This is regarded as a symbolic sacrifice in memory of Christ's death, and some Christians continue to follow this practice every Friday. Fish may be eaten instead. However, as in many other religions, the requirement for fasting is lifted during hospitalization (Carson, 1989). An example where this is essential is in relation to the potential effects of fasting on Type 1 Diabetes, where there is a risk of a hypoglycaemic (low blood sugar) coma (Morris and Worth, 2006).

Different groups of Christians 'behave differently at the time of death' (Neuberger, 1994). For example, patients from an Orthodox Church may wish to keep a family icon with them at all times. However, Neuberger (1994) points out that these icons are often of monetary as well as personal value, which could make it difficult to keep them safe in a hospital environment. She suggests that sensitivity to the patient's needs in such cases is important.

For nurses involved in family planning services or working in gynaecology wards, the rules with regard to contraception and termination of pregnancy are of particular significance. Schott and Henley (1996, p. 297) state that 'The Roman Catholic Church forbids all artificial contraception, including sterilisation, on the grounds that it interferes with God's natural law. Contraception using the safe period (rhythm method) is permitted'.

Termination of pregnancy is viewed by practising Catholics as murder and a mortal sin. Practising Anglicans also believe strongly that abortion is wrong, but like many Catholic women today some will agree to a termination if the baby has a serious congenital abnormality, or if they have been subjected to rape.

Reflective exercise

1. Find out the current position of the Nursing and Midwifery Council in the UK with regard to nurses and their personal religious objections to taking part in the termination of pregnancy and the care of women in the preoperative and postoperative period.
2. Discuss your findings with colleagues from different cultures and religious backgrounds.

Your discussion will probably have revealed significant individual and cultural differences. However, it is important to remember that, as a nurse or healthcare practitioner, you are bound by a professional code of conduct that gives guidance on how you should act in your role. Your personal beliefs may conflict with professional expectations in situations such as participating in the termination of pregnancy. This leads some nurses, once qualified, deliberately to choose not to work in clinical areas where they would experience such conflict.

Key points

1. Christians belong to many different churches (e.g. Roman Catholic, Baptist, Church of England).
2. Prayer is important to practising Christians during periods of crisis and illness.
3. Many Christians carry or wear jewellery which has religious significance (e.g. St Christopher medallion).

Islam

Islam is one the world's major religions; it is the religion of Muslims. There are many different Muslim sects, and it is important to be aware of this, especially as some are stricter in their practices than others. The two main branches are Sunni Muslims and Shia Muslims. According to Henley (1982), Sunni Muslims believe that 'every Muslim has an equal status before God', whereas the Shia Muslims believe that there is 'a continuous line of divinely designated charismatic leaders'. Being a Muslim involves obeying the rules which practising Muslims have to follow in all aspects of their life (Henley, 1982); it is therefore not just a religion but a way of life. Muslims believe that the Prophet Mohammed is the messenger of the one and only God, and that they must observe the five main duties or pillars of Islam: 'faith, prayer at five set times every day, giving alms, fasting during the month of Ramadan and making a pilgrimage to the sacred city of Makka [Mecca] in Saudi Arabia' (Schott and Henley, 1996, p. 313).

The Muslim Holy Book is the Qur'an (Koran), which according to McDermott and Ahsan (1993) is:

> the foundation and the mainstay of Muslim life; it binds Muslims together, gives them a distinct identity and fashions their history and culture. It deals with all the important aspects of human life, the relationships between God and man, between man and man, and between man and society, including ethics, jurisprudence, social justice, political principles, law, morality, trade and commerce.

(McDermott and Ahsan, 1993, p. 20)

The Muslim community in the UK is largely Asian, originating mainly from Pakistan, Bangladesh and India, although some also originate from East Africa. The main Muslim groups, together with their first language (Henley, 1982) are listed in Box 4.3.

Box 4.3 *Muslim groups and their first language (adapted from Henley, 1982, p. 9)*

Pakistan Muslims come from Mirpur District (first language, Punjabi–Mirpur dialect), Punjab province (Punjabi)

Bangladesh Muslims come from Syhet District (first language, Bengali– Syheti dialect)

Indian Muslims come from Gujarat State, especially the Kutch region (first language, Gujarati or Kutch dialect)

Muslims from other areas of India often speak Urdu as their first language

---

The main place of worship is the mosque, and some NHS Trusts provide a small mosque or prayer room within their hospital. The mosque is mainly a place of worship for men; it is also used for teaching children. In the UK the Imam is in charge of each mosque. He also teaches the children as well as overseeing all religious functions and offering pastoral support to those who may be ill and have no family.

Muslims have to adhere to certain food restrictions as laid down in the Holy Qur'an. They do not eat pork or anything made from it or its products. Other meat is acceptable provided that it is 'halal' (i.e. killed according to Islamic law). This involves cutting an animal's throat and consecrating it in the name of Allah. If halal meat cannot be provided in hospital, Muslims will eat a vegetarian diet. Jewish kosher food is an acceptable alternative, as this is killed in the same way. Alcohol in any form is forbidden. Every adult Muslim is expected to pray at five set times each day: 'after dawn, around noon, in the mid-afternoon, early evening (after sunset) and at night' (Henley, 1982).

Muslims are required to wash before praying and they must face Mecca during prayers. Washing is of special significance to Muslim patients, and in particular it should be noted that they are unable to pray if they have not washed themselves after urination or defecation. This is especially important for those patients who are unable to get out of bed. However, there are exemptions from the five daily prayers, including all patients who are seriously ill and women up to 40 days after childbirth and during menstruation, as they are considered unclean at these times.

The Muslim holy day is Friday (Raza or Siyan). There are certain times of the year when fasting is also compulsory and considered to be a form of worship. This means abstaining from taking food between dawn and dusk. This main compulsory fasting time is at Ramadan, the dates of which may vary from year to year in accordance with the time of the new moon. This makes it difficult to predict in advance when Muslim healthcare workers may require special leave arrangements. This is more important if it occurs during the summer months, when the period of fasting is longer than in the winter months. Towns and cities where there are significant Muslim communities very often publish the dates of Ramadan in their local newspapers. The end of Ramadan is marked by the festival of Eid-ul-Fitr (oftened shortened to Eid). The word Eid means 'anniversary' and, after the first prayers, the day is spent visiting relatives and friends and exchanging gifts. Muslims also pay the Sadaqah al-Fitr (welfare due) for the poor (McDermott and Ahsan, 1993). In addition, those who can afford to are encouraged to make a pilgrimage to Mecca (Haj) at least once during their lifetime.

Reflective exercise

1. Discuss with a Muslim colleague or student:
   (i) how they manage to work and cope with the fasting period at Ramadan;
   (ii) how they celebrate the festival of Eid-ul-Fitr.
2. Find out about other Muslim festivals and their meaning.

Effects of Islamic beliefs on healthcare practice

As modesty is an obligation of Islam, nakedness and exposure of the body can be very distressing to both men and women. If at all possible, Muslim patients should be examined by a doctor or nurse of the same sex as themselves (e.g. during childbirth or gynaecological examination), and similarly 'diseases which require examination of the male genitalia and anus are likely to cause acute embarrassment when performed by a female doctor'; (McDermott and Ahsan, 1993, p. 60). It is important to be aware of and responsive to the need for prayers, and the fact that associated bathing or washing will be important (for a discussion of death rituals, see Chapter 10).

There are certain issues which should be considered during pregnancy and childbirth which have a religious significance. Schott and Henley (1996) highlight the following:

- **Labour:** a few Muslim women may be reluctant to use narcotic methods of pain relief on religious grounds as narcotics are forbidden in the Qur'an except in cases of overriding medical need.

- **Immediately after the birth:** many Muslim parents consider it very important that a baby should be washed immediately after the birth to get rid of any impurity … Some may be distressed if the baby is given to them unwashed and may not want to hold or feed the baby until he or she has been cleaned properly.

(Schott and Henley, 1996, p. 320)

McDermott and Ahsan (1993) also explain in the Islam Foundation Muslim Guide another Islamic practice which is of major importance to Muslims, namely that of saying the adhan (call to prayer) into the ears of the baby immediately after childbirth:

> The whole "ceremony" does not take more than 3–4 minutes; either the father or any member of the family stands in front of the baby and calls out the adhan in the ear of the baby as a mark of blessing. Sometimes members of the family prefer to bring along a learned member from the Muslim community to give the adhan for the child. The hospital authorities are not always aware of this Islamic religious custom, and often appear reluctant to allow a person other than the husband to visit the baby outside the visiting hours of the hospital. Muslims will be grateful if the parents are allowed to invite one other person to perform this brief ceremony – simple and short yet very essential for Muslims.
>
> *(McDermott and Ashan, 1993, p. 62)*

Reflective exercise

1. Consider how a midwife can demonstrate cultural awareness and respect for the Muslim faith at the time of labour.
2. Find out your local maternity department policy with regard to the Islamic practice of saying the 'adhan'.

Key points

1. Muslims believe that the Prophet Mohammed is the messenger of Allah, the one and only God.
2. The Qur'an (Muslim holy book) is the guide to Muslim life.
3. Washing and modesty have religious as well as practical significance.

Hinduism

Hinduism is not only a religion but also a whole way of life for a large number of people from India. Unlike other religions and belief systems, it has 'no single founder or major prophet from whom all events are dated' (Henley, 1983b) and no single holy book to which Hindus can refer. However, the most popular book is the Bhagavad Gita. There is a fundamental belief in the Hindu Dharma (ways of conduct or laws of nature) and a belief that God is One and is called by different names. They also believe that this God can take many forms – male, female or animal.

The three main Hindu gods are 'Brahma, the Creator, symbolizing creative power, Vishnu, the Preserver, who preserves and maintains what has been created, and Shiva, the Destroyer, who brings all things to an end' (Henley, 1983b, p. 3).

These three gods represent the Hindu belief that everything in the universe is in a constant eternal cycle. Because of this, Hindus believe in reincarnation and that their eternal soul (atman) does not die but is reborn again in another body.

Most Hindus are from India, and the main groups in the UK are listed in Box 4.4.

> **Box 4.4 The main Hindu groups in the UK and their first language**
>
> Gujarat (first language, Gujarati)
> Punjab (first language, Punjabi or Hindi)
> Small groups from Delhi (first language, Hindi or Punjabi)
> West Bengal (first language, Bengali)
> Kerala (first language, Malayali)
> Tamil Nadu (first language, Tamil)

Karmi also informs us that:

> every Hindu is born into a caste which is determined by individual karma in a previous life.
> This reflects the central Hindu tenet of reward for good deeds and punishment for wickedness.
> Orthodox Hindus believe that a person's karma is permanent and cannot be altered, and
> disapprove of the mixing of castes through contact in any form. The caste system continues to
> exert a strong influence in Indian society as well as among Indians in Britain, particularly
> when marriage partners are chosen.
>
> *(Karmi, 1996, p. 20)*

The four castes are:

- the Brahmins (highest caste);
- the Kshatriyas;
- the Vaishyas;
- the Shudras (the lowest caste).

There are also individuals with no caste who are known as the Outcastes or Untouchables. These
people undertake work that is considered to be 'spiritually polluting, such as cleaning streets and
lavatories and dealing with dead animals' (Schott and Henley, 1996).

Effects of Hindu beliefs on healthcare practices

In order to understand how the Hindu religion and way of life influence the care that is given to
patients in hospital, consider the following Case Study.

Case study

Shri Rajkumar Sharma, a 55-year-old man, is to be admitted to hospital for removal
of the prostate gland. He is accompanied by his wife and son, who inform the Ward
Sister that it is Diwali, the Hindu Festival of Lights, in 2 days' time.

As the nurse who will be caring for him, you will need to undertake an assessment of
his needs in order to plan culturally appropriate care. The following factors will
require specific consideration on his admission to hospital:

continued

Case study

1. the Hindu naming system;
2. specific dietary needs;
3. specific personal cleansing and dressing needs;
4. religious practices whilst in hospital.

The following information will help you to make an informed decision.

Hindu naming system

The first point to note is the man's name. 'Shri' is the equivalent of Mr (if the person was a woman it would be Shrimati – Mrs). Rajkumar – Raj is the man's personal name and Kumar is his middle name (only used with his first name and not normally used on its own).

Sharma is the surname or family name. This is often a caste name. Many Hindu families in the UK share the same caste or family name (Henley, 1983b) because most of them originate from the same geographical areas in India (i.e. Gujarat and Punjab). The family name of Patel is therefore very common.

However, it is very important to remember that according to Hindu custom only the first and middle name will be given (e.g. Rajkumar). This could be wrongly recorded (e.g. Kumar being identified as the surname). It is therefore important to ask for the first name, middle name and surname for recording purposes. When asked for her name as 'next of kin', his wife will include her husband's name after her own first and middle name (e.g. Lakshmidevi Rajkumar Sharma).

This naming system is most important when patients on a ward have the same family name (e.g. Sharma or Patel) (see Chapter 9 for a discussion of children's names).

Dietary needs

Hindus believe that all living things are sacred, and most will not eat meat or meat products. In addition, many Hindus will not eat fish or eggs. The cow is considered to be sacred, and dairy produce is only acceptable if it contains no animal fat. Some Hindus will eat meat but not beef or pork. The pig is considered to be an unclean animal.

It will be important to check whether Mr Sharma is able to read English in order to understand the menu sheets, and that any questions he may have about the content of the hospital food or how it is prepared are answered truthfully. Many older people refuse to eat any hospital food, preferring their meals to be brought into hospital by relatives. If this is the case, it is important that nurses or the dietician ensure that foods prohibited on medical grounds are made known to them (see Chapter 9 for a further discussion of food preferences).

Personal cleansing and dressing needs

Mr Sharma may wear a kameez (a loose shirt with or without a collar) and trousers with a drawstring (pyjama). If he is a high caste (Brahmin) he may also wear a sacred thread (janeu) which consists of white cotton thread with three strands and is worn over the right shoulder and round the body. This must not be removed unless it is absolutely necessary. The head is considered to be the most sacred part of the body and the feet the dirtiest. Therefore, when putting his clothes in his bedside locker, it is important not to store his shoes in the same place.

Washing in running water is very important to Hindus. Mr Sharma will be unable to do this for himself in the immediate postoperative period, and he will need help with it, as until he has washed in this way he will be unable to eat or drink.

Having a catheter will be a potential source of embarrassment to him: urine is considered to be polluting and he may be upset by having to look at the catheter bag. During visiting hours he could sit in a chair and the catheter bag could be covered up by a blanket. All body products and fluids that leave the body are considered polluting (i.e. urine, faeces, saliva, menstrual blood, mucus, sweat and semen). It will be important for Mr Sharma if all matters related to his surgery and its after-effects can be discussed with either a male doctor or a male nurse (see Chapter 8 for men's health care issues).

Hindu religious practices

Hindus have a chosen god whom they worship, and every home has a prayer room (puja). The Bhagavad Gita (holy book) must be kept clean and safe if it is brought into hospital. It is usually wrapped in a cotton or silk cloth for protection (Henley, 1983b).

Mr Sharma will be able to attend the hospital temple (if one is available) before going to theatre if he wishes, and could be taken there when he is well enough postoperatively. If unable to attend a temple, privacy could be ensured for prayer by pulling the bed curtains around him.

There are no set times for prayer, although many Hindus pray first thing in the morning, around midday and in the evening. Holy days and festivals will be celebrated according to the main god that Hindus worship. The two main festivals are Holi and Diwali:

- Holi – Hindu spring festival (February/March);
- Diwali – five-day festival of light and the goddess Lakshmi – the Goddess of Good Fortune and Prosperity (October/November).

It would be good practice, whenever possible, to take these important festivals into consideration when planning patient hospital admissions.

> **Key points**
>
> 1. Hindus belong to one of four main castes or one outcaste.
> 2. Hindu religion does not allow the eating of pork or beef, as the pig is considered to be an unclean animal and the cow is regarded as a sacred one.
> 3. The Hindu religion has no single founder or major prophet.

CONCLUSION

As can be seen from this brief introduction to some of the world's major religions, their impact on health care is significant. An awareness of their meaning and importance for patients and clients and their families should therefore be an essential part of the induction of staff within healthcare environments. The Patient's Charter standard (Department of Health, 1991) and its recommended guidelines on privacy, dignity and religious and cultural beliefs should therefore be compulsory reading within any planned induction programme.

> ### Reflective exercise
>
> 1. Obtain and read a copy of your NHS Trust/Health Board guidelines for good practice with regard to the religious, cultural and spiritual needs of patients.
> 2. Discuss with your colleagues how these are being implemented in your workplace.
> 3. If a student, consider how your university supports the religious and cultural needs of its students and staff.

CHAPTER SUMMARY

1. Religion plays a significant role in the health and well-being of patients.
2. Nurses need to be sensitive to the religious practices of patients when they are ill.
3. Healthcare trusts are responsible for implementing Patient Charter standards that take into consideration the privacy, dignity and religious and cultural beliefs of patients.
4. *The Code: Standards of Conduct, Performance and Ethics for Nurses and Midwives* (Nursing and Midwifery Council, 2008) acknowledges the importance of the spiritual and religious beliefs of patients and their carers.

FURTHER READING

Andrews M M and Boyle J S (2008) *Transcultural concepts in nursing care*, 5th edn., Wolters Kluwer Health/J B Lippincott, Philadelphia.
This book offers a broad introduction to transcultural care and includes an excellent chapter on religion, culture and nursing.

Burnard P and Gill P (2008) *Culture, communication and nursing*. Pearson Education, Harlow.
This book includes a short chapter on beliefs and religion.

Kirkwood N A (2005) *A hospital handbook on multiculturalism and religion*, 2nd edn. Morehouse, London.
This book offers practical guidance on a wide range of religions and related practices.

McSherry W (2007) *The meaning of spirituality and spiritual care within nursing and health care practice*. Quay Books, London.

Mootoo J S (2005) *A guide to cultural and spiritual awareness*. RCN Publishing Company, London.
This book offers guidance for nurses on spiritual and cultural beliefs of a wide selection of different religions and cultures.

Sampson C (1982) *The neglected ethic*. McGraw–Hill, Maidenhead.

Although not a current text, this book still offers a valuable insight into the spiritual and cultural beliefs of patients and the associated decisions required by healthcare practitioners.

WEBSITES

http://www.bbc.co.uk/religion/religions

This is a BBC website devoted to all aspects of religious beliefs. It has a large number of resources, including pictures of different religious practices at weddings, pilgrimage to Haj and Muslim prayer movements. There are also some quizzes that test your knowledge of various different religions and practices.

**http://www.dh.gov.uk/en/Publicationsandstatistics/Publications/
PublicationsPolicyAndGuidance/DH_093133**

This is a direct web link to *Religion or belief: A practical guide for the NHS* (Department of Health, 2009).

http://www.mfghc.com/resources/resources_73.htm.

This website includes a guide called *The religious, spiritual and cultural needs of patients* (a guide and reference document for Staff at the Derby Hospitals NHS Foundation Trust).

http://www.rcseng.ac.uk/publications/docs/jehovahs_witness.html

This is a useful website for the code of practice for the surgical management of Jehovah's Witnesses (The Royal College of Surgeons of England).

http://www.scottishinterfaithcouncil.org/resources/Religion+and+Belief.pdf

This website links to a report on religious beliefs on health care in Scotland by the Scottish Inter-faith Council.

http://www.sikhchaplaincy.org.uk/default.htm

This site has some excellent booklets and leaflets about caring for Sikh patients and is the page for the Sikh Chaplaincy in the UK.

5 Cultural care: knowledge and skills for implementation in practice

Karen Holland

INTRODUCTION

This chapter examines the nature of the knowledge and skills required for implementing cultural care in nursing practice. Nursing theories and models that have been developed specifically to guide nurses in their cultural assessment of patient needs will also be explored. A case study approach will enable nurses to test out the model frameworks that they use for the assessment of individual cultural needs and the implementation of culturally appropriate care.

This chapter will focus on the following issues:

1. developments that promote culturally sensitive nursing practice;
2. cultural awareness;
3. cultural knowledge;
4. cultural care and interventions:

(a) Leininger's model of transcultural care diversity and universality;
(b) Giger and Davidhizar's model of transcultural nursing assessment and intervention;
(c) Purnell's model of cultural competence;
(d) Littlewood's anthropological nursing model;
(e) Papadopoulos, Tilki and Taylor's model of transcultural skills development;
(f) Roper, Logan and Tierney's model of nursing.

Before examining the nature of knowledge and skills required for cultural care, two questions need to be considered. First, why is cultural care an important issue for healthcare professionals? Second, what are the rights of patients and their families with regard to receiving care that is culturally appropriate? (It is recommended that Chapter 1 be read first as this introduces the reader to many of the issues that will be explored in this chapter.)

For nurses in the UK, the importance was highlighted in the UKCC code of professional practice (United Kingdom Central Council for Nursing, Midwifery and Health Visiting, 1992), which stated that they should 'recognise and respect the uniqueness and dignity of each patient and client and respond to their need for care, irrespective of their ethnic origin, religious beliefs, personal attributes, the nature of their health problems or any other factor'.

The most recent UK Nursing and Midwifery Council (NMC) Code, *The Code – Standards of Conduct, Performance and Ethics for Nurses and Midwives* (Nursing and Midwifery Council,

2008), however, appears to assume that ethnicity and cultural awareness has been internalized by nurses and midwives, for example:

> **Make the care of people your first concern, treating them as individuals and respecting their dignity.**
>
> - **You must treat people as individuals and respect their dignity**
> - **You must not discriminate in any way against those in your care**
> - **You must treat people kindly and considerately**
> - **You must act as an advocate for those in your care, helping them to access relevant health and social care, information and support**

The current NMC standards for pre-registration nursing education (Nursing and Midwifery Council, 2004) focus on anti-discriminatory practice in relation to beliefs and culture, as well as culture in its broadest sense:

> **NMC outcomes to be achieved for entry to the branch programme**
>
> > **Practise in a fair and anti-discriminatory way, acknowledging the differences in beliefs and cultural practices of individuals or groups (p. 27, Professional and ethical practice)**
> >
> > **Provide a rationale for the nursing care delivered which takes account of social, cultural, spiritual, legal, political and economic influence (p. 30, Care delivery)**

Those for pre-registration midwifery education (Nursing and Midwifery Council, 2009) are more explicit and reference to cultural beliefs can be found throughout many of the standards. For example:

> **Practise in a way which respects, promotes and supports individuals' rights, interests, preferences, beliefs and cultures. This includes:**
>
> - **offering culturally sensitive family planning advice**
> - **ensuring that women's labour is consistent with their religious and cultural beliefs and preferences**
> - **the different roles and relationships in families, and reflecting different religious and cultural beliefs, preferences and experiences**
>
> *(NMC Standard – Domain: Professional and ethical practice)*

This makes it clear that student midwives will need to be given every opportunity to gain an understanding of the way culture and religion affects any care delivered in partnership with women.

In New Zealand the Nursing Council has developed specific guidelines, for both nursing education and practice, in relation to cultural issues; this is directly linked to the wider societal changes in New Zealand with regard to the Maori people (Nursing Council of New Zealand, 2005). This is the adoption of a cultural safety model into all curricula; the revised model for teaching this in nursing programmes includes teaching about the Treaty of Waitangi and Maori health as separate but inter-linked issues.

Their definition of cultural safety is:

> **The effective nursing practice of a person or family from another culture, and is determined by that person or family. Culture includes but is not restricted to, age or generation; gender; sexual orientation; occupation and socioeconomic status; ethnic origin or migrant experience; religious or spiritual belief; and disability.**
>
> **The nurse delivering the nursing service will have undertaken a process of reflection on his or her own cultural identity and will recognise the impact that his or her personal culture has on his or her professional practice. Unsafe cultural practice comprises any action which diminishes, demeans or disempowers the cultural identity and wellbeing of the individual.**
>
> *(Nursing Council of New Zealand, 2005, p. 4)*

The concept of cultural safety is also implicit in midwifery curricula and competencies (Midwifery Council of New Zealand, 2007).

Care that acknowledges the culture and ethnic background of the individual takes into account the beliefs and way of life that are shared by members of the same cultural groups (see also Chapter 1). These beliefs extend to all areas of daily living, including those related to health and illness. Although many of these will be common to all members of a cultural group, it is important to remember that even within cultures each person is an individual.

The Patient's Charter Standard in relation to religious and cultural beliefs (Department of Health, 1996) states that 'all health services should make provision so that proper consideration is shown to you, for example, by ensuring that your privacy, dignity and religious and cultural beliefs are respected', and the recent publication of a guide on religion and belief by the Department of Health (2009) appears to extend beyond that of the cultural needs of patients to also take account of the religious and cultural needs of its staff. It recognizes the need for religious observance of holy days by staff and how this could be accommodated through the use of the multi-faith event calendar and year planner to provide advanced warning for those completing duty rotas. This kind of development clearly acknowledges the need for all staff working in the NHS to know what such events may mean to individuals and to the patients in their care, who will also require consideration of such holy days whether as a hospital inpatient or in their own homes.

How, then, have nurses contributed to ensuring care that takes into account the cultural and ethnic background of their patients and clients?

Reflective exercise

1. Consider your own beliefs about religious and cultural needs and how this has had an impact on how you have experienced being a student or working as a qualified member of staff.
2. What knowledge and skills would you consider essential to being able to work in a culturally competent or culturally aware way?

The following sections should help you with these two questions and will consider past and present developments and evidence available in relation to nursing practice.

DEVELOPMENTS THAT PROMOTE CULTURALLY SENSITIVE NURSING PRACTICE

Within nursing and other healthcare professions there have been attempts to address issues related to cultural healthcare. This has been mainly in response to the needs of those societies across the world that are becoming increasingly multicultural in their constitution. The effect of this change has been to create a different set of healthcare needs, which then require healthcare delivery systems that will ensure culturally appropriate and relevant care.

Within the nursing profession, one such attempt has been the development of transcultural nursing care (TCN) – a concept that was relatively new to nursing in the UK (Weller, 1991) when we wrote the first edition. This has now changed in terms of availability of information about cultural care in the NHS and to some extent in the UK nursing literature (Nairn *et al.,* 2004; Darvill, 2003). Despite this, making sure that curricula include cultural competency statements is not always visible in the evidence base for nurse education. Lauder *et al.* (2008) in an evaluation study of pre-registration nursing and midwifery education programmes in Scotland found, for example, that 'students (nursing and midwifery) were given exposure to the issues rather than any competency development' and commented that 'work needs to be undertaken to ensure that the provision of education in responding to the needs of the increasingly ethnically diverse community, develops consistently to meet local needs' (Lauder *et al.*, 2008, p. 196).

In relation to transcultural nursing as a way forward for nursing practice and education, the main advocate and developer of the transcultural nursing model has been Madeleine Leininger, an American nurse anthropologist, who has undertaken extensive cultural and ethnographic studies in an attempt to determine the nature of 'culture-specific and cultural universal nursing care practices' (Leininger, 1978b). She believed that 'today's world situation and concern for the welfare of mankind is challenging us to understand the culture concept' (Leininger, 1978b), and that nurses and other healthcare professionals in their role as carers have an obligation to try to understand the meaning of being a 'cultural individual'. Leininger (1978b) claims to be the originator of what she calls 'the sub-field of transcultural nursing', and she believes this to be an essential prerequisite for effective nursing practice, and that nurses learn about those cultures for which they care. She has written extensively about transcultural nursing (Leininger, 1978a, 1985, 1989a, 1989b, 1990, 1994, 1998, 2002) and in the USA she was the founder and first editor of the *Journal of Transcultural Nursing* which is now a leading journal for this field of nursing (http://tcn.sagepub.com/). Leininger's definition of this subfield of nursing is:

> the comparative study and analysis of different cultures and subcultures in the world with respect to their caring behaviour, nursing care, and health–illness values, beliefs and patterns of behaviour with the goal of generating scientific and humanistic knowledge in order to provide culture-specific and culture universal nursing care practices.
>
> *(Leininger, 1978b, p. 8)*

Herberg has a similar view, that transcultural nursing is:

> concerned with the provision of nursing to the needs of individuals, families and groups. Such individuals, families or groups often represent diverse cultural populations within society, as well as between societies.
>
> *(Herberg, 1995, p. 3)*

However, transcultural nursing care has both advocates and critics within the nursing profession. James believed that Leininger's 'establishing transcultural nursing as a speciality has made it an elitist area' of practice (James, 1995). Bruni (1988) believed that as a result of focusing on culture as the means of 'determining patterns of behaviour', other important variables such as class and gender are left out of important healthcare-related discussions and decisions. Bruni cited the healthcare problems and situation of the Australian Aborigines as an illustration, whereby:

> the culturalist explanation focuses on the inability of the people to relinquish their traditional ways. The force of strength of traditional beliefs and practices is seen to prevent their successful adoption of Western practices.
>
> *(Bruni, 1988, p. 29)*

The subsequent lack of success in implementing healthcare programmes is then blamed on the fact that the Australian Aborigines want to adhere to their traditional explanations of ill health. However, when the Aboriginal people took charge of their own healthcare services, which recognized both gender and class inequalities, a much more successful outcome was achieved with regard to health education and health care (Bennett, 1988).

The health of Australian Aborigines nevertheless remains of concern and the rates of illness amongst them are higher than any other group of people in Australia (see the list of websites at end of this chapter).

On a more general level, a study by Pinikahana *et al.* (2003) found that, regardless of what was advocated in practice, in nursing education in Australia the inclusion of transcultural issues in the curriculum, focusing on how different cultures may respond to different situations, often did not prepare students enough for meeting the complexity of health needs of a multicultural society. This seems to reflect the findings of a study by Lauder *et al.* (2008) in the UK. The government of South Australia however now have a Nursing and Midwifery Strategy (SA Health, 2008) for Aboriginal healthcare which includes an educational strand and key outcomes.

Cortis (1993), an advocate of the implementation of TCN in the UK at that time, discussed some of the issues that are problematic with regard to the concept of culture within health care. He cited Bottomley's (1981) view that 'the study of culture can be interpreted as a mechanism for avoiding the real issue which is racism', and that there is an additional problem of stereotyping culture through focusing on its own potentially static and universal nature (e.g. African culture). However, Stokes believes that:

> whilst the intentions of the transcultural nursing movement may be honourable, the reality is that a new group of so-called 'experts' will not replace the need for well-prepared and informed nurses who are able to plan care from basic principles.
>
> *(Stokes, 1991, p. 42)*

Wilkins (1993), in an extensive literature review of transcultural nursing, takes a similar view and concludes that there 'could well be a danger in discussing culture-specific nursing care', and that nurses should be taught cultural awareness and sensitivity that acknowledges the uniqueness of the individual. This view appears to be a strong recommendation in both UK and USA literature on what nurses need to be encouraged to learn in order to care for a multicultural community.

A small study by Megson (2007) reported on how students, on a combined learning disability/ social work undergraduate programme, gained more awareness of ethnicity and culture through examining aspects of their own ethnic identity, but that issues regarding multicultural learning remained unresolved. In particular, there was a message for educators 'against choosing learning environments that feel right and comfortable for them as they may be creating learning environments based on their own cultural norms and not one that is multicultural' (Megson, 2007, p. 115).

Serrant-Green's (2001) view is that 'transcultural nursing needs to be embedded in the clinical education of nurses so that they are able to detect signs, symptoms and presentations of disease in all patients, irrespective of ethnic group or skin colour' and that 'if nurse educators continue to isolate transcultural issues to concerns about communication and adhere to the "menus" approach to teaching, there will continue to be negative consequences for the provision of clinical care for minority ethnic patients and a failure to "value diversity" in the education of the profession'.

These issues were also highlighted in a study by Tuohy *et al.* (2008) who explored the 'educational needs of nurses when nursing people of a different culture in Ireland'. One of their recommendations was 'to review nursing curricula and increase transcultural nursing education at both pre and post registration level'.

The general theme that nursing education is not preparing students for working in a multi-cultural society is not unique to the UK (Gebru and Willman, 2003), and a study in Sweden (Gebru and Willman, 2009) highlighted that, according to Momeni *et al.* (2008), 'there was still a need to develop curricula in Swedish nursing programmes that enable nursing students to become culturally competent'. Ensuring that educators, both in the university and practice contexts, have the requisite knowledge and skills themselves to deliver learning experiences which integrate the wider cultural and ethnic perspective is an issue that is not widely explored but one that is vital if students are to engage with multicultural communities. In addition there is a need to increase the evaluation and research of how nurses and other healthcare professionals utilize cultural competency in their work, both in their care of patients and their families and also with each other. One such study was undertaken by Fleming *et al.* (2008) in examining 'the influence of culture on diabetes self-management in Gujarati Muslim men in the northwest of England'.

CULTURAL AWARENESS

In order to provide culturally appropriate and sensitive care, we take a similar broad view but suggest that there is a need for two levels of knowledge, namely specialist expertise in one or more cultures and a general awareness of many cultures. For example, in certain parts of the UK (e.g. rural Wales), caring for a patient from Japan is a rare occurrence. However, caring for Gypsy Travellers may be a regular event and demonstrates the fact that the nurse will require a more in-depth knowledge of this cultural group and their way of life over time, in order to care for them. For example a study by Parry *et al.* (2004) highlighted many issues of relevance to nurses and healthcare workers, in particular those working in a community setting.

An awareness of the need for cultural sensitivity when caring for a Japanese patient is also essential, however, because of global travel and work. Both Japanese and Gypsy Traveller cultures have belief systems with complex pollution taboos in relation to the body. For the Gypsy Travellers 'the primary distinction is between washing objects for the inner body and the washing of the outer body. Food, eating utensils and tea towels for drying them must never be washed in a bowl used for washing the hands, the rest of the body or clothing' (Okley, 1983, p. 81). An example of the conflict caused by lack of understanding on the part of a Gorgio (Gypsy name for a non-Gypsy or a Gadje as noted by Vivian and Dundes 2004) health visitor, is cited by Okley:

> **A Gorgio health visitor discovered that a traveller had a deep cut in his foot. Well versed in Gorgio germ theory, she grabbed the first bowl she saw inside the trailer – the washing-up bowl – poured in disinfectant and water and bathed the man's foot in it. Afterwards the travellers threw away the bowl and recounted the incident with disgust. The bowl was permanently mochadi (ritually polluted).**
>
> *(Okley, 1983, p. 81)*

Vivian and Dundes (2004) also point out, however, that 'the proper term to use to refer to the Gypsies is 'Roma'' and that 'to the Roma, the term Gypsy is offensive and derogatory because it misrepresents the Romani heritage'.

In Japanese culture, 'outside' is associated with dirt and impurity and 'inside' with cleanliness and purity. For the Japanese, 'hospital, where the dirt of others is concentrated, is one of the dirtiest places' (Ohnuki-Tierney, 1984). It is important to understand this belief should you be required to care for a Japanese person who has been taken ill on holiday in the UK. For the same reason if a nurse were to visit a Japanese patient in their own home it would be appropriate to ask whether they should remove their shoes prior to entering.

Brink (1984) has stated that there is a need for nurses to be able to access easily transferable information about cultures, such as the above examples, from an anthropological standpoint. She believes that 'nurses are inherently pragmatic' and 'will want to read what they can use' (Brink, 1984). In other words, they may find a great deal of literature about different cultures very interesting, but unless they can use it at the point of contact with the patients it will be of little value to them. An ethnographic study of Punjabi families by Dobson (1986) provides an example of how an understanding of culture and family systems could help health visitors in their postnatal visits to Punjabi mothers. Some of the families followed the Sikh religion and others followed Islam, but 'a Punjabi culture pervaded and unified both groups' (Dobson, 1991).

It is important therefore that we do not stereotype individuals according to their culture. Individuals can belong to one culture (e.g. Punjabi) yet may have different religious beliefs from one another (e.g. Sikhism and Islam). These examples demonstrate the complexity of knowledge that is required to ensure culturally appropriate care that also meets individual needs.

Key points

1. The NMC Code (2008) and the Department of Health (2008) in their *Confidence in Caring* report recognize the importance of care that is culturally appropriate.
2. An increasing number of nurses and other healthcare professionals are becoming proactive in promoting cultural and racial awareness.
3. Transcultural nursing as a specialist field of nursing practice is not widely promoted in the UK.

CULTURAL KNOWLEDGE

Watkins (1997) reminds us that Kuhn (1970) and Polanyi (1958) identified two types of knowledge, namely 'knowing how' and 'knowing that'. According to Manley (1997), this 'know how' knowledge is usually acquired through practice and experience and often cannot be theoretically accounted for by 'know that' knowledge, which is synonymous with practical knowledge. However, 'know that' knowledge encompasses theoretical knowledge such as that found in textbooks (Manley, 1997). However, it is important to remember that in nursing practice these two types of knowledge are not regarded as separate but rather as interlinked, with one informing the other. Weller provided a case study to demonstrate this.

Case study

Mr C is in a surgical ward recovering from a prostatectomy. His primary nurse is trying to arrange a good oral fluid intake and takes care to explain why this is necessary. However, Mr C, who is of Chinese origin, consistently refuses to take the cold drinks he is offered.

Explanation

The drinking of 'cold fluid' does not fit in with Mr C's ideas of a humoral system of beliefs about health and healing. Surgery is considered a 'hot' condition and the drinking of cold water unhealthy and to be avoided at this time. In this situation, a flask of warm tea at the bedside would be acceptable.

(Source: Weller, 1991, p. 31)

We can use these types of knowledge to determine what cultural knowledge may be required by community nurses to care for the patient in the following case study.

Case study

Cheung-Ng Wai-Yung, an elderly Chinese woman, has moved to Manchester to live with her unmarried daughter, Chung Mee-Ling. She has registered with a new GP and it has been discovered that she requires an initial visit for continuing care for a chronic leg ulcer. The district nurse will need to undertake an assessment of Mrs Cheung's needs.

Examples of 'know that' knowledge required to carry out this process would include the following:

1. Understanding the naming systems of Chinese culture in order to ensure respect for the individual and accurate recording of the patient's name.

   According to Schott and Henley (1996):

   In traditional Chinese naming systems the family name comes first, followed by a two-part personal name always used together (or occasionally a single personal). In many families the first part of the personal name is shared by all the sons, and another by all the daughters. A woman does not change her name on marriage. She usually adds her husband's family name

before her own e.g. Cheung is the husband's family name. Chinese Christians may have a Christian personal name as well.

(Schott and Henley, 1996, p. 110)

2. A knowledge of Mrs Cheung's religious beliefs: she does not have a Christian name, therefore she followed the traditional Chinese society beliefs based on the philosophy of Confucianism, Taoism or Buddhism.

   (a) **Confucianism:** this philosophy emphasizes 'social harmony, through a code of personal and social conduct' (Schott and Henley, 1996), stressing many virtues such as honesty, respect for older people and traditions.

   (b) **Taoism:** this philosophy 'stresses the perfection and beauty of nature and the importance of achieving purity and union with the natural world through meditation' (Schott and Henley, 1996). Harmony may be achieved by avoiding conflict and confrontation.

   (c) **Buddhism:** this philosophy is 'concerned with achieving an understanding of the human situation and the means whereby suffering and death can be transcended so that a new state of being is achieved' (Schott and Henley, 1996). This philosophy is characterized by a belief in reincarnation.

3. 'Know how' knowledge, such as communication, (Burnard and Gill, 2008) may be used by nurses alongside the 'know that' knowledge related to Chinese culture to plan care that is essential both for Mrs Cheung's physical health problem and for her personal well-being. McGee (1992) recorded a nurse–patient interaction that illustrates this. The scenario described was that of a Chinese woman admitted to hospital after a car accident. The patient refuses pain relief, 'yet she is clearly in pain. What the nurse has not taken into account is her personal philosophy. The patient knows that physical pain is a sign that something is wrong with her body – its natural balance and harmony have been disturbed and must be restored' (McGee, 1992, p. 2). However, the nurse's explanation of the effect of the medication has made the patient believe that it will make her drowsy, causing further disharmony in her body. Thus communication between the nurse and patient has not been effective.

Mrs Cheung may also practise Chinese traditional medicine, which is based on achieving a state of physical and mental balance (yin and yang) within the body. This may be important in the nursing care plan related to the chronic leg ulcer which will require treatment from the district nurse. Finn and Lee (1996) report that in China both healthcare systems coexist (see also Chapters 2 and 3 for additional discussion of this topic).

Reflective exercise

1. Reflect on the care that you have given to patients from different cultures.
2. How would knowledge of their cultural background and religious beliefs help you to assess their individual needs?

> **3.** Consider one situation where you have had to care for a patient from a different culture and find out information about their belief system and culturally specific practices. Make notes and key points which will be valuable to you in a future encounter with someone from that culture or with those same beliefs. If a student, you could undertake this as part of a learning outcome for a clinical placement.

CULTURAL ASSESSMENT AND CARE INTERVENTIONS

In order to provide care, the nurse requires not only knowledge related to the culture of the patient but also knowledge that enables the nurse to provide the care. The nursing process offers a problem-solving framework for care planning and delivery. This involves four main responsibilities for the nurse, namely assessment of patient needs and subsequent planning, implementation and evaluation of the care (Holland *et al.*, 2008).

In order to ensure that the nurse assesses the needs of the individual patient in a systematic way there are numerous nursing models (frameworks) which organizations have utilized in their nursing care documentation (patient-record systems). Some of these are now being incorporated into the development of Integrated Care Pathways documentation, which uses the multi-disciplinary contribution to patient care (Stead and Huckle, 1997; Atwal and Caldwell, 2002). There are a few theoretical frameworks that have been developed specifically for cultural care, the most well known being Madeleine Leininger's 'Sunrise' model of transcultural care diversity and universality. However, a range of nursing theorists advocate that nurses should ensure their understanding of cultural needs (Roper *et al.*, 1996). This section will examine six nursing models that identify the need for cultural awareness and cultural knowledge.

Leininger's model of transcultural care diversity and universality

Leininger (1985) states that:

> The theory of transcultural care diversity and universality explains and predicts human care patterns of cultures and nursing care practices. It can explain and predict factors that influence care, health and nursing care. Folk, professional and nursing care values, beliefs and practices, as well as multicultural norms, can be identified and explained by the theory. From these knowledge sources three kinds of culturally based nursing care actions are predicted to be congruent with and beneficial to clients. They are:
>
> a. cultural care preservation (maintenance);
>
> b. cultural care accommodation (negotiation);
>
> c. cultural care re-patterning (restructuring).
>
> *(Leininger, 1985, p. 210)*

Leininger's model of care attempts to establish a theory of care as it is perceived by individuals, cultures and nurses in order to be able to use these constructs to care for people from different cultural groups. Her model has four levels of analysis (of needs) which should be taken into account when planning patient care, and is similar to other models in this respect. For example, Roper *et al.* (1996) identified five factors that influence activities of living that need to be accounted for during the individual care assessment, planning, implementation and evaluation process (i.e. biological, psychological, sociocultural, environmental and politico-economic factors).

Leininger's four levels of needs analysis are interpreted as follows:

- **Level 1:** social systems and social structures which include technological factors, religious and philosophical factors, kinship and social factors, cultural values and beliefs, politico-legal factors, economic factors and educational factors. It takes into account both language and environment contexts.

- **Level 2:** the nature of care and health in different healthcare systems.

- **Level 3:** the folk, professional and nursing subsystems.

- **Level 4:** the development and application of all the data collected in terms of delivering nursing care (Leininger, 1985).

These four levels of assessment are then linked to three main aspects of nursing care:

- Maintenance – those cultural behaviours that help individuals to preserve and maintain positive health and caring lifestyles.

- Accommodation – those helping behaviours that reflect ways of adapting or adjusting to individual health and caring lifestyles.

- Restructuring – new ways of helping clients to change health or lifestyles that are meaningful to them (Leininger, 1985).

This approach is viewed by Leininger (1985) as offering culturally competent (nursing) care. It is not apparent from searching the literature whether or not there are examples of this model being used in UK nursing practice. However, there was evidence of how it had been used as part of a wider analysis of transcultural models, in order to identify a new model for cultural competence for primary care nurses in their management of asylum applicants in Scotland (Quickfail, 2004).

There is evidence of this approach in other cultures. For example, Finn and Lee (1996) have used the model to help them to gain an understanding of the Chinese 'world view, cultural values and health care systems' which they would need to provide culturally appropriate care for individuals from a Chinese culture. Rather than use it to plan care, Gebru *et al.* (2007) used the model to evaluate whether nursing and medical documentation actually reflected the cultural background of their patients. They found that although the care was not 'culturally congruent', 'the nursing care was based on cultural assessment, as the documentation related to kinship and social factors, ethnohistory, language and educational factors' (Gebru *et al.*, 2007, p.2064). However, it appears that despite its use in the USA as a framework for nursing care, its use is limited in the UK.

Giger and Davidhizar's model of transcultural nursing assessment and intervention

Giger and Davidhizar (2004) offer a completely different approach in focusing on a framework for 'cultural assessment and intervention techniques'. This is based on the use of six 'cultural phenomena' that they believe are in evidence in all cultural groups (see Box 5.1).

Box 5.1 Giger and Davidhizar's six cultural phenomena

Communication
Space
Social organization
Time
Environmental control
Biological variation

Each of these phenomena will be defined in terms of its significance both within and across cultures.

Communication

The importance of communication in a nurse–patient relationship is viewed in relation to both verbal and non-verbal forms, especially during the assessment process. In particular, they state that 'nurses must have an awareness of how an individual, although speaking the same language, may differ in communication patterns and understandings as a result of cultural orientation' (Giger and Davidhizar, 2004, p. 22).

Space

This is defined in terms of personal, tactile and visual space, which is an area within the nurse–patient relationship that is not always given credence in terms of cultural care practices.

Giger and Davidhizar (2004) cite Hall's (1966b) view of personal space in a Western culture as having three dimensions, namely 'the intimate zone (0–18 inches), the personal zone (18 inches to 3 feet) and the social or public zone (3–6 feet)'. These zones are linked to different types of activities in different cultures. For example, touching (intimate zone) between individuals of the same sex in Arab cultures could be misinterpreted if it was attempted in a more reserved culture such as that of North America.

Social organization

This phenomenon is explained in terms of the role of the family in society and social structures. Giger and Davidhizar (2004, p. 65) believe that 'patterns of cultural behaviour are learned through a process called enculturation which involves acquiring knowledge and internalising values'.

Time

This phenomenon is a relatively unexplored area within the assessment process. However, in many cultures the concept of time is managed differently. Social time reflects the 'patterns and orientations that relate to social processes and to the conceptualisation and ordering of social life' (Giger and Davidhizar, 2004, p. 103). Cultural perceptions of time determine how people live and conduct their daily activities.

Environmental control

This cultural phenomenon is viewed as 'the ability of an individual or persons from a particular cultural group to plan activities that control nature ... [it] also refers to the individual's perception of ability to direct factors in the environment' (Giger and Davidhizar, 2004, p. 121). This is illustrated by how individuals determine whether to use Western medical healthcare practices or folk medicine.

Biological variation

This phenomenon is linked to epidemiological differences between cultures and the ways in which their biological structure and systems influence their response to health and illness. An example is the need for nurses to make an accurate observational assessment of skin colour changes (e.g. cyanosis or jaundice) (Giger and Davidhizar, 2004).

These six phenomena are then used to offer culturally appropriate care to individuals from different cultures. Examples of individual cultures that are examined in this way include American Eskimos (Yipik and Inupiat), Navajo Indians and Vietnamese Americans. Each has different concepts of illness which can influence the way in which they manage healthcare situations. There may be misunderstandings about treatments, as in the following Vietnamese examples:

> Drawing blood for diagnostic purposes may cause a crisis for a Vietnamese American patient. The patient may complain, although often not to the healthcare workers, of feeling weak and tired for varying periods following the procedure. Such symptoms may last for months. A Vietnamese American patient may feel that any body tissue or fluid removed cannot be replaced and that once it is removed, the body will continue to suffer the loss, not only in this life but in the next life as well.
>
> Giving flowers to the sick is a practice that may surprise and upset a Vietnamese American patient who has not been given an explanation of this practice. In Vietnam, flowers are usually reserved for the rites of the dead.
>
> *(Giger and Davidhizar, 2004, p. 472)*

Purnell's model of cultural competence

Purnell and Paulanka (2008) offer a similar model for cultural competence, which is based on 12 domains (of culture) that are essential for assessing the ethno-cultural attributes of an individual, family or group, namely:

1. overview, inhabited localities and topography;
2. communication;
3. family roles and organization;
4. work-force issues;
5. bicultural ecology;
6. high-risk health behaviours;

7. nutrition;
8. pregnancy and child-bearing practices;
9. death rituals;
10. spirituality;
11. healthcare practices;
12. healthcare practitioners.

These 12 domains are then used as a framework for identifying specific cultural issues in relation to different cultures within the USA (e.g. Amish, Irish-Americans, Chinese-Americans). Purnell (2009) has also published a guide to culturally competent care which although focused on multi-cultural USA does have value in other countries in relation to information offered regarding a large number of different cultural groups such as people of Iranian heritage (p. 215) and people of Irish heritage (p. 230). There is an associated website (http://davisplus.fadavis.com), which has additional resources.

Littlewood's anthropological nursing model within the nursing process framework

Although this is not a nursing model in the traditional sense, it does raise issues of the importance of another discipline which could influence the nursing care of a patient. Littlewood (1989) proposed a model for nursing which utilized knowledge from anthropology – a discipline which, like nursing, views the individual as a 'holistic being'. Her main premise was that when using the nursing process, nurses need to pay more attention to 'lay concepts of health and causation of illness' in order to ensure that both they and the patients are working together towards the same goal. The role of the nurse as someone who can mediate between the patient and the doctor to ensure culturally appropriate care is also considered to be important. Littlewood used the model to show how medical anthropology could be used as part of the nursing process. The focus is very much on the importance of taking account of 'lay concepts of health and causation of illness' (Littlewood, 1989). In particular, she stresses its importance at the assessment stage of the nursing process. She identified her framework as a 'generalised nursing model within the nursing process framework'.

The case example she used to illustrate the model was that of a woman with high blood pressure during pregnancy. Examples of questions/care patterns using the nursing process framework include the following:

- **Assessment:** what does the patient regard as the cause of her presenting problems and debility? What does she feel are the disturbances in terms of basic physiological needs?
- **Planning:** care is then planned which takes into account other help (e.g. alternative or complementary therapy).
- **Interventions:** nursing care/treatment is carried out as negotiated with the patient, including other 'healers'.
- **Evaluation:** does the person feel healed? The main point is that the care is patient-centred rather than professional.

The premise made by Littlewood (1989) that anthropology has much to offer nurses in their care of patients is one that we entirely support. However, there is insufficient detail within Littlewood's paper describing the proposed framework to support its application in practice by nurses. For the nurse to have some knowledge of the nature of anthropology as it relates to health and illness and healthcare practices in different cultures is a potential challenge (see Chapters 2 and 3 for information relating to health and illness beliefs). However, the introduction of anthropology to the nursing curriculum in the UK has not been as focused as in the USA, where nurses are encouraged to undertake postgraduate and doctoral studies in anthropology as part of the transcultural nursing movement led by Madeleine Leininger, who is herself an anthropologist (see above). In considering her model for nursing, it is clear that it is very much influenced by the discipline of anthropology.

Papadopoulos, Tilki and Taylor's model of developing cultural competence

Papadopoulos, Tilki and Taylor recommended using a

> model for transcultural care that is underpinned by the principles of anti-oppressive practice; the successful application of this model depends on the commitment by the whole organisation not just by those who deliver hands-on care.
>
> *(Papadopoulos et al., 1998, p. 175).*

Their model was called the transcultural skills development model, and it was built around four stages:

- cultural awareness;
- cultural knowledge;
- cultural sensitivity;
- cultural competence.

For each stage they built in a set of exercises that the reader could pursue in order to obtain a more detailed knowledge of different cultures. One exercise used 'ethno-history', and cited as an example the former Yugoslavia as an area from which refugees have arrived in the UK. The importance of understanding the culture of the refugees is relevant from both physical and mental health perspectives. Culture shock and the effects of being displaced from their own country may be mixed with the after-effects of mental and physical trauma. This could result in severe stress and communication problems. An understanding of how these people came to be refugees is therefore crucial to helping them. This example illustrates the need for an awareness of cultures other than those that are established in the UK.

The achievement of cultural competence is dependent on the healthcare practitioners addressing 'prejudice, discrimination and inequalities': i.e. practice which is 'anti-discrimination and anti-oppressive' (Papadopoulos et al., 1998). Since 1998 the model has been developed further (Papadopoulos, 2006), but has retained the four essential elements of cultural awareness, competence, knowledge and sensitivity (Papadopoulos, 2006), and is named as a model for developing cultural competence. Papadopoulos (2006) also recommends the model for assessing the cultural competence of researchers, by utilizing the four elements to assess whether studies actually take account of cultural issues such as 'cultural self-awareness' in interviewing others of a different culture.

Roper, Logan and Tierney's model of nursing

A nursing model that is familiar to most nurses in the UK is Roper, Logan and Tierney's model based on the activities of living (Roper *et al.*, 1996; Holland *et al.*, 2008). This model identifies factors which affect 12 activities that they consider to be a part of every individual's daily living. These are:

- maintaining a safe environment;
- communicating;
- breathing;
- eating and drinking;
- elimination;
- personal cleansing and dressing;
- controlling body temperature;
- mobilizing;
- working and playing;
- expressing sexuality;
- sleep;
- dying.

Although cultural perspectives are promoted in relation to each activity of living, the model does not offer specific examples to illustrate its application to different cultural groups. However, the model framework could be used in much the same way as Purnell's model of competence, using the 12 activities of living to analyse individual cultures. It would be important, however, that this does not become a 'recipe' approach to individualized care, but could offer guidance to practitioners to consider key issues when assessing someone's needs and planning and carrying out care.

An example of its use 'transculturally' can be seen in the experience of Heslop (1991) working in a Tibetan refugee settlement in Northern India. She undertook an assessment of the activities of daily living of a young Tibetan child called Tensin using Roper *et al.*'s model of nursing. The boy's father, Sonan, by using these activities as a guide, was able to identify the child's problems in relation to the poliomyelitis from which he was suffering. A plan of care was then implemented and evaluated. An understanding and awareness of the family's beliefs in Tibetan medicine and Buddhism had been an essential prerequisite to the provision of holistic care.

However, there is a danger of using cultural assessment guides as check-lists (Fleming *et al.*, 2008), and Mulhall (1994) believes that it is important to ensure that nurses take into account how patients 'perceive and interpret sickness in terms of their own symbolic systems'. One way of doing this could be through undertaking research that takes into account the 'insider's' experience of their culture and illness. For example, a study by Payne-Jackson (1999) of adult-onset diabetes in Jamaica shows how a community training programme is being established to ensure that conflict between the biomedical and folk models of illness will be reduced. The researcher gained an 'insider' cultural perspective on how adult Jamaicans perceived diabetes and how they managed their own treatment.

1. Identify the knowledge and skills that you will need to undertake an assessment that is culturally appropriate for all patients.
2. Discuss with your colleagues how you can help one another to understand more about different cultures, their health and illness beliefs and how their religion can influence the care they require (see Appendices for further information about the influence of religion on healthcare practices).

The following Case Study may be of value in helping you to identify some of these issues.

Case study

Mrs Amina Begum, a 45-year-old woman, is admitted to Ward 5 in a large district general hospital for investigations related to a persistent cough, increased sputum and loss of weight. She has also become very tired and unable to undertake her normal household activities. She has recently returned from a visit to her relatives in Pakistan and was persuaded to consult her GP by her sister, who had noticed her increasing health problems. The GP sent her to a consultant physician who, following preliminary tests, felt that it was necessary to admit her to hospital.

On arrival at the ward Mrs Begum is accompanied by her daughter, who explains that this is her mother's first visit to hospital and although she is able to converse in English, she does not always hear properly and therefore may not understand the questions asked or information given to her. Her daughter informs the staff nurse that her mother is waiting for a new hearing-aid but is unable to use sign language. The staff nurse, after introducing himself, asks how Mrs Begum wishes to be addressed, and is told that Amina would be acceptable during her stay in hospital. The nurse then undertakes a full assessment of her needs and enquires whether Amina has any food preferences and any personal cleansing and dressing requirements. The nurse informs Amina and her daughter that shower and bidet facilities are available on the ward and that her cultural dietary needs would be met. As weight loss is a problem, Amina will need to have additional supplements to ensure adequate nutrition. After this initial assessment, both women are taken round the ward and shown the day-room and dining-room, but this tires Amina, who begins to cough, and the nurse notices blood on the tissue used (adapted from Holland, 1996).

Using a model of nursing of your choice, assess Amina Begum's specific cultural needs during her first week in hospital.

Listed below are some of the specific cultural needs that you may have considered if you used a nursing model such as that of Roper *et al.* (1996). A similar example using the Roper *et al.* model of nursing, of a Muslim lady named Razia Bibi, can be seen in Holland *et al.* (2008).

1. **Communication:** this patient has no difficulty in either speaking or understanding English. However, she has a hearing problem which could affect the nurse's perceptions of her ability to communicate effectively.
2. **Eating and drinking:** she will need an appropriate diet (e.g. Muslim diet). She may eat halal meat or be a vegetarian.
3. **Elimination:** she will require facilities for washing after elimination (e.g. bidet or shower facilities).
4. **Personal cleansing and dressing:** she may wish to wear her own clothes (e.g. shalwar kameez). These are worn day and night. She may also wear a long scarf, chuni or dupatta, particularly when being visited by strangers, older people or men (Henley, 1982).
5. **Expressing sexuality:** this includes aspects such as body image, weight loss and religious preferences. She might not be happy about a male nurse caring for her, especially if she needs to discuss matters of a personal or intimate nature.

If nurses are to be sensitive to the needs of patients from different cultures, they need to be able to:

- assess and identify the specific cultural needs of their patients and how these would affect their other needs;
- understand the cultural background of their patients;
- plan interventions with the patient (as necessary) which take into account their cultural care needs;
- have skills and knowledge to enable them to intervene on their behalf or access others in the wider community who can do so;
- manage care for a number of different cultural groups.

CONCLUSION

The implementation of cultural care is dependent on many factors, including the nurse's own personal beliefs and practices. Prejudice and racist behaviour have no place in the delivery of culturally sensitive and appropriate care. When using frameworks for care assessment it is also essential to ensure the individuality of the patient and not be influenced by cultural and religious stereotypes. This is implicit within the nurse's NMC Code.

FURTHER READING

Jirwe M (2008) *Cultural competence in nursing*. Karolinska Institute, (ISBN 978-91-7409-153-3; Accessed online August 11 2009 via Google Scholar).
A thesis which explored the meaning of cultural competence and how it was understood by nurses, student nurses, nurse teachers and researchers.

Burnard P and Gill P (2008) *Culture, communication and nursing*. Pearson Education, Harlow.
This book offers valuable insight and guidance on many issues related to culture and communication and how these can be integrated into nursing.

Spector R E (2009) *Cultural diversity in health and illness*, 7th edn. Pearson Prentice Hall, New Jersey.
This book focuses on multicultural America but offers an insight into cultural knowledge that has world-wide application. It also has a companion website at: http://www.prenhall.com/spector.

Government of South Australia (2008) *Aboriginal nursing and midwifery strategy, Nursing and Midwifery Office*. SA Health http://www.nursingsa.com/office_pub.php (Accessed October 16 2009).
This is a strategy for improving access to a career pathway in nursing and midwifery for Aboriginal people.

WEBSITES

http://www.betterhealth.vic.gov.au/bhcv2/bhcarticles.nsf/pages/Aboriginal_health_issues?open
This website offers an insight into the issues related to Aboriginal health.

http://www.culturediversity.org/cultcomp.htm
This is the website for transcultural nursing, with a number of case studies, resources and other links.

http://davisplus.fadavis.com/landing_page.cfm?publication_id=2417

This website has resources linked to Purnell and Pulanka (2008) and Purnell (2009).

http://diss.kib.ki.se/2008/978-91-7409-153-3/thesis.pdf

This website offers an insight into Aboriginal culture and health and has statistical data related to a number of health issues affecting Aboriginal cultures.

http://www.gypsy-traveller.org/health/health-status

This website offers an insight into a range of issues, including health and education related to Gypsy Travellers in the UK.

http://www.nurseinfo.com.au/becoming/aboriginalhealth

This website offers an insight into a range of topics and resources for those considering becoming a nurse in Australia.

6 Culture and mental health

Christine Hogg

INTRODUCTION

Mental health problems are common and occur in all cultures and societies. Emotions such as distress, anger and grief are universal, and most people will experience them at some time in their life. However, the way in which emotional or psychological distress is manifested varies not only from person to person but also from culture to culture.

This chapter will explore the following issues:

- concepts of normality and abnormality;
- transcultural psychiatry;
- culture-bound syndromes;
- culture in care and treatment;
- intercultural communication;
- using interpreters in mental health;
- racism and intercultural communication.

Finally, a Case Study will explore the skills that are necessary for caring for a person from another culture who has mental health problems.

CONCEPTS OF NORMALITY AND ABNORMALITY

Culture determines what is perceived to be normal and abnormal within society. However, like the term 'health', the term 'normal' has different meanings in different contexts. The concept of normality is based on a shared set of beliefs and values that provide us with codes of behaviour. These principles guide how we speak, communicate, dress, eat, drink, pray and conduct ourselves in day-to-day life. In Western culture, for example, it is traditional for people to wear black clothes at funerals, and indeed the colour black is generally associated with death and mourning. This behaviour conveys to others the message that you are respectful of the dead person you are mourning. People may flout conventions, but generally they are aware of what usually constitutes socially acceptable behaviour and codes of conduct at important times.

Behaviours that appear abnormal at certain times may be regarded as normal at others. For example, it is acceptable for men to dress as women at fancy-dress parties, pantomimes or carnivals. Normality is therefore a value judgement: it is a relative concept that depends on who is making the judgement and the context in which that judgement is occurring. As members of a culture we are continually making judgements about normality that are dependent on many factors.

In the 1970s it was considered abnormal (or even deviant) for men to wear make-up in the UK. However, in the early 1980s it became acceptable and even fashionable for pop stars such as the 'New Romantics' to wear make-up. By contrast, in African and Australian Aboriginal cultures, men adorn their bodies with paint and/or jewellery for ceremonial occasions.

Reflective exercise

1. Think of other events in your life when convention is disregarded and behaviours are changed deliberately (e.g. Hallowe'en).
2. How would you explain them to someone outside your culture?

Codes of behaviour are constantly changing, and normality seems to depend not only on who we are and where we live, but also on where we are in history. Normality is not a neutral term. It is difficult to prove and also hard to define. Rosenhan (1973, p. 250) states that: 'What is viewed as normal in one culture may be seen as quite aberrant in another. Thus notions of normality and abnormality may not be quite as accurate as people believe they are'.

Rosenhan's classic research in 1973 demonstrates the difficulties that are encountered in ascribing normal and abnormal labels to behaviours. In this experiment, eight mentally healthy people gained secret admission to 12 different hospitals. The 'pseudopatients' arrived at hospital complaining of hearing voices but reported a stable personal life that lacked any other 'symptoms'. On admission to the psychiatric ward the pseudopatients stopped simulating any symptoms of abnormality and maintained ordinary behaviour. It was then left to these patients to try to obtain discharge from hospital by convincing the staff that they were not mentally ill. This proved to be a difficult task. The pseudopatients were designated as 'in remission' when they were ready for discharge, and the experiment was not detected by staff. Interestingly, it was common for the 'genuine' patients to detect the pseudopatients' sanity, and comments such as 'You're not crazy ... you're checking up on the hospital' were made. Behaviour that would not be questioned outside a psychiatric hospital (e.g. note-taking), was pathologized as abnormal behaviour inside the hospital. One nurse wrote in the nursing records 'Patient engages in writing behaviour'. Rosenhan (1973) comments as follows:

> Once a person is designated as abnormal, all of his other behaviours and characteristics are coloured by that label. Indeed, that label is so powerful that many of the pseudopatients' normal behaviours were overlooked entirely or profoundly misinterpreted.
>
> *(Rosenhan, 1973, p. 253)*

Reflective exercise

Rosenhan's research was conducted in the early 1970s in the USA.
1. What are the implications of this study for mental health services in the UK today?
2. Do you think that this experiment could be replicated today? Give reasons for your answer.

Rosenhan's experiment is a sharp reminder that perceptions of normality inside a psychiatric hospital may be skewed and instead we may search for mental illness, often when it does not exist. Both this issue and the problems of interpretation of behaviours will be discussed in more detail later in this chapter.

In 1988, Loring and Powell published the findings of a study examining the diagnostic approaches of 290 American psychiatrists. All were given similar information about clients except for details about gender and race. The study ensured that each group of clinicians evaluated a white female, a white male, a black male and a black female. Using standardized diagnostic criteria (DSM-III: The American Psychiatric Association's Diagnostic and Statistic Manual of Mental Disorders, 1980 revision), the researchers examined how race affected diagnosis. Generally, black clients were given a diagnosis of schizophrenia more frequently than white clients, and all of the psychiatrists were willing to label the black client as more dangerous than the white client, despite the fact that they were displaying the same behaviour. A similar study undertaken in 1990 by Lewis *et al.* in the UK revealed that African-Caribbean clients were judged to be potentially more violent than their white counterparts. It may be argued therefore that judgements about mental health may be influenced not only by who is making the judgement, but also by culturally determined ideas about race and gender.

Key points

1. Normal and abnormal behaviours are culturally determined and shaped.
2. Behaviours that appear normal in some contexts may be deemed abnormal in others.
3. Research evidence has demonstrated that normality is often subjectively determined in mental health.

TRANSCULTURAL PSYCHIATRY

The science of psychiatry developed in parallel with colonialism and slavery, when myths about race were common and pervaded European society. These beliefs were dominated by the notion that Europeans – that is, 'white' people – were naturally superior. A desire to emulate the contemporary popular biological sciences gave rise to much theorizing about mental illness. For example, slaves were considered to be vulnerable to mental illness and the term 'drapetomania' was used to describe a condition characterized by the 'irresistible urge amongst slaves to run away from plantations' (Littlewood and Lipsedge, 2001). Indeed, slavery provided a rich source of data for the science of psychiatry, and this was often used as a rationale to retain the practice of slavery.

At the end of the nineteenth century the myth that the brains of black people were smaller than those of white people was accepted, and the famous psychologist Stanley Hall described Asians, Chinese, Africans and Native Americans as psychologically 'adolescent races' (Fernando, 2002). Black people were perceived as possessing limited capacity for growth and as having abnormal personalities. These theories have since been discredited but they continue to pervade the mental health system.

Even today the causes and prevalence of mental illness in minority ethnic populations remain controversial. Of particular concern is the high rate of schizophrenia among African-Caribbean populations in the UK, and the high rate of suicide and self-harm among South Asian women and Irish people. Patients from all minority groups are more likely to be misdiagnosed and misunderstood in mental health services. They are more likely to be prescribed drugs and electro-convulsive therapy (ECT) and less likely to receive 'talking' treatments, such as psychotherapy and counselling (National Institute for Mental Health in England (NIMHE), 2004).

The relationship between mental health and migration is often a source of debate in psychiatry. In general, research has demonstrated higher levels of mental illness among migrant populations than in indigenous populations.

There appear to be two broad hypotheses to explain this phenomenon. The first of these is the selection hypothesis. Cox (1977) argues that certain mental disorders incite their victims to migrate. These may be people who are restless or unstable, or who have poor social networks and are thus able to migrate more easily. A study by Shaechter (1965) examined the mental health of migrants to Australia. It found that 45.5 per cent of non-white British female immigrants who were admitted to a psychiatric hospital within 3 years of migration had had an established mental illness prior to migration. In addition, when a 'suspected' mental illness was added, the rate increased to 68.2 per cent.

The alternative theory is the 'stress' hypothesis. It is argued that a high rate of mental illness among migrants is primarily caused by the stress of migration. The new migrant may have to deal with uncertainty, isolation, loss of family and friends, helplessness and in some cases open hostility from the host population (Cox, 1977).

However, Littlewood and Lipsedge (2001) argue that higher levels of mental illness among migrant populations are complex and probably result from an interplay of many factors, including both the stress hypothesis and the selection hypothesis. The detrimental effects of racism and discrimination may force migrants to experience material and environmental deprivation (e.g. overcrowding, lack of amenities, poor housing conditions), which in themselves may precipitate mental health problems. Language difficulties may also be significant. In a study in Newcastle, Wright (1983) found that 58 per cent of Pakistani women spoke little or no English and were completely illiterate.

However, Helman (2007) indicates that different migrant groups may have specific difficulties. Littlewood and Lipsedge (2001) note that West African students appear to be particularly vulnerable to mental health problems owing to dissatisfaction with food, the climate, discrimination and economic difficulties in the UK. Those migrants with low rates of mental illness (Chinese, Italians and Indians) seem to have a greater determination to migrate, migrate for economic reasons, intend to return home and have a high level of entrepreneurial activity. Thus it appears that money protects against the stress of migration (Bhugra and Ayonrinde 2004).

In contrast, refugees and people who are forced to leave their homes against their wishes may be more vulnerable to mental health problems.

Without doubt, factors such as dislocation from the native community, transition to new communities and rejection by the host community may also cause stress in individuals who may or may not be psychologically vulnerable.

In mental health care, nurses may encounter behaviours that are acceptable in other societies but which could be interpreted as signs of mental illness. An example of this is obeah – a prevalent belief among people from rural and sometimes urban communities of Africa and Asia. Obeah centres on the premise that it is possible to influence the health or well-being of another person by action at a distance. Victims of obeah may believe that illness is caused by a curse being placed on them. Treatment may involve traditional healers who are able to lift the curse (e.g. with counter-magic). An illustration can be seen in the following brief Case Study.

Case study

Mrs S, a 39-year-old woman, had emigrated from Trinidad. She was admitted to hospital after becoming increasingly hostile and angry and refusing to eat or drink. Mrs S reported that she believed an obeah curse had been placed on her. She was diagnosed with severe depression and was detained under the Mental Health Act for her own protection and for treatment. She did not respond to the treatment, and a traditional healer was consulted who lifted the curse. Mrs S responded immediately. She began to eat and drink within a day, and she became calmer and less agitated. She was discharged within a week of her admission to hospital.

CULTURE-BOUND SYNDROMES

Culture-bound disorders or syndromes are illnesses found in particular cultures. Each culture-bound disorder has a particular set of symptoms and changes in behaviour that are recognized as abnormal by members of the cultural group that it affects. Often culture-bound syndromes are a way of communicating distress or resolving interpersonal difficulties. An example in Western culture is agoraphobia, in which affected individuals may refuse to leave the home because of acute anxiety or fear. Other culture-bound syndromes are listed in Box 6.1.

Box 6.1 Culture-bound syndromes

- Amok: a spree of sudden violent attacks on people or animals that affects men in Malaysia. The expression 'running amok' is taken from this syndrome.
- The evil eye: a belief in some cultures that illness is caused by the state of a jealous person. It may be found in the Middle East, in Europe and North Africa and in Hispanic cultures.
- Susto: found in Hispanic cultures and is a belief in the loss of the soul after a frightening event, leading to unhappiness and sickness. People may also complain of loss of appetite, sleep disturbance and listlessness. It may be described as 'magical

continued

Box 6.1 *Culture-bound syndromes (continued)*

fright'. A curandero or folk healer may coax the soul back to the patient's body using massage and other treatments.

- Koro: found in males in Asian cultures, particularly South East Asia. There is a belief that the genitals are withdrawing into the abdomen or body and that this may cause death. It may cause individuals to become very distressed.
- Shinkeishitsu: a form of anxiety and obsessional neurosis found in young Japanese people.
- Hsieh Ping: a trance-like state found in Chinese cultures where a person believes that he or she is possessed by dead relatives and friends that have been offended.
- Wild man syndrome: found in the Gurumba of New Guinea. It occurs in young men during the long betrothal. Men may start running round the village attacking neighbours and stealing objects.
- Zar: reported in North Africa and the Middle East and is a form of spirit possession involving dissociative episodes and socially inappropriate behaviour.

From Helman (2007), Swartz (2000) and Littlewood and Lipsedge (2001).

Western or European culture-bound syndromes

The term 'culture-bound syndrome' can be criticized on the grounds that it is ethnocentric in that it implies that other cultures may exhibit strange behaviours that are not apparent in 'Western society'. However, some behaviours that are exhibited in Western cultures may themselves appear bizarre or odd in other cultures. Examples of culture-bound symptoms as defined by MacLachlan (1997) are listed in Box 6.2.

Box 6.2 *Western culture-bound syndromes*

- Anorexia nervosa: a syndrome characterized by refusing food until one becomes extremely emaciated, sometimes to the point of death
- Agoraphobia: the fear of leaving a restricted area, characterized by mood disturbance and panic. It may also be (mis)termed 'the housewives' disease'
- Kleptomania: a condition in which people steal goods from shops when they are capable of paying for them. It may be associated with anxiety or depression

These expressions of emotional distress may appear bizarre or strange to members of other cultures but are recognized in Western cultures as mental health problems. MacLachlan (1997) has discussed the issues related to eating disorders, which are classically perceived as 'Western' disorders. However, there are indications that anorexia nervosa is increasing in incidence among young Asian women in different countries (Miller and Pumariega, 2001; Soh *et al.*, 2006). MacLachlan (1997) argued that an Asian girl who develops an 'English disorder' could be demonstrating her identity with England and thus rejecting her Asian heritage and cultural traditions.

ISSUES IN CARE AND TREATMENT

In mental health care, most attention has focused on the elevated rates of schizophrenia diagnosed in Caribbean populations. Initially, high rates were attributed to factors relating to migration, but studies have shown that the rates are actually higher among UK-born people of Caribbean origin (McGovern and Cope, 1987; see website list at end of chapter for NHS Evidence – Ethnicity and Health 2009).

There are several possible explanations for such high rates of schizophrenia (London, 1986; Harrison *et al.*, 1988; Lloyd, 1993; Littlewood and Lipsedge, 2001):

- **biological/genetic:** black people are more 'prone' to schizophrenia because of their physical make-up;
- **economic deprivation:** e.g. the effects of living in inner-city areas with poor housing and high levels of unemployment;
- **psychological:** e.g. having to cope with racism, discrimination and harassment on a day-to-day basis;
- **service-related:** accuracy in diagnosing, labelling and stereotyping behaviours, types of services offered, and the relevance and suitability of those services.

Once in contact with psychiatric services it appears that their problems are compounded. For example, it has been shown that people from black and minority ethnic communities are:

- less likely to have contact with the GP prior to admission to hospital (Cope, 1989; W Koffman *et al.*, 1997; Bhui and Bhugra, 2002; Health Care Commission, 2008);
- more likely to be detained by the police to a 'place of safety' under the Mental Health Act (MHA) (Moodley and Thornicroft, 1988; Bhui and Bhugra, 2002). This is a particular issue for African Caribbean and Irish people and may be because they do not receive adequate care in primary health services and thus detention by the police is the first point of contact as 'help';
- up to three times more likely to be admitted or detained compulsorily under the MHA (Littlewood, 1986; Health Care Commission, 2008; Coid *et al.*, 2000; National Institute for Mental Health in England, 2004);
- more likely to be diagnosed as violent and to be detained in locked wards, secure units and special hospitals (McGovern and Cope, 1987; Coid *et al.*, 2000);
- more likely to be placed in 'seclusion' or isolation (Health Care Commission, 2008);
- more likely to receive 'physical treatments' (e.g. medication and ECT (Littlewood and Lipsedge, 2001)) and less likely to be offered talking treatments (e.g. psychotherapy and counselling; (Moodley and Perkins, 1991));
- likely to spend longer periods in hospital than their caucasian counterparts and less likely to have their social care and psychological needs addressed in their treatment (National Institute for Mental Health in England, 2004; Health Care Commission, 2008).

Commentators on these figures point out that data from hospital admissions are notoriously problematic, and that they may reflect the policies and attitudes of the health professionals instead of the prevalence of disease. Sashidharan and Francis (1993) argue that most studies have been undertaken in large, inner-city hospitals. They indicate that there is an ethnic drift to inner-city areas of mentally ill people, so the figures are naturally artificially high. Finally, many studies fail to take into account the fact that schizophrenia itself is linked to social and economic deprivation, to which black and minority ethnic groups are more vulnerable owing to the effects of racism and discrimination.

This data indicates concerning trends in mental health care for the African-Caribbean population. Pilgrim and Rogers (1993) offered a number of possible explanations for these trends. They argued that young black people spend a greater part of their social lives in public places, so are more visible and hence more vulnerable to police attention. They may also be stereotyped by the police as more violent and dangerous than their white counterparts. When a mental illness is indicated, they may therefore be considered 'doubly dangerous'.

This issue is further exacerbated by African-Caribbean people's mistrust of the psychiatric services because of fear of racism and mistreatment, which may prevent them from accessing services at an early stage of the illness. Pilgrim and Rogers (1993) argue that mainstream psychiatric services may be perceived as part of larger social control networks, such as the police, which serve to repress black people.

The plight of young black men in psychiatric services was highlighted by the case of David Bennett. David 'Rocky' Bennett was a 38-year-old African-Caribbean man who died in a medium secure unit after being restrained by staff. The inquiry into his death highlighted that greater numbers of black and minority ethnic (BME) people were diagnosed with schizophrenia and were given higher doses of medication than caucasians with similar health problems. The report recommended, among other findings, that all staff in mental health care should receive cultural awareness training and that the Care Programme Approach (CPA) care plan should include details of each patient's ethnic origin (Norfolk *et al.*, 2003).

The survey 'Breaking the Circles of Fear' (Sainsbury Centre for Mental Health, 2002) of over 200 black service users, carers and professionals and police found that stereotypical views of black people, racism and cultural ignorance were prevalent in mental health services. These factors are responsible for stopping BME groups engaging with treatment and accessing support. Services were generally seen as inhumane and unhelpful and sometimes inappropriate. Primary care was seen as lacking and acute care as unhelpful in enabling people to recover from mental health problems. Many people spoke of their fear of being admitted to hospitals, which were viewed as being similar to prisons.

One of the recommendations of the report was that there should be a range of organizations that act as 'gateways' to services and thus help to build bridges between communities and mental health services. This might lead to people from BME communities to become more involved in and less fearful of services. The report also suggests that inequality is an issue of customer care rather than ethnicity and there is a need for people to be treated with respect and dignity.

In a similar vein the report 'Inside Outside' (National Institute for Mental Health in England, 2004) focused on making services non-discriminatory to ensure that organizations work towards racial equality and cultural and ethnic diversity. The report stressed the need to develop a mental health workforce capable of delivering effective mental health services to a multicultural population. It also stressed the need for building capacity within communities and the voluntary sector for dealing with mental disorder.

'Delivering Race Equality in Mental Health Care' (Department of Health, 2005), is a 5-year action plan designed to tackle race inequalities in mental health care in England and Wales that builds on the 'Inside Outside' report. It is based on the themes of improved services between community engagement and better information. The plan aims to improve the quality of care and indicates the need for a reduction in the use of seclusion and compulsory detention. The plan also describes an improvement in the provision of effective therapies and a more active role for BME communities. A key outcome measure for the programme is route of admission to hospital. Since 2005 a yearly census of inpatient units – the 'Count Me In' – has monitored the statistics on the inpatient populations by gathering information on the ethnicity of patient populations (Health Care Commission, 2008).

Higher rates of schizophrenia among African-Caribbean populations are of great concern. However, of equal concern are the high levels of suicide and self-harm among black and minority ethnic groups. Raleigh and Balarajan's (1992) research indicated that with the exception of African-Caribbean-born people and men born on the Indian subcontinent, suicide rates are higher than for the general population. Of particular concern are the high rates of suicide, para-suicide and self-injury among young South Asian women and Irish people. (Leavey, 1999; Raleigh and Balarajan, 1992; Department of Health, 2001; National Institute for Mental Health in England, 2004). Raleigh and Balarajan (1992) indicate that the suicide rate in women in the 20–49 years age-group born in the Indian subcontinent is 21 per cent higher than that in the general population. In the 24 years age-group it is almost three times higher.

A group often overlooked in mental health care are Irish people. Irish people may be excluded from discussions about inequality and discrimination in health care perhaps because they are predominantly and ostensibly a 'white' community. In the 2001 census approximately 691 000 people in England identified themselves as 'white Irish' – this represents 1 per cent of the population.

Erens *et al.* (2001) note that some groups of Irish people (older people, particularly homeless men, people with alcohol problems and the Irish Travelling Community) do not access primary care because of stereotyping, perceived hostility and lack of confidence.

Migration to the UK was a feature of Irish life in post-war Britain. Many Irish migrants were young, single and female and were typically employed in nursing or domestic service. In post-war society prejudice and discrimination was rife, with signs advertising accommodation saying 'No Blacks, No dogs, No Irish' common. In the 1970s and 1980s political conflict in Northern Ireland (often referred to as the 'Troubles') led to negative stereotypes of Irish people and often they were subject to hostility, mistrust and abuse (Kelleher and Cahill, 2004). Stereotypes of Irish people led to some people changing their accents to disguise their identity. Irish populations in the UK tend to be older and single, and poor housing facilities and homelessness are particular issues. Irish communities also have higher rates of physical health problems and disabilities, which in turn may lead to mental health problems.

There are higher rates of mental health problems in Irish populations, above the rates of other migrant groups (Sproston and Nazroo, 2002). Suicide rates are higher particularly among Irish Travelling communities and in particular among men (Commission for Racial Equality, 2004). Like other minority ethnic groups, mental health issues may be related to discrimination, unemployment, poor housing and homelessness. There is also evidence to suggest that Irish people have difficulty in accessing help in primary care (Tilki, 2000). It is suggested that problems with accents may hamper care, that Irish culture may not be understood or that Irish people may be stereotyped as alcoholics. There may be higher rates of alcohol abuse but sometimes there may be self-medication of alcohol to cope with depression or other problems. There is some suggestion that GPs may fail to deal with mental health issues underlying alcohol problems, such as depression and anxiety, and that the Irish people are disproportionately labelled as having problems with alcohol abuse because of their cultural identity (Erens *et al.*, 2001).

In a study by Parry *et al.* (2004) examining health issues in Gypsy and Travelling communities, mental health issues were recognized and discussed at length. Many people reported that they had experienced depression or had a relative with depression. The report also noted that many people tried to keep this hidden: 'I said I felt great and happy and all that, you know, gave them a bluff'.

The specific problems encountered by young South Asian women are largely labelled as 'culture conflict'. D'Alessio (1993) claimed that young women in Asian families are often in conflict with their parents and families, and thus generational clashes occur. Young Asian women who are born and raised in the UK may be exposed to an ethos at school which espouses the value of individual advancement and self-fulfilment by means of education and a career. However, this may be in direct conflict with the values they encounter at home, which stress the importance of the home, collective family life and marriage. The family may value submissiveness and loyalty to family above all else. When young Asian women go to school and mix with young white women of their own age, they will be subject to all the usual peer pressures of adolescence. Young women may, for example, wish to reject the tradition of arranged marriage and may demand greater freedom, such as the right to pursue a career and choose a partner themselves.

However, it is important not to stereotype and label their distress as simply 'rebellion'. The danger here is that mental health nurses may view rebellion and the rejection of traditional ways of life as 'good' or healthy. Individualism may be perceived as the norm in Western cultures but it may be viewed as selfish in other cultures, inevitably leading to direct confrontation. Rejection of one's family values may be regarded as a part of growing up to others, but may lead the young Asian woman in particular to feel even more isolated, thus exacerbating her emotional distress (Yazdani, 1998).

Webb-Johnson (1992) argues that conflict between generations exists in all societies and nearly all cultures, not least in the indigenous UK population. Moreover, many South Asian women find the idea of arranged marriage acceptable. Certainly the issues are more complex than mere oppression and culture clashes. For example, to what extent do racism and isolation play a part in poor mental health? There are other cultures and religions where young teenage women are subject to a high degree of parental control (e.g. in Orthodox Jewish communities), yet the incidence of suicide and self-harm is apparently not as high. Another common stereotype that pervades mental health issues is that Asian people and others from non-Western cultures somatize psychological distress. Somatization is defined by Lipowski (1988) as:

> **... a tendency to experience and communicate somatic distress and symptoms unaccounted for by pathological findings, to attribute them to physical illness, and to seek medical help for them.**
>
> *(Lipowski, 1988, p. 1359)*

This leads to the assumption that people from the Indian subcontinent in particular communicate emotional distress in physical terms. Another prevalent stereotype is that South Asian people are not 'psychologically minded' and are therefore unsuitable candidates for certain therapeutic interventions, such as the psychotherapies. However, a study by Belliappa (1991) refutes this notion. This study, which was conducted in Haringey in North London, consisted of in-depth interviews into the lives of South Asian people. It revealed that they expressed major concerns and distress about their lives. The men, for example, identified distress caused by feeling the effects of powerlessness and racism, while the women were most affected by feelings of isolation. In this study, 82 per cent of individuals could identify concerns and 23 per cent reported experiencing emotional distress. A high percentage of people talked openly and readily about their concerns, which contradicts the stereotype of Asian people being 'psychologically tough' or unable to recognize or believe in mental distress.

The study also highlighted the fact that only 3 per cent of individuals perceived the health services to be a possible source of support. Other sources of support were also lacking. Only 13 per cent of people regarded the family as a source of support, and then only for concerns relating to childcare. None of the people with marital problems felt that the family was an appropriate source of help for their difficulties. This suggests that there is a large gap in the support available to South Asian people who are experiencing severe distress. Following the recent death of her husband, another woman described her health in the following way:

> Since my husband's death, I have been feeling very poorly with dizziness, aches and pains. I feel this has been caused by sorrow and loneliness.'

> *(Belliappa, 1991, p. 41)*

The term somatization is therefore misleading, and may be used either to minimize or to discredit a person's distress. Moreover, it might be suggested that somatization is not restricted to other cultures but is actually present in our own. Western biomedical models of health do not recognize the relationship between mind and body. However, Eastern medicines do not isolate the mind and body, but regard them as interdependent. Thus it may appear quite logical for people to express their distress in different ways and for them to refer to parts of the body as being affected.

In a study in 1996, Fenton and Sadiq-Sanster interviewed a group of South Asian women to elicit their beliefs and views about mental health and emotional distress. In this study, the women did not use conventional terms such as 'depression', but used other expressions instead. Many of the women referred to the heart when describing emotional distress:

> My heart kept falling and falling ... I felt as if my head was about to burst. The life would go out of my heart. My heart has taken many shocks. I'd get up in the morning and feel as if something heavy was resting on my heart.

> *(Fenton and Sadiq-Sanster, 1996, p. 75)*

Another phrase that was commonly used in the study was 'thinking too much' as the key description of illness. Fenton and Sadiq-Sanster (1996) argue that the women in the study were describing a syndrome of mental distress in which a number of symptoms correspond to those of depression.

The notion of expressing emotional distress in physical terms is not uncommon in UK culture and throughout the English language. For example, we use expressions such as 'a heavy heart' or 'feeling gutted' or 'feeling empty inside' to denote extreme distress. We commonly have physical reactions to emotional distress or anxiety (e.g. feeling nauseous before an important event or needing to urinate when anxious).

Reflective exercise

Consider the issues with regard to culture and mental health problems and undertake a search of the NHS Evidence: Ethnicity and Health website for information related to men, women, young adults and children (http://www.library.nhs.uk/ethnicity).

INTERCULTURAL COMMUNICATION

Effective communication skills are essential when caring for people with mental health problems, and especially when helping someone from another culture or minority ethnic group. When considering the issues related to intercultural communication, perhaps the greatest challenge of all is that of language barriers. However, communication requires knowledge about the person's culture as well as their language.

For example, Schott and Henley (1996) argue that:

> Every language is part of a culture and has its own cultural feature. It is often assumed that it is easy to communicate with clients whose first language is not English but who speak English well. In fact, people who retain features of their mother tongue that clash with those of English often unintentionally cause offence or give the wrong impression. Such misunderstandings can be difficult to overcome because they are often subtle and unrecognised.
>
> *(Schott and Henley, 1996, p. 69)*

Language consists of more than just groups of words. For example, as children we learn to speak in certain ways with particular dialects, rhythms and mannerisms that may be unique to our culture and even to our own family or peer group. From our own ethnocentric group perspective some language and communication practices may appear strange, alien or even a symptom of mental disturbance. For example, in British English it is customary to indicate emotions such as anger by emphasizing specific words within a sentence. However, in other cultures this may be interpreted as merely stressing something important. In other cultures people may speak quietly to signify importance, or alternatively they may slow down and lower their voice (Mares *et al.*, 1985).

Inevitably, such subtle linguistic differences may be misinterpreted in mental health. For example, people who speak quickly and/or loudly may have their behaviour interpreted as a symptom of hypomania or grandiosity. Alternatively, people who speak slowly or quietly may be labelled as depressed, shy or anxious.

The amount of eye contact that is made may also differ in other cultures. In Western culture, looking people directly in the eye may denote honesty and straightforwardness, but in other cultures it may be interpreted as challenging and rude. In Arabic cultures, people like to share a great deal of eye contact, and not to do so may be interpreted as disrespectful. However, in South Asian cultures and in Australian Aboriginal cultures direct eye contact is generally regarded as aggressive or even confrontational.

Linguistic conventions are often very complex and subtle, and again require a deal of understanding and consideration. The convention in English of saying 'please' and 'thank you' presents problems for some languages. For example, in Urdu there is no equivalent for these terms, and instead they are built into the verb. This may be interpreted as hostility or rudeness. However, sometimes it is not just a linguistic difference, but also a cultural one. In North America, for example, it is considered vulgar to use the word 'toilet', and people prefer to use the word 'bathroom' instead. By contrast, North Americans use the term 'fanny' to refer to one's backside, whereas in British English it is a slang word used to denote the female genitalia.

Schott and Henley (1996) stress that when people cannot be understood they may begin to feel nervous and anxious, and will inevitably become sensitive to the non-verbal signals of others. They may remain quite passive and silent, avoid eye contact, and avoid initiating conversations or prolonging them. They may also give simple yet inaccurate answers (e.g. 'yes' to everything) simply because they cannot explain themselves. Finally, they may avoid situations that they find difficult to cope with. For someone who is already distressed, these difficulties may compound their feelings of inadequacy and low self-esteem. Furthermore, behaviours such as passivity may be misinterpreted as depression, social avoidance or anxiety.

In 1992 Perry highlighted the need for greater sensitivity and self-awareness when caring for someone from a black or minority ethnic population. Of particular importance is the need for white staff to recognize and confront the overt and covert messages about black people from their own culture. These may often result in the internalization of negative feelings.

Perry (1992) makes the following points:

> **When a white mental health worker becomes involved therapeutically with a black client, he or she carries a legacy, which affects the context and outcome of that relationship. How can workers begin to discuss how powerlessness and racism affect mental health unless they have already acknowledged and begun to deal with their own prejudices? Without such preparation there is danger that the power imbalance experienced by black people in society will be reproduced in the "therapeutic relationship" and the client's mental health will suffer. The client may become angry and demoralised and feel the therapist does not listen and is incapable of empathising with his or her problem. The therapist may be unaware of the dynamics behind the apparent 'failure' and so will conclude that black clients are not receptive to counselling.**

(Perry, 1992, p. 63)

Thus, unless attention is paid to language and communication needs, clients from a different background are at risk of receiving inadequate or inappropriate care, and health service staff may make decisions based on inadequate information.

Corsellis and Crichton (1994) argue that service provision needs two elements: first, reliable channels of communication, and second, the delivery through these of a service that is appropriate to the background and needs of the individual. More specifically, they advocate more mental health professionals that have a second language and/or interpreters that hold a qualification in mental health.

USING INTERPRETERS IN MENTAL HEALTH

Undertaking skilled assessment and treatment in mental health through an interpreter or translator can be problematic. Communication is subtle, as cues come not just from the actual words used but also from non-verbal communication and the tone and meanings of specific words.

Belliappa's survey in 1991 revealed that language and communication barriers play a significant part in preventing people from using existing services. For people whose first language is not English this has clear implications. For example, when people are unwell, and particularly when they are distressed, they often revert to their mother tongue to express themselves.

The provision of interpreters may be central to clients receiving good-quality care. In reality, partners, other relatives, friends and even children may carry out interpreting services. In some cases delicate and sensitive information is conveyed, and this may result in embarrassment and compound the client's distress. In some situations this may result in people withholding vital information. One nurse recounted the following experience:

> It was a Saturday night when Mrs A was admitted to the ward. Try as I could there were no interpreters available. Mrs A was very upset, crying and threatening to harm herself, and we were worried about her safety. As a last resort, it was decided to ask Mrs A's teenage daughter to interpret for us. It turned out that Mr A had been having an affair and that the family business had been in some trouble for some time. Mrs A's daughter didn't know about this situation, and you can imagine her shock and disbelief. It taught me a big lesson. Children, whatever their age and the situation, shouldn't be used in this way – they have a right to be protected just as people have a right to have their feelings kept confidential. In that situation we ended up with the daughter in a terrible state as well as the mother. From then on we made sure that there was always someone on call to interpret for us, but it's a shame that a teenager had to undergo so much trauma because of our inadequate services.

Henley and Schott (1999) state that effective interpreting requires someone that:

- is trained and experienced;
- is fluent in both English and the patient's mother tongue;
- is able to understand medical terminology and what the health professional is trying to achieve;
- both the health professional and the patient can trust.

Webb-Johnson (1992) argues that interpreters must be considered a central rather than a peripheral part of the services and that there is an urgent need to raise the status of this activity within the NHS.

> In an interpreting situation, however, a literal translation of the words is not sufficient. Words are culturally loaded and have different meanings and concepts in different languages. The interpreter, therefore, has to decode within the cultural context what is being expressed behind the words in order to communicate the full message to the professional.
>
> *(Webb-Johnson, 1992, p. 86)*

Interpreting services also need to adhere to confidentiality codes, which are of special significance when interpreters are recruited from the local community. Breaches in confidentiality may result in members of the community rejecting interpreters that belong to the same community at interviews (Webb-Johnson, 1992).

Using interpreters in mental health services requires sensitivity and commitment. It is an aspect of mental health care that may not take priority when funding is limited. However, if people are to receive care that is individualized and comprehensive, then interpreting services must become a central part of care for individuals whose communication skills may be compromised by language barriers.

RACISM AND INTERCULTURAL COMMUNICATION

People from black and minority ethnic groups/communities may already face racism and hostility because of physical differences, and this may be compounded by the stigma of having a mental health problem. Mental illness, particularly schizophrenia, is synonymous with the notion of danger, and the association between black people and violence perpetuates this stereotype. This double discrimination may actually prove to be of greater disadvantage for women – that is, being black, having a mental illness and being female (i.e. more likely to be diagnosed with a mental illness).

However, central to these issues are the effects of racism on mental health. The extent to which racism contributes to mental health is an important question, but one which may get overlooked. For example, racism is a contributing factor to the maintenance of social and economic deprivation, which is itself a contributing factor in poor mental health. Moreover, as Fernando (1986) has argued, racism itself causes depression by knocking self-esteem, which may evoke a sense of helplessness and powerlessness in the individual.

Thomas (1992) argues that being black affects people's psychological development in the same way as being male or female. The ways in which people behave and respond towards us shape us as individuals and influence our sense of self.

A black colleague related the following incident:

> I can be in a good mood, going to work in the morning full of the joys of spring, minding my own business, when something can upset me. It's usually a chance remark or something stupid that people say or do. Like the other day. I went into a shop to buy a paper; the woman served everyone else in the queue and deliberately left me till last. She didn't speak to me or give me any eye contact, I could tell that she resented me; she was so cold and stand-offish. By the time I got to work I felt like the pits. It's not the direct in-your-face abuse that gets you down, I can cope with that. It's the subtle things that aren't always obvious to everyone else – they're the worst.

The detrimental effects of overt and covert racism and the undermining effect that this may have on a day-to-day level may cause people immeasurable distress. In mental health services there has been a trend to promote services that are 'colour-blind' in their approach. Colour-blind care and treatment assume that everyone is equal and therefore that everyone should be treated in the same way, irrespective of culture, race or ethnicity. At the heart of this notion is equality, but in reality it may, paradoxically, result in everyone being treated as 'white', leading to inequality. It assumes that everyone should adapt to the dominant culture, taking on the values, beliefs and behaviours of that culture. For example, there is a belief (reported anecdotally) that women in traditional South Asian communities would be happier if they learned to 'stick up for themselves' – that is, learned to be more assertive and behave like 'us Westerners'. In other words, they would be more acceptable (and therefore receive more sympathy) if they became 'like us'.

The colour-blind approach does not take into account the damaging and destructive psychological effects of racism; neither does it acknowledge or value the cultural context, background and lifestyle of the client.

By contrast, therefore, it may be argued that transcultural therapy and counselling are more appropriate and therapeutic. Transcultural therapy addresses the limitations of Western models of therapy, which may separate the mind and body and may not address or recognize the power of racism and the different contexts of people's lives. It also addresses the issues of racism that may occur within a therapeutic relationship.

Thomas (1992) argues that ideas about white superiority and white supremacy form part of the fabric of the UK, and that they play a part in the way in which white people relate to non-white people. Thomas (1992) also states that:

> **Subtle racism attaches to a system of assumptions and negative stereotypes about black people that is counter-therapeutic. Racism, whenever it arises, denies the black person individual characteristics seen as normal or ordinary, which white people are held to possess.**
>
> *(Thomas, 1992, p. 134)*

Within a therapeutic relationship is an unequal relationship between, for example, a white therapist and a black client. This imbalance of power needs to be addressed through the process of race awareness training, through clinical supervision and by self-awareness and self-knowledge.

In contrast, where the client and the nurse/therapist have similar backgrounds and cultures, socio-cultural factors may be taken for granted. Counselling may be an example of this. In Western cultures the individual is placed at the centre of the therapeutic process, and choice and empowerment may be given a high priority. However, in Eastern cultures people may view themselves and their whole identity in terms of the family. The pursuit of individual goals may conflict directly with the wishes and/or needs of the family, and this may in turn cause tension, antagonism and further distress, and possibly even a deterioration in the person's mental state.

However a report by the Joseph Rowntree Foundation (2008) demonstrates that although the uptake of counselling is still low for South Asian people, those that had used it found it to be beneficial. They seemed to derive increased self-esteem and a feeling of comfort from counselling. Factors that were important included the opportunity to communicate in one's own language, the opportunity to speak with someone of their own gender (particularly for women) and someone from the same community/ethnic background.

In many Eastern cultures great importance may be attached to a person's relationships with others. Kuo and Kavanagh (1994) discussed Chinese beliefs about and perspectives on mental health. For example, interpersonal relationships may be held together by a hierarchy of social roles that tend to restrict personal choice and individual action while promoting a group response over individual action. For example, Confucian philosophy demands that people behave in certain ways according to their own social status, valuing compliance and self-control in order to avoid conflict. In Chinese traditional medicine, the concept of balance and the dual forces of yin and yang are central to good mental health. Kuo and Kavanagh suggest that:

In conventional thinking, harmonious personal relationships are the basis of psychosocial equilibrium. The keys to survival, peace and happiness are harmony, interdependence and loyalty.

(Kuo and Kavanagh, 1994, p. 555)

They go on to stress that these values are in sharp contrast to American culture, which is frequently characterized by competitiveness, independence and change. It is argued that interventions may need to focus on interpersonal relationships, adjustment to others' expectations, and negotiation skills.

Communication skills in mental health are perhaps the most important means of enabling people to gain a sense of self and to communicate and express their distress. In working with those from other cultures, who may speak a different language or who may have different ways of communicating, nurses may be faced with unique challenges. However, this challenge may present opportunities to improve nurses' skills in communication and self-awareness. Consider the following Case Study.

Case study

Yusuf is a 19-year-old man in the first year of a course in chemistry at the local university. He lives with his mother and father, who describe him as a quiet but polite young man. He is the second eldest of four children, two of whom live at home. Yusuf has been spending long periods at home in his bedroom, locked away from the family. His father, who is a devout Muslim, says that Yusuf is becoming obsessed with religion and he feels that his son is becoming very distant and difficult to talk to. Yusuf has grown a beard and started to wear traditional Islamic dress, whereas previously he had been wearing Western clothes. He prays every 4 hours, getting up in the night. The only time he leaves the house is to attend the Mosque. He rarely spends time with his younger brothers and sister (something he used to do), and this morning he hit his 14-year-old sister, Jasmine, saying that she was 'Satan's daughter'. His mother and father are extremely distressed, saying that they are in despair. His mother speaks a little English and is crying quietly.

continued

How would you ensure effective and therapeutic communication?

Use the following points to help you to make informed decisions.

- Find a quiet place to meet. It would be preferable to assess Yusuf at home and to meet him in his own environment (e.g. to assess how he lives and how he gets along with his family).
- It would be useful to speak to both parents, so it may be necessary to get a link worker with a good knowledge of mental health to speak with Yusuf's mother as well as his father.
- A broad mental health assessment will be needed, taking into account Yusuf's religious and spiritual needs. This may include information gleaned from his parents.
- Assess his physical state (e.g. sleep, appetite, and signs of recent weight loss).
- Assess his social interactions. Does he still have friends? Does he still mix with his peer group? How has he been coping at university? How does he spend the day?
- Assess his psychological state. What is his explanation of recent events and circumstances? Why did he hit his sister? Why does he believe that she is 'Satan's daughter'? Does he have thoughts of harming himself or anyone else? Does he hear voices? Does he feel that he has special powers? Does he feel that he is being controlled by anything or anyone?
- It is vital to elicit from the family whether they feel that Yusuf's behaviour is appropriate for a young man of his age, and how they feel about his behaviour in terms of his religious beliefs and practices. Has anyone else in the community commented on his behaviour? Has anyone spoken to the elders in the Mosque? What are their views?
- It may be useful to ask his father if he had similar problems or patterns of behaviour in his youth? Is it usual in his peer group?
- Is there any mental illness in the family? What are the family's views on mental illness?
- Ask Yusuf what importance religion plays in his life. Has anything significant changed in his life recently? Has he felt stressed in any way? Has he suffered any threats or persecutions recently in his life? Is anyone intimidating him?

If Yusuf is admitted to hospital, the following points may assist his stay there.

- He needs appropriate care to accommodate his religious beliefs. For example, he will need somewhere quiet and private to pray. It may be relevant to ask the family to bring in appropriate articles such as a prayer mat, a compass, a copy of the Qur'an, and clothing for him to wear in accordance with his religious needs.
- He will also need an appropriate diet and should be offered a choice of halal food.
- He will need to be offered appropriate facilities for personal hygiene (i.e. running water to wash with, a jug for washing after using the toilet, and the opportunity to wash before praying).

continued

- He may feel uncomfortable mixing closely with women and may find it easier to relate to a male key worker. Be aware that he is likely to find hospital a strange and disorientating environment. He may also be vulnerable to exploitation and may need some degree of protection. His key worker needs to engage the family in order to inform them and discuss Yusuf's progress and care.
- Yusuf may wish to receive spiritual guidance while he is in hospital. With his permission, it may be useful to contact leaders at the Mosque who will be able to maintain contact with him. The key worker and other staff may need to give Yusuf the opportunity to discuss his spiritual needs and beliefs.
- Key workers need to be aware that Yusuf's parents may be consulting traditional healers and/or alternative medicines from home (i.e. Pakistan or within the community).
- Yusuf's parents and family need to be kept fully informed of his progress and must be given opportunities to express their concerns and fears for their son.
- The key worker needs to ensure that Yusuf has time and space to consider his spiritual needs.

CONCLUSION

The relationship between culture, race and ethnicity and mental health is both controversial and fraught with difficulties. Central to these difficulties are the issues related to racism and discrimination, and some argue that the starting point for the provision of transcultural care in mental health is to challenge oppressive and discriminatory practice in Western psychiatry (Fernando, 1991). However, mental health nurses are in an ideal position to promote the needs of patients from other cultures. They are often in close proximity to patients, and their capacity to form close, long-standing relationships with patients and their families can play a central role in helping to provide holistic and sensitive care. However, at the heart of this undertaking is the need for nurses to understand and confront overt and covert racism in mental health and psychiatry. Central to this is the need for self-reflection and an honest approach to one's own prejudices and preconceived ideas. In mental health nursing this premise is perhaps underpinned by the promotion of such practices as clinical supervision and the concept of self-awareness. However, when considering transcultural mental health issues, there needs to be sensitivity and it is sometimes necessary to suspend and challenge our ideas about normality. Thus, if we are to provide quality services that are appropriate and responsive to people's needs, we must listen and involve people in those services, in addition to being willing to learn and understand the world from someone else's perspective.

CHAPTER SUMMARY

1. Mental health problems occur in all cultures, but are manifested differently and are culturally determined.
2. Good communication skills are essential for caring for people with mental health problems, and thus interpreting and translating services are needed as a priority.
3. Nurses need to be sensitive to issues relating to prejudice and stereotyping of people from black and minority ethnic groups with mental health problems.

FURTHER READING

Bhui K and Bhugra D (1999) Pharmacotherapy across ethnic and cultural boundaries. *Mental Health Practice* **2**, 10–14.
  An extremely useful and interesting article that examines psychotropic medication and minority ethnic groups.

Hussain A (2001) Islamic beliefs and mental health. *Mental Health Nursing* **21**, 6–9.
  This article explores Islamic perspectives on mental health. It is interesting and informative.

Salas S (2004) Sensitising mental health professionals to Islam. *The Foundation of Nursing Studies Dissemination Series* **2**(5), http://www.fons.org.
  This paper discusses a project in London which aimed to enhance the knowledge of practitioners in relation to Islam. It is a comprehensive and enlightening study that approaches the issues around culturally sensitive care with some creativity and innovation.

Endrawes G, O'Brien L and Wilkes L (2007) Mental illness and Egyptian families. *International Journal of Mental Health Nursing* **16**, 178–87.
  This article discusses Egyptians' beliefs about mental illness and looks at how families cope with a mental illness in the family. It also describes the Zar cult and the belief in the evil eye, magic and evil possession.

Littlewood R (1998) *The butterfly and the serpent. Essays in psychiatry, race and religion.* Free Association Books, London.
  This is an extremely interesting and in-depth analysis of transcultural psychiatry from an anthropological perspective.

WEBSITES

http://www.library.nhs.uk/ethnicity
  Pages for NHS Evidence – Ethnicity and Health 2009. This website cites the best evidence in relation to healthcare needs for migrant and minority ethnic groups.

http://www.mmha.org.au/

Multicultural Mental Health Australia. This is a very interesting and informative website that aims to build greater awareness of the issues in relation to mental health for people from culturally and linguistically diverse backgrounds.

http://bmementalhealth.org.uk

National BME Mental Health network. This network aims to address the needs of people with mental health needs from BME backgrounds.

http://www.mentalhealthcare.org.uk

This website provides a range of different information sources on mental health problems experienced by adults as well as young people.

7 Women and health care in a multicultural society

Karen Holland

INTRODUCTION

Women have significant roles in most societies as mothers, carers and workers. For example, they represent the majority of the nursing work-force and they also provide the majority of care as mothers and informal carers (Trevelyan, 1994; Buchan *et al.*, 2008). However, in most societies women do not experience equality with men in many areas of their daily lives, and often this will influence how they experience and receive health care.

This chapter focuses on women's healthcare in a multicultural society. The importance of men's healthcare is acknowledged as being of equal importance (and will be discussed in Chapter 8) but the potential impact of women's health and health problems significantly influences the lives of others, particularly their role in child care and as mothers.

> ### The chapter will focus on the following specific issues:
>
> - the role of women in society;
> - women as carers in society;
> - cultural beliefs and the needs of women;
> - women and the need to maintain privacy and dignity;
> - the effects of women's role and cultural beliefs on their health and health care.

THE ROLE OF WOMEN IN SOCIETY

Events such as man-made and natural disasters (e.g. war, earthquakes), the increasing longevity of women and changing family structures have influenced the role that women play in their own cultural groups and in society. Consider, for example, the changing role of women in society in the UK. Owing to factors such as unemployment and increased divorce rates, many women in traditional UK culture have now become the main breadwinner, with more men adopting a child-caring role. However, traditional social norms still do not view this as 'normal' behaviour within a nuclear family structure. As a result of changing family patterns and the need for many men and women to move away from their locality during the past century, there are no longer the same extended family support networks. By contrast, in some other cultures, there are extended families that give women a great deal of support.

However, Schott and Henley (1996) point out that even this is no longer guaranteed, especially if families are separated geographically, and that a stereotype of extended family support could prevent adequate services being provided for different cultural groups. They cite an example from a Bradford study (Gatrad, 1994) which found that South Asian mothers who wanted and needed help from Social Services were less likely to receive it than English mothers. However, a recent report by the National Society for the Prevention of Cruelty to Children (NSPCC) notes that with regard to issues of domestic violence, this extended family (i.e. the women) will not always intervene or support the woman who may need help, encouraging them to stay in their abusive marriage rather than leave it (Izzidien, 2008). Izzidien (2008) states, however, that when the family condemned the actions of the perpetrator and sympathised with the women, they were a great source of help'.

Hendry (1999) cites an example of the Pakistani community, where this extended family network includes a group of individuals known as the biradari, commonly translated as 'relations'. This group is a central support network for girls when they get married, and is reinforced by 'arranged marriages between members of the same biradari, very often between first cousins' (Hendry, 1999; see Chapter 9 for further information). For young British-Pakistani men in Bradford, however, 'biridari (clan) networks no longer had the centrality they once enjoyed, as there were now other ways to gain support, understanding and group identification' (Alam and Husband, 2006).

Reflective exercise

1. Consider your own family structure. What kind is it?
2. Discuss with a colleague from another culture what kind of support networks exist in their family structure.
3. Compare the way in which women receive or give support to family members.

Within society motherhood is viewed as the natural role for women, and in the UK 'the status of mothers is generally low in comparison to some other cultures and countries' (Schott and Henley, 1996). However, Bowler (1993) does point out that our understanding of 'normal' motherhood is based on Western white middle-class behaviours. Phoenix and Woollett (1991), cited by Bowler (1993), believe that it is this view that has helped to ensure that when we talk about what is right or wrong about women's role in bringing up children, anything that does not fit into this traditional pattern is not 'normal'.

Marriage patterns are also linked to the role of women in society. Many couples marry their own choice of partner, but some cultures have arranged marriages and/or very strict prohibitions about partners. For example, a student nurse from a Muslim culture gave the following history:

> My parents are letting me do this course because I want to be a nurse and help people from my own culture. However, once I finish, I am expected to get married to someone they arrange for me to marry, and unless he supports me to carry on working I won't be able to.

This student did in fact complete her course, but because of her marriage was unable to register as a qualified nurse. She subsequently divorced her husband and trained for another care profession.

This type of example was also seen in a study by Dyson *et al.* (2008), which explored the experiences of a group of South Asian student nurses. They found that 'negotiating marriage' was 'one of the most significant themes in the study' whereby 'students talked of negotiating with their parents, for the most part with fathers, to be allowed to study or work before returning home to be married' (Dyson *et al.*, 2008, p. 169). They also highlighted the issue of 'not bringing shame' on their families and as one student explained:

> If I find someone at University then he would have to be the same religion and the same caste
> and come from a good background – that's not a big issue – as long as he's the same religion.
> My parents would be disappointed if he wasn't because it's society – and they would talk and
> parents can't seem to handle that gossip and they care what people think. The biggest sin, as
> an Asian girl, would be to bring shame on your family.

> *(Student 5, Dyson et al., 2008)*

Marriage across cultures is also discouraged by other societies. For example, Gypsy Travellers are not allowed to marry a Gorgio (an outsider or non-gypsy), as marriage relates to purity of the race and blood (Okley, 1983); neither are they allowed to marry first cousins. The latter prohibition is in complete contrast to other cultures. For example, in Islamic law, first cousins are allowed to marry one another (Henley, 1982). This is permitted by the Qur'an. The issue of first cousin marriages was a topic raised in the House of Lords in April 2008 in relation to genetic risks and the response to one question related to the role of health professionals and genetic counsellors:

> Lord Darzi of Denham: My Lords, the noble Baroness makes an important point. I would like to
> put on record the Government's commitment to this. The role of the healthcare professional
> and of the Government is to provide support and advice to empower people to make informed
> choices based on clear information and advice. The healthcare professional's role is to allow
> the individual to assess these risks and to make their own decisions about what to do; it is not
> to tell them who they should marry. As a result the Government have made a significant
> investment in this field, not only in the training of genetic counsellors but in changing the
> curriculum of primary care colleagues with the collaboration of the Royal College of General
> Practitioners. We will see more and more genetic knowledge being disseminated through
> postgraduate education.

> *(Parliamentary Business, Hansard, April 21, 2008; http://www.parliament.uk)*

(See Appendix 4 for further information on Islamic religious beliefs and practices.)

It is also important to understand the role that women play in marriage in different cultures. In Hindu culture women often undertake vows, the purpose of which is:

> to attain the grace of a deity for a specific objective – whether for the care, protection and
> well-being of the family or specific members by acquiring merit with God, for personal
> satisfaction and the "goodness of God", through devotion and discipline, or to achieve a
> particular wish, often in times of family or personal crisis or during episodes of illness.

> *(McDonald, 1997, p. 141)*

One such ritual is described as follows:

> Jaya parvati vrat is a ritual performed by women for five years after marriage in order to ensure the health and longevity of their husbands, and to protect their own state as an auspicious married woman.

(McDonald, 1997, p. 141)

The annual ritual lasts for five days and consists of fasting and worship. McDonald (1997) found that among the Gujarati women in her study, many still believed that they were subordinate to their husbands in certain aspects of their lives. If a woman had been widowed, she was traditionally viewed as bringing bad luck or being 'the cause of the evil eye' (McDonald, 1997), and it is still a tradition for a widow to remove all of her marriage jewellery. She may not put the vermilion mark in her hair parting or wear brightly coloured saris, as these are symbolic of her married status. A similar ritual is Sitala Satam, which takes place in July or August and involves both fasting and eating cold food (McDonald, 1997). Many childhood diseases are associated with the goddess Sitala, who, unless worshipped properly, brings illness into the community. The ritual is for the protection of children and to ensure their good health. Failing to worship the gods and goddesses is often viewed as the cause of illness and 'infertility in women' (McDonald, 1997).

Reflective exercise

1. Consider your own personal experiences. What role do women play within your family?
2. How is the role of women as workers, mothers and carers viewed in your culture?
3. If you are a woman, what role conflict have you experienced in relation to the above?

You may have concluded that in your culture men and women are considered to have equal status in the family and at work. In other cultures the roles of men and women may differ from this, with women taking the major role in child care and the home, and men having the major role as 'breadwinner'. However, in the UK this traditional male role is being taken on by women in all cultures for economic reasons (e.g. male unemployment). This is often in addition to their roles as wife and mother, which can cause increased role conflict and stress for women as they try to manage both successfully.

WOMEN AS CARERS IN SOCIETY

Caring is traditionally viewed as the role of women, which Colliere (1986) believed was not considered to be valuable or of great necessity to society. Although this may appear to be a very sweeping statement, let us consider how nursing as a caring profession is viewed in some societies. Most nurses are women, and Davies (1995) reported that in 1988 only 9 per cent of nurses working in the NHS were men. In 1998 this number had increased to 10.5 per cent: 44 557 out of a total of 421 749 (Department of Health, 1998). In 2006–7 90 per cent of entrants into UK pre-registration nursing programmes were women (National Nursing Research Unit, 2009), and the policy report concluded that 'men could be a significant recruitment pool in the future if barriers to male recruitment could be overcome'.

The image of nursing as a profession for women has tended to persist, even though the NHS has attempted to change this in order to aid the recruitment of nurses. The status of nurses and that of women in society have also been identified as being very closely linked (Davies, 1995). This was observed in a study by Mizuno-Lewis and McAllister (2006) on the issue of how Japanese nurses take leave from their work and the impact that their culture has on whether they do or not. They point out that there is gender inequality in Japan and that 'there remains a profound belief that the Japanese man should go out to work while the woman should stay home and look after the house and children' (Mizuno-Lewis and McAllister, 2006 p. 275). Although there is some change in this belief, men's careers are seen to be the priority but when women are working (i.e. nursing), their culture with its strong work ethic does not enable them to take sick leave nor many holidays (33 per cent are reported to take less than five days annual leave a year). The paper reports on the case of a young female nurse who died of a subarachnoid haemorrhage and a dispute whereby there was an attempt by her parents to prove that it was caused by Karoshi (death by overwork). It appears that the nurse 'was allegedly forced to work more than 80 hours of overtime per month'. No final outcome was reported, but the authors concluded that there was a need for 'Japanese nursing ... to benefit from preparatory education that teaches students about ... emancipation of women and the need to change traditional values about not taking leave and the value of a balanced approach to work' (Mizuno-Lewis and McAllister, 2006, p. 279).

Wolf (1986) found that there was also a relationship between nurses' work being regarded as sacred and profane. Nurses were perceived as being involved in both 'dirty work', such as handling body excreta with its pollution image, and sacred work, such as 'administering to the sick', with its religious symbolism (Wolf, 1986). These images have a major influence on the position and status of nurses world-wide.

In Japan, for example, nurses have a relatively low status because of their association with pollution and illness (Hendry and Martinez, 1991). According to Tierney and Tierney (1994), 'nurses in Japan are regarded as having a "3K" job – kitsui (hard), kitanai (dirty) and kiken (dangerous)'. Similar findings have been reported with regard to nursing in India (Nandi, 1977; Somjee, 1991). A study by Zaman (2009) reported that 'nurses in Bangladesh rarely touch the patient; the relatives of the patient do all the "body work" and play the role of nurses'. It was also reported that:

> The negative opinion of nursing also comes from the existing religious notions in Bangladesh. In this context, the nursing profession is considered socially low because of Hindu ideas about the caste system and because of Islamic notions about decent moral conduct for women.
>
> *(Zaman, 2009, p. 373)*

Reflective exercise

1. How often have you heard the same kind of views being expressed about nursing in the UK? Ask some of your non-nursing friends how many of them would consider nursing as an occupation and why.
2. Ask your non-nursing friends what their image of female and male nurses is, and how both professional (nurses and other healthcare occupations) and lay (non-healthcare worker) caring is viewed.
3. Compare these with the earlier comments on Japanese nurses.

In Japan, as in the UK, there has been an increase in the number of women going out to work (Tierney and Tierney, 1994), which is now creating a problem with regard to care for the elderly in traditional extended families. Atkin and Rollings (1993) have reported on one of several studies which have examined this informal carer role within black and minority ethnic communities. A study by McCalman in 1990 cited by Atkin and Rollings (1993) found that of 34 carers living in the London Borough of Southwark:

> **All the carers looked after a close relative; just over half [of carers] – a parent, step-parent or parent in law, one-third a spouse and just over an eighth a grandparent. Twenty-one carers were female.**
>
> *(Atkin and Rollings, 1993, p. 12)*

Atkin and Rollings also point out from their research that 'the supportive extended family network is largely a myth' and that there are many Asian people now living on their own (Atkin and Rollings, 1993). A study by Walker in 1987 also revealed that 'out of 15 Asian families caring for a child with severe learning difficulty – the mother always assumed responsibility for all aspects of care' (Atkin and Rollings, 1993). This predominantly female role was also identified by Poonia and Ward (1990), who discussed the value of such initiatives as the 'Give Mum A Break' service in Bradford or 'Contact a Family' in the London Boroughs of Lewisham and Southall. These schemes ensured that women caring for children with severe learning difficulties, who are especially vulnerable to isolation and depression, are given a 'lifeline'.

A recent report by the Foundation for People with Learning Disabilities (Towers, 2009), however, found that fathers of children with learning disabilities wanted more involvement in looking after their children but also recommended that more support was required for them to maintain their health and well-being where they were very involved in the caring role. Further information on matters relating to minority ethnic communities and people with learning disabilities can be found in the website list at the end of this chapter.

In one Case Study, Davis and Choudhury (1988) analysed an Asian family and the ways in which healthcare professionals helped them. They demonstrate how their interventions reduced the possible plight of the woman carer. However, this Asian woman's situation was made doubly stressful because she was from a different culture and was unable to communicate in the language of the caring profession.

Case study

The family lived in a fourth-floor council flat where the lift was frequently broken. This was intimidating, as is often the case in housing in inner cities. Mrs B was 45 years old and had two sons (aged 12 and 16 years) and a daughter with Down syndrome (aged 11 months) living with her. At the first meeting, Mrs B appeared bewildered, lonely, distraught and unable to cope with the problems facing her, including the recent sudden death of her husband, her daughter's Down syndrome, her own ill health, her inability to speak English, her fear of leaving the flat, her enforced separation from her other children in Bangladesh, the absence of a support system (family or friends) and her extreme poverty. (From Davis and Choudhury, 1988, p. 48.)

continued

Reflection point

Imagine that you are a member of the community team who is assigned to helping this woman. What cultural factors would you have to consider in order to establish an understanding of her situation?

Mrs B was helped over a period of 12 months, and she eventually became more independent and had started to make friends. The main source of help was a Parent Advisor Scheme set up to help the families of children with special needs (Davis and Choudhury, 1988). The scheme has trained counsellors who speak the same language as the families and can thus offer support through communication; it also involves a team of healthcare and education professionals. This planned support is based on trust and effective communication.

Poonia and Ward (1990) also highlight the fears of many parents of dependent children who may require additional care outside the home. These are especially focused on their concerns that the children's cultural needs will not be met. They cite the experience of Mr and Mrs Rafiq, who were unhappy that 'their son Nadeen was unable to pray during Ramadan as they would like when he attended a local scheme' (Poonia and Ward, 1990).

This scenario could apply to any parents from any culture, but it is clear from the literature that there is a perceived inequality in the services provided for families from minority ethnic communities (Ellahi and Hatfield, 1992; Rickford, 1992). Other studies and similar evidence can be found on the NHS Evidence – Ethnicity and Health website (see website list at the end of this chapter).

Key points

1. Caring for others is traditionally viewed in many cultures as being the role of women.
2. The status of nurses in society is very much linked to that of women.
3. The literature indicates that communication between carers and health and social care professionals has to be effective if care is to reflect multicultural needs.

CULTURAL BELIEFS AND THE NEEDS OF WOMEN

An understanding of individual and cultural beliefs about menstruation, pregnancy and childbirth, for example, can be considered essential to an understanding of women's health care in a multicultural society.

In many cultures, women who are menstruating are considered to be polluted and 'dirty'. For example, Jewish law states that while a woman has any vaginal blood loss, and for seven days after the loss ends, touch between her and her husband is forbidden (Schott and Henley, 1996). There is no contact between Orthodox Jewish couples until the woman has had no bleeding for seven clear days, at which time they go to the 'mikvah' (a special bath-house attached to the synagogue) for a ritual cleansing bath. The couple can then resume contact. This belief that women are unclean during menstruation is also found in Muslim, Hindu, Sikh and Gypsy–Traveller culture.

Muslim women are also considered to be unclean for 40 days after giving birth. During this time they do not fast, say their daily prayers or touch the Holy Qu'ran (Henley, 1982). Sexual intercourse during menstruation is strictly forbidden in all of these cultures. These beliefs could explain why many men do not touch their wives during labour (it is not because they are uncaring towards them). Japanese women do not bathe or wash their hair during menstruation, and 'there are beauticians who make sure their customers are not menstruating before they will agree to wash their hair' (Ohnuki-Tierney, 1984, p. 28).

The onset of menstruation is not only evidence that reproductive activity has started in the body but is also a symbol of having reached maturity as a woman. Helman (2007) cites a study undertaken by Skultans (1970), who found that some women in a South Wales mining village believed that menstruation and the 'monthly flow' had a positive value in terms of their health (i.e. that getting rid of 'bad' blood was a means of purging one's body). Standing (1980) also reported that many of the women in Skultan's study believed that menstrual blood was poisonous, even at the menopause, and that 'menopausal women were told not to touch red meat because it might go off or to make bread because the dough would not rise'. Gypsy Traveller women are considered impure or 'Mochadi' during both menstruation and pregnancy (Vernon, 1994). These are cross-cultural beliefs and an example illustrating this can be found in Wogeo Island, New Guinea, where any woman who is menstruating is kept in seclusion in her own hut and 'must not come into contact with people or property while she is in this condition, nor touch the food of her husband lest he die' (La Fontaine, 1985). A recent study of menstrual hygiene and management in adolescent school girls in Nepal (WaterAid, 2009) also highlighted the beliefs of the 'polluting touch' and the equally polluting potential of the 'menstrual cloth' but many of the girls were beginning to challenge the rituals surrounding menstruation. One participant offered the following explanation:

> **I grew up being told of what to do and what not to do. I know of what I am supposed to do ... but then when no one is around I do everything that I am not supposed to ... I touch water, I touch food in the kitchen, I enter every room ... I have also touched many fruit trees and none of them have wilted so I think it is not true.**

(WaterAid, 2009, p. 11)

Reflective exercise

Reflect on your own experiences of menstruation.

1. If you are a man, identify what you were told about the experience of menstruation and who told you. How has it influenced your care of women?
2. If you are a woman, identify how menstruation is viewed in your culture and how it has influenced your life.

Understanding the different cultural practices in relation to menstruation is important for any nurse, but it is essential for those working in women's healthcare. For example, to be able to offer advice to women who have had investigations for menstrual problems, knowledge of cultural beliefs and practices will be necessary in order to establish an effective nurse–patient relationship. Consider the following Case Study.

A 38-year-old woman from an Orthodox Jewish family is admitted to hospital for a hysterectomy (removal of the uterus).

You are required to discuss with her the effects of the surgery.

Points to consider
1. How may she view the fact that she will no longer menstruate?
2. Will this affect her relationship with her husband?
3. What knowledge of the Jewish religion and beliefs will be required for you to be able to discuss possible future health problems with her?
4. Consider the same scenario for women of different cultures.

If you are working in a women's healthcare ward or department, you could develop a resource pack that focuses specifically on multicultural care issues. Although this could be perceived as a 'recipe'-type approach, it remains one of the most effective ways of acquiring accessible information which can then be supported by other resources. (See Holland, 2008, for another Case Study of a Muslim woman who was admitted to hospital for a hysterectomy.)

Key points

1. Individual and cultural beliefs with regard to menstruation, pregnancy and childbirth need to be understood in order to offer women's health care that is culturally sensitive.
2. Women who are menstruating or who have given birth are considered to be 'unclean' and polluted in many cultures.
3. Many cultural practices with regard to menstruation, pregnancy and childbirth have a religious significance.

WOMEN AND THE NEED TO MAINTAIN PRIVACY AND DIGNITY

The way in which women dress can be linked to their relationship with men. For example Muslim women wear clothes that cover their whole body except for their hands. This clothing is known as chador in Iran and parts of Arabia, and consists of a long black dress or skirt and blouse and a black veil. Many of these women also wear a covering to their eyes and nose. In Pakistan, women wear a shalwar (trousers), kameez (shirt) and a long scarf (chuni or dupatta) that covers their head and their mouth and nose. When women are waiting for an X-ray, for example, the exposure of their legs and arms can be very embarrassing and upsetting. It is important that both nurses and other healthcare professionals are aware of this in order to ensure that the woman's dignity is maintained. Consider the following Case Study.

A 40-year-old married Muslim woman is admitted to an intensive-care unit (ICU) in a critical state. She is unconscious and receiving artificial ventilation. The other four patients in the unit are all men.

How would you ensure that her privacy and dignity are maintained while relatives are visiting her and the other patients?

Points to consider
1. The role of the nurse as advocate for the unconscious patient.
2. The needs of the relatives and of the healthcare team.
3. The position of women in Muslim culture.
4. The traditional dress and customs of Muslim women.

Gerrish *et al.* (1996b) highlighted the lack of respect for maintaining dignity as perceived by users of healthcare services, which in many instances was caused by a lack of cultural knowledge on the part of the healthcare professionals. One example was related by a Gujarati women's group that was interviewed during this study:

> Many women felt that there was insufficient privacy in getting changed or going for operations. One woman in hospital for suspected appendicitis had a finger thrust up her anus without explanation. She only found out later that this was a test for appendicitis. She was absolutely devastated, but the nurses just didn't seem to notice. When her husband came in later, she completely broke down (BG6).

(Gerrish et al., 1996b, p. 44)

Nurses are bound by a professional code (Nursing and Midwifery Council, 2008), which stresses the importance of respecting the dignity of patients and clients. To ensure that this happens, nurses need to be aware of the potential cultural needs of all individuals in their care. To avoid cultural misunderstandings such as the example highlighted above, the nursing team on the ward concerned could have provided patient information explaining the investigations and treatment in relation to the patient's illness in different languages. Many nursing-focused information packages for patients are now written in different languages but it is important, regardless of the language involved, to ensure that patients are able to read it. Some healthcare organizations provide the information in different formats such as audio tapes or a CD-ROM to ensure patients have the information required.

Reflective exercise

1. Identify how you currently explain to any patient or client the nature of intrusive investigations or treatments to be carried out either by yourself or by others.
2. Following this, undertake a similar exercise but focus on the culture-specific needs of those patients and clients with whom you are in most contact.
3. Determine a plan of action to ensure that your care in relation to maintaining privacy and dignity is culturally focused.

THE EFFECT OF WOMEN'S ROLE AND CULTURAL BELIEFS ON THEIR HEALTH AND HEALTH CARE

The 'low' status afforded to women in some societies is reflected in how girl and boy babies are viewed and in some parts of the world 'infanticide of female babies still persists, especially in rural areas' (Helman, 2007).

Trevelyan (1994) reported that in societies where 'there is a strong son preference' the following trends are likely:

> Girls get a smaller percentage of their food needs satisfied than boys do, and boys tend to get the more nutritious food. In one region of India, for example, girls are more than four times as likely to be malnourished as boys.

> Boys are breastfed longer. When the baby is a girl, the mother may interrupt breastfeeding to become pregnant and try for a boy.

> Boys are more often taken for medical care when they are sick and more money is spent on doctors' fees and medicine for them. According to UNICEF, for example, in one paediatric unit of a hospital in the North-West Frontier province of Pakistan in 1989, out of a total of 1233 patients, only 424 were girls.

> *(Trevelyan, 1994, p. 49)*

Explanations for this preference stem mainly from cultural and economic sources, and Trevelyan (1994) cites the work of Smyke (1991), who creates a link with this continued devaluing of women's place because they are women. Smyke (1991) believes that this: 'has a profound influence on many women's attitudes towards their own health and their bodies. They accept ill health, pain and suffering rather than finding out if there is something they could do about it' (Trevelyan, 1994, p. 50).

When women from different countries then find themselves living in Western cultures where they still adhere to such beliefs, it becomes clear why they may not use the available healthcare services.

A conflict sometimes arises between first-, second- and third-generation members of minority cultures when exposure to the 'main culture' enables women to consider alternative cultural views. Depression and suicide become common. Schreiber *et al.* (1998) highlight issues such as this in their study of how black West Indian women in Canada manage depression in a Eurocentric society. They were reluctant to seek help for their problems because of the strong stigma attached to mental illness.

One cultural practice that has had a major impact on women's health in some societies is that of female genital mutilation (FGM) (sometimes called female circumcision). According to Schott and Henley (1996) there are three types of FGM:

1. Removal of the clitoral hood – this is the only type that can correctly be called circumcision.

2. Excision of the clitoris and part or all of the labia minora (clitoridectomy).

3. Infibulation – the most extensive form of FGM in which the clitoris and the labia minora are removed and the labia majora are reduced and then stitched together, leaving a small

opening so that urine and menstrual fluid can escape. Occasionally infibulation is performed over an intact clitoris.

(Schott and Henley, 1996, p. 213)

Female genital mutilation is performed at different ages, from very young babies (e.g. in Ethiopia) to just before puberty (e.g. in West Africa). It does not appear to be an Islamic requirement, as it is not mentioned in the Qur'an (Trevelyan, 1994; Schott and Henley, 1996) and has no health benefits whatsoever. Trevelyan (1994) cites the severe immediate and long-term complications of this procedure. These include:

- **immediate complications:** severe bleeding and shock; infections; death;
- **long-term complications:** recurrent urinary tract infections; chronic pelvic infection; painful intercourse; menopausal problems;
- **complications during pregnancy and delivery:** vaginal delivery may be impossible; passing a urinary catheter is impossible.

Consider the following Case Study.

Case study

You are working on a gynaecology ward and a young Somalian woman is admitted with severe right-sided abdominal pain. The doctor suspects that it is either appendicitis or an ectopic pregnancy, but the woman has refused to be examined by him. The link worker has obtained information from her mother that she is not married and has never had a 'proper period'. She has also found out that this young woman has had problems with passing urine since she arrived in the UK as a child. She is extremely distressed and in severe pain.

Reflection points
1. What are your priorities with regard to helping this young woman?
2. What knowledge would you need to be able to identify her potential problems?
3. Examine your own beliefs and feelings if it is discovered that she has had some type of female genital mutilation procedure performed on her.

The Royal College of Nursing in the UK has produced excellent guidance for nurses (Royal College of Nursing, 2006) which will help you to understand more about this problem and how to answer these questions and more (see also the website list at the end of this chapter). The World Health Organization (WHO) has other information related to this topic (see website list at the end of this chapter).

The way in which health professionals project their own personal beliefs is crucial to the care that individuals and their families receive. Bowler (1993) undertook a small-scale ethnographic study of women's maternity experiences in a hospital in the south of England, and although it is acknowledged that this study is not representative of all midwives or nurses, it does illustrate an example of stereotyped images influencing care. She identified four main themes that stereotyped

Asian women: 'the difficulty of communication, the women's lack of compliance with care and abuse of the service, their tendency to "make a fuss about nothing" and their lack of normal maternal instinct' (Bowler, 1993, p. 160).

These stereotypes resulted in inappropriate care. Because communication was problematic, given that many of the women did not speak English, some of the midwives told Bowler (1993) that 'they were unable to have a "proper relationship" with them, and that having a "good relationship" with a mother was reported as an important part of a midwife's role'. This example could apply to any care worker relationship in which the patient or client does not speak English.

The stereotypes that emerged from the midwives' perceptions of the women's lack of compliance with care stemmed from their ideas about family planning and fertility. The fact that many of the women did have large families led the midwives to believe that they were uninterested in contraceptives, yet it was clear to Bowler (1993) that many women did use them but were embarrassed to discuss the issues, or had language or translation difficulties. However, Parsons *et al.* (1993) stated that little information was available nationally about the contraceptive practices and needs of people in minority ethnic groups.

> ### Reflective exercise
>
> 1. Imagine that you are responsible for setting up a family planning service for a multicultural community. You will be expected to offer an advisory service for both men and women.
> 2. Identify the cultural issues that will need to be taken into account if the service is to be successful.
> 3. Identify which cultural and religious groups would not use this service.

The theme that Bowler (1993) identified as 'making a fuss about nothing' is also a stereotypical image that will be familiar to some readers. When questioned by Bowler (1993) about the needs of different women, a typical response was 'Well, these Asian women you're interested in have very low pain thresholds. It can make it very difficult to care for them'. A phrase used by midwives in relation to the last theme of 'lack of maternal instinct' was that 'they're not the same as us', which was attributed in part to their 'large numbers of children and "unhealthy" preference for sons' (Bowler, 1993).

The latter issue is very significant to Muslim women, as male children are considered extremely important in Islamic culture.

This issue has already been highlighted by Trevelyan (1994), and it is important to remember that women who have just given birth to girl babies may be extremely distressed not only by the birth, but also by their fears about not giving birth to a boy.

The theme of 'lack of maternal instinct' can be seen in the following Case Study, and it also results from a lack of cultural understanding of 'bonding' practices among mothers who have just given birth.

A Vietnamese woman, after giving birth to a son, refused to cuddle him, but she willingly provided minimal care such as feeding and changing his diaper [nappy]. The nurse, feeling sorry for the baby, picked him up, cuddled him and stroked the top of his head. Both the mother and her husband became visibly upset. This apparent neglectful behaviour does not reflect poor bonding, but instead indicates a cultural belief and tradition. Many people in rural areas of Vietnam believe in spirits. They believe that these spirits are attracted to infants and are likely to steal them (by inducing death). The parents do everything possible not to attract attention to their newborn; for this reason infants are not cuddled or fussed over. This apparent lack of interest reflects an intense love and concern for the child, not neglect. Not only did the nurse attract attention to the infant, but also she touched him in a taboo area. Southeast Asians view the head as private and personal; it is seen as the seat of the soul and is not to be touched.

Reflective exercise

1. Reflect on your own experience of childbirth or that of a family member. Discuss with a colleague from another culture their experiences, and compare the two.
2. What similarities and differences were there? What were the cultural reasons, if any, for these?

Childbirth is associated with long-term health problems as well as those of an immediate nature. For example, a study conducted by Hagger in 1994 illustrates the way in which a change in cultural lifestyle has influenced patterns of health norms. There appeared to be an increase in the number of Bangladeshi women with continence problems following pregnancy and childbirth in the UK, whereas those women who had given birth to their children in Bangladesh and received traditional postnatal care often did not have these problems (Hagger, 1994). If the cultural reasons for this are examined, we can see that:

> Traditional postnatal care involves 40 days' rest, during which time relations take over domestic duties, the diet is light, there is no sexual intercourse, breastfeeding is common and compression bandages are often used – also it is usual to squat over a hole to urinate. Squatting instead of sitting on chairs, and regular swimming, also help to strengthen pelvic floor muscles.

(Hagger, 1994, p. 72)

However, in the UK few of these traditional practices can be undertaken, with the result that there is now an increasing number of Bangladeshi women with incontinence problems.

Schytt (2006), in her study on women's health after childbirth, also found similar issues with Swedish women, together with a range of other problems such as perineal pain and sexual problems.

A study by Ross *et al.* (1998) of the way in which women in rural Bangladesh view their health priorities illustrates the need for improved understanding of women's cultural healthcare needs. The study found that, despite appreciating that their health problems could become chronic if left untreated, these women were reluctant to seek early treatment. Even when they did so, it was very often the traditional healers whom they consulted initially.

One example they referred to is described in the following Case Study.

Case study

A 24-year-old Bangladeshi woman had a persistent vaginal discharge. She believed that her husband was aware of her problem as he had once bought her medicine from a chemist in the bazaar. However, it was ineffective, and her health continued to fail during her second pregnancy because of her discharge. Her second daughter is now 4 months old. Her health has been even more compromised because, with the second pregnancy, she is experiencing paddaphul (uterine prolapse). This made intercourse very difficult, 'even more so than before' (Ross *et al.*, 1998). Unfortunately, the woman's husband then left her and the children. However, the young woman continued to live with her mother-in-law.

Reflection points

1. If this young woman had been English (non-minority ethnic culture), how different would her experience have been?
2. How can the experience of this young woman be of value with regard to understanding the heath care needs of Bangladeshi women in the UK?

CONCLUSION

Being a woman in different societies has many similarities with regard to biological functions such as menstruation, pregnancy and childbirth. However, the influence of cultural beliefs on these life events ensures that they are unique not only to the individual but also to the cultural community. It is important that, when caring for women in a multicultural society, healthcare professionals are 'culturally prepared' in order to ensure that they provide non-discriminatory practice and understanding.

CHAPTER SUMMARY

1. A woman's health status has a major effect on the health and well-being of her family.
2. Women make a significant contribution to care as both professional and lay carers.
3. Menstruation, pregnancy and childbirth are 'normal' life events for women. However, the significance of each of these in different cultures will vary according to both health beliefs and religious practices.

FURTHER READING

Ahmed S (2009) *Seen and not heard: voices of young British muslims.* Policy Research Centre, Islamic Foundation, Leicester.

This report highlights the lives of young Asian men and women in Britain, and in particular their views on issues such as gender and identity.

Davies C (1995) *Gender and the professional predicament in nursing.* Open University Press, Buckingham.

This book explores the status of nursing as a profession in the context of gender and the status of women in society.

Riska E and Wegar K (1993) *Gender, work and medicine.* Sage Publications, London.

A sociological account of the division of labour in medicine and its relationship with nursing and midwifery.

Schott J and Henley A (1996) *Culture, religion and childbearing in a multiracial society.* Butterworth-Heinemann, Oxford.

This book, although published in 1996, still offers health professionals a specific insight into the major issues related to childbearing and how culture and religion impact on this experience.

WEBSITES

http://www.globalhealth.org/womens_health/

This website is the Global Health Council where there is not only information and resources about women's health internationally but also a range of other topics such as sexual and reproductive health.

http://www.harpweb.org.uk/

This website is the Health for Asylum Seekers and Refugees Portal and is a key resource site for healthcare professionals working with asylum seekers. This is an excellent site for women's health-related resources and information.

http://www.intute.ac.uk

This website includes a section on women and health and has links to a vast array of other internet sites as well as tutorials on how to use the internet for nurses and midwives.

http://www.learningdisabilities.org.uk/

For information on matters relating to minority ethnic communities and people with learning disabilities.

http://www.lgfl.net/lgfl/leas/tower.../JG%20Guidebook%202.pdf

This website links to a guide for healthcare staff and other professionals to help them understand more about the Gypsy/Traveller/Roma culture.

http://www.library.nhs.uk/ETHNICITY/ViewResource.aspx?resID=296479

This is the NHS Evidence – Ethnicity and Health website and hosts resources and links to articles, reports and related websites.

http://www.nspcc.org.uk/Inform/.../ICantTellFullReport_wdf57889.pdf

This is the direct web-link to a report by the report: 'I can't tell people what is happening at home', Domestic abuse within South Asian communities: the specific needs of women, children and young people' (Izzidien, 2008).

http://www.rcn.org.uk

The Royal College of Nursing has produced excellent guidance for nurses on genital mutilation which will help you to understand more about this subject.

http://www.who.int/mediacentre/factsheets/fs241/en/

World Health Organization information related to female genital mutilation.

8 Men and health care in a multicultural society

Karen Holland

INTRODUCTION

Men's healthcare is acknowledged as being equal in importance to women's (see Chapter 7), and while in the past the impact of men's health problems may not have been as apparent, in today's society this is no longer the case. Men in many cultures, for example, are more involved in child care and in many instances women have taken over the man's traditional role as the main breadwinner in the family. At the same time there has also been an increase in the number of men entering nursing and other healthcare professions, although nursing in the main remains a female-dominated profession.

> **This chapter will focus on issues in men's health care in a multicultural society:**
>
> - the role of men in society;
> - men as carers in society;
> - men in nursing;
> - the effects of men's role and cultural beliefs on their health and health care.

THE ROLE OF MEN IN SOCIETY

The society or country that you live in will have an effect on the role that men have, and considering that for many of us society is now multicultural, it is important that we do not take an ethnocentric view of this role. Traditionally, in the UK, the main role for men in society was that of the main provider or 'breadwinner', being responsible for earning the main income to support his family. Although this has altered owing to economic and political change, resulting in male unemployment for many, there still remains in many families the traditional scenario of men going out to work and women staying home to look after the children. This view in the 1990s was the cause of 'a great deal of discussion, debate and reflection on what it meant to be a 'man' in the modern world and how this might influence health practices' (Robertson and Williamson, 2005). Robertson and Williamson (2005) concluded that it was not just being men that accounted for differences in 'men's health outcomes and practices' but that 'other aspects of identity, such as sexuality, disability, ethnicity and social class' were just as important 'if not more so'.

Men are socialized in many cultures to be masculine with expectations of behaviour associated with that status. According to White (2002) this issue of 'masculinity' is central to the discussion of the current state of men's health and 'we need to consider the variety of ways in which masculinity is constructed in the course of day to day living'. Basically, he states that this is considered in terms of specific behaviours, whereby :

> ... men are meant to be stoical, unemotional, rational, virile, independent, sexually active and physically strong (as indications of their dominant social position and role) while women are presented as essentially fragile, emotional, irrational, dependent, sexually submissive and physically weak (and hence suited to their socially sub-ordinate position and role in society).

(White 2002, p. 274)

Reflective exercise

Consider this explanation and how you view men and women in these terms. Are there any circumstances where you have seen this stereotype of men and women? Consider situations where the opposite has been the case.

For certain cultures these kinds of specific behaviours are more anticipated than others and this will have an impact, as we will see later, on how nurses and healthcare professionals engage with men in relation to their health behaviours and practices, as well as how they relate to the women in their lives (see Chapter 7).

So how are men viewed in different societies? Rather than single out specific cultures in relation to the division between men and women, the differences will be illustrated throughout each section of this chapter as appropriate. The role of men in most societies is inextricably linked with their health-related behaviours and practices as well as how men view the health professions as possible employment opportunities. In most societies there is a division of labour between men and women in looking after children, working and the organization of family structures. In addition, there are cultures where men or women undertake both traditional roles in same-sex relationships, and in many developed countries this has had a major effect on many aspects of the health of men and women.

Despite the Civil Partnership Act 2004 (Her Majesty's Stationery Office, 2004) in the UK where significant changes were made with regard to legal responsibilities of partners, for example State Pension entitlement, there remain areas of confusion in decisions about health issues. Ensuring being named as next of kin if a person is ill is one area where there is a change, and King and Bartlett (2006) pointed out that the discriminatory use of the term 'nearest relative' in current mental health law was also being addressed in the new Mental Health Act in the UK, important in decision-making regarding the detention of individuals. King and Bartlett (2006) indicate that same-sex civil partnerships may also have a positive benefit on health through increasing stability in relationships and lessening contact with multiple partners with its associated risk of sexual infections. They also note that as 'same sex unions constitute a new social form, which poses challenges for health staff', training may be required to enable staff to work effectively, especially, one assumes, in relation to the rights of partners in decision-making.

Consider your own family structure.
1. What role do (or did) your parents undertake?
2. Was it any different from any of your friends and if yes in what way?
3. Who undertook the main employment role and how did that affect responsibilities for care roles?
4. Discuss with others their experiences and how understanding about various ways of living helps you to undertake your care role.
5. Read the following paragraphs and consider whether any of the issues raised were also found in your families.

Henley (1982) noted that in Muslim culture the family was central and that the man, especially a son, is 'considered responsible for the care and support of their parents as they grow older' and that 'when a son marries he and his wife often remain with his parents and bring up their children there'. Although shared decision-making might occur within the home, 'in most matters outside the home a Muslim woman should always be under the protection and guardianship of a man: her father, her husband or her sons, if she is a widow'(Henley, 1982). This role requires understanding by the nurse, especially if a Muslim woman has to be admitted to hospital or visit her GP, as she may be seen to defer to her husband at all times. Consider the following scenario described by Galanti (2008).

Case study

A 19-year-old Saudi Arabian woman named Sheida Nazih had just given birth. Her husband, Abdul, had been away on business during most of their 10-month marriage but brought her to the United States to have their baby. He moved into the hospital room with Sheida immediately after she gave birth. He kept the door to their room shut and questioned everyone who entered, including the nurses. The nurses were not happy with this procedure but felt they had no choice except to comply. Although Sheida could speak some English, the only time she would speak directly to the nurses was when Abdul was out of the room. Otherwise, he answered all questions addressed to her. He also decided when she would eat and bathe. As leader of the family, Abdul felt it was his role to act as intermediary between his wife and the world.

Although this scenario took place in another country with a different healthcare system (USA), it gives us an insight into the perceived role of the man in an Islamic country with regard to his responsibility to his wife. It is important to recognize this as a possibility rather than consider that the man does not wish his wife to talk to the nurses about their relationship or home life. Galanti (2008) described another scenario where the husband was clearly abusing the wife, and that not letting her speak was a possible indication of not wishing the medical and nursing staff to find out. She cautions that 'health care providers should not jump to unwarranted conclusions based on that evidence alone' (Galanti, 2008).

Men's role in childbirth and child care is also an important area of family life where cultural differences predominate. However, even in cultures where traditionally it is seen as the man's role to earn income to provide for the family, there are some notable changes when it comes to helping with child care. A study by Turan *et al.* (2001) of men's involvement in perinatal health in Katamandu found that new fathers were now playing a more significant role in their child care than was traditionally the case. However it remained the woman's role to undertake the housework as seen in this narrative:

> now that we have a child, I take care of the baby when I come home from work so that my wife can easily do her housework ... there is a little bit more sharing than before.
>
> *(new father, Turan* et al. *2001, p. 116)*

Social stigma in relation to helping their wives was identified in a study of Nepalese husbands' involvement in maternal health (Mullany, 2006), where husbands who did help their wives were made fun of by others in their community:

> I know society criticizes me when I carry the water container and let my wife walk empty handed or let her stay in bed. When I bring my vegetables and help my wife my community makes fun of me saying that I work for a woman.
>
> *(a 24 year old service industry worker, Mullany, 2006, p. 2801)*

This same study raised many other issues which have an impact on men's role in perinatal health, and concluded that it was important to differentiate between situations where women required or expected the help of their husbands in communicating with health professionals as part of a loving relationship and that of men opting out of sharing as they considered it to be a woman's role. Hoga *et al.* (2001) used Leininger's theory of Culture Care Diversity and Universality (Leininger, 1991) to recommend to nurses how to integrate 'men's worldview of reproductive health values and lifeways' into care.

Leininger (1991) proposed three different kinds of action to guide decisions by nurses: cultural care preservation or maintenance, accommodation or negotiation and repatterning (or restructuring). In relation to preservation, Hoga *et al.* (2001) recommended that nurses ensure that they take account of the man's views and beliefs about reproductive health care practices and not to 'assume an ethnocentric view'. They suggested that care of the women should 'target increased male participation' (cultural care accommodation) and offered the example of 'extending hours of home care services to accommodate men's work schedule'. In relation to repatterning of reproductive health practices they suggested that men, once educated themselves, should be encouraged to be involved in 'teaching other men about sexuality and sex education' to alleviate the 'myths about vasectomy, condom use, and STD [sexually transmitted disease] and HIV/AIDS transmission'. The education of men in relation to their role in society, concerning women generally and wives in particular, was also the focus of a successful programme on men's sexual and reproductive health in Northern Namibia (Mufune, 2009), leading to a change in many of the men's views of their wives 'not simply as appendages of their husbands[,] and that women are not quite as inferior as their culture had taught them to believe'.

MEN AS CARERS IN SOCIETY

Men can be occupied in caring for others within their own families or others (informal or lay carer), or in professions which care for others in a formal way, such as a nurse or physiotherapist. According to Arber and Gilbert (1989) 'men make a larger contribution to caring than is often recognised' and this is borne out in the 2001 Census data (see Box 8.1).

Box 8.1 Carers UK – Policy Briefing (January 2009)

The 2001 Census shows that women are more likely to be carers than men. Across the UK there are 3 400 000 female carers (58 per cent of carers) and 2 460 000 male carers (42 per cent).

Women have a 50:50 chance of providing care by the time they are 59 years old compared with men who have the same chance by the time they are 75 years old. Women are more likely to give up work in order to care (It could be you, Carers UK, 2000).

Caring varies between ethnic groups. Bangladeshi and Pakistani men and women are three times more likely to provide care compared with their white British counterparts (Who cares wins, statistical analysis of the Census, Carers UK, 2001).

Although this Census reports that there are more women than men carers, there is still a significant number of men carers. A reason given by Arber and Gilbert (1989) for the increase was that there was an increasing number of men looking after elderly spouses or parents who may be severely disabled in some way. They did not focus on any particular ethnic group. A report published by the Afyia Trust for National Black Carers and Carers Workers Network (2008) highlights the distinct lack of 'baseline data available regarding the numbers, role and experiences of carers within black and minority ethnic communities'. The Afyia Trust also offers an excellent guide for people working with black carers (National Black Carers Network, 2002).

Reflective exercise

If you are a student nurse, how many male carers have you met during your clinical placements in a community setting? What was their role as carer? Were any of them child carers (i.e. caring for children)?

The 2001 Census figures noted that there were 174 995 young people under the age of 18 years who provide care and 13 029 of these were providing care for 50 hours or more per week (Carers UK, 2009). Doran *et al.* (2003) conducted an analysis of some of this data to determine issues of carers' well-being. They found that many 'children and pensioners were not in good health themselves' and considered that this was of some concern.

If there has been an increase in the number of men caring in the community, has there been a parallel increase in men becoming professional carers in occupations such as nursing?

MEN IN NURSING

Whittock and Leonard (2003) point out that despite the historical position of men in nursing in the UK that 'numbers of registered male nurses have seldom exceeded 10 per cent of the total'. In a UK Parliament (House of Commons) question time, the issue was raised of men entering the nursing profession as a career. A response from the Secretary of State for Health noted that there had in fact been an increase between 2004 and 2006 (see Table 8.1). Whittock and Leonard (2003) provided preliminary evidence of key themes as to why men chose nursing as a career, such as influence of family members who were in the same career and having 'experienced some form of caring situation, usually in a family capacity', but concluded that careers advice was lacking for young men with regard to nursing. The NHS Careers website (see website list at the end of this chapter) has three life stories of men in nursing and reflects the drive to encourage more men to make nursing a career. Duffin (2009), in a recent opinion-seeking paper on the benefit of male nurses to the profession, found that there were still concerns by some organizations, The Patients Association being one, and cite the director of that organization as saying that:

> **Many older female patients would feel vulnerable and uncomfortable if there were only male nurses on a ward, especially if there were gynaecological issues.**
>
> *(Duffin, 2009, p. 13)*

This comment is also reflective of cultural concerns generally in relation to being cared for by both male and female nurses when sensitive issues need to be discussed. However, in support of more men in nursing he stated that the union Unite had recently 'submitted evidence to the Prime Minister's Commission on the Future of Nursing and Midwifery drawing on the under-representation of men in the profession' and that it hoped that 'the Commission will suggest that the image of men in nursing needs a boost when it reports its findings next year' (Duffin, 2009).

Entwistle (2004) explored the place of men within nursing in New Zealand and among his conclusions was the fact that 'men who choose nursing as a career risk challenging the traditional roles of their gender stereotype'. Loughrey (2008) also considered gender issues in his study in Ireland, which was aimed at obtaining data to help recruit more men into the nursing profession. Although it was a small study it did indicate that there was more of a tendency towards traits considered as female in the men but 'considering that gender is strongly influenced by culture' deemed it important to undertake further study into men in caring roles in order to influence future policy. A study carried out in Israel (Romem and Anson, 2005) to determine why men choose nursing as a profession found that 'it seems that nursing appeals more to men who do not

Table 8.1 Qualified Nursing, Midwifery and Health-Visiting staff – broken down by gender

2006				Percentage	
	Male	Female	Unknown	Male	Female
All qualified nursing, midwifery and health visiting staff	38 242	304 942	31 354	11.1	88.9
Nurse consultant	136	654	—	17.2	82.8
Modern matron	204	1 767	11	10.4	89.6
Manager	1 303	5 707	148	18.6	81.4
Registered nurse – children	531	11 710	955	4.3	95.7
Registered midwife	176	22 937	1356	0.8	99.2
Health visitor	176	11 507	351	1.5	98.5
District nurse (1st level)	418	9 239	351	4.3	95.7
District nurse (2nd level)	65	1 101	96	5.6	94.4
School nurse	9	1 100	20	0.8	99.2
Other 1st level	34 283	229 596	26 690	13.0	87.0
Other 2nd level	921	9 279	1 375	9.0	91.0

Table from Hansard (House of Commons Daily Debates) 21 May 2007 (Written Answers – Health – Nurses) See website list for source url. (Reproduced with permission from the Office of Public Sector Information 2009: www.opsi.gov.uk.)

belong to the mainstream of the Israeli society, i.e. immigrants and ethnic minorities'. They concluded that because these two groups found challenges and difficulties in 'the educational system and labour market' that the 'nursing profession enables them to obtain an academic degree which is highly regarded in Israeli society, ensures steady job opportunities and steady income'.

The theme of 'guarantee of work' was also predominant in a study of Turkish male nursing students (Kulakac *et al.*, 2009), as was the fact that in Turkish culture caring was traditionally a woman's role.

Objections to male nurses caring for women patients together with perceptions by others that male nurses must be homosexual (Evans, 2002; Kulakac *et al.*, 2009) are two other areas that are predominant in the literature on men in nursing. Kulakac *et al.* (2009) found that some of the male student nurse participants in their study 'indicated that they would reject a male nurse who would attempt to care for their female relatives', and that this objection, as in Evans' (2002) study, was based on the fact that they considered male touch to carry sexual connotation when applied to women. Keogh and Gleeson (2006) in their study on male and female student nurses found that this was a major concern in caring for both adult and mental health patients. They offer examples of the students' concerns:

> Obviously the big thing that I am highly aware is the gender of the patient ... I steer clear of female patients because I am just very aware of allegations ... it's just something that I am very uncomfortable if I am left on my own with a female patient (RPN 3).

It makes no difference because anything, a touch, can be interpreted in the wrong way so I would always have someone with me ... and I'll be very careful of that because in this day and age you just have to watch yourself (RGN 2).

(Keogh and Gleeson, 2006. p. 173)

Inoue *et al.* (2006) also found that 'providing intimate care for women clients was a challenging experience for male nurses' and concluded that 'nurse educators should assist male nurses to be better prepared to interact with women clients in various settings'.

Given the worldwide need for an increase in the number of nurses in the future, owing mainly to the ageing workforce, there are already indications of increases in the number of male nurses internationally. It is, however, important to consider the effect of this on the nature of caring interventions they may be required to undertake and the possible educational implications for nursing curricula in the future.

Reflective exercise

1. Consider the issues raised in this section on men in nursing. What have your experiences been during clinical placements?
2. If you are a male student nurse, which field of practice (branch) are you undertaking and why did you choose that one? How do you think your chosen field of practice is portrayed in the media or literature?
3. If you are a female student nurse, answer the same questions, then discuss with your male nurse colleagues their experiences of being a male nurse caring for female and male patients.

Key points

1. There has been an increase in the number of men in caring roles within the community in the UK.
2. The number of men choosing to register as qualified nurses has more or less remained around 10 per cent of the total nursing population in the UK.
3. Although men are still choosing nursing as a career there remains a need to keep promoting it as a career for men worldwide.

THE EFFECTS OF MEN'S ROLE AND CULTURAL BELIEFS ON THEIR HEALTH AND HEALTH CARE

It is recognized that in many countries the life expectancy of men is lower than that of women (Sun and Liu, 2007; Nuttall, 2008; Men's Health Forum, 2009) and the reasons for this are varied. White and Cash (2003) noted that there were differences between countries in Europe 'in the impact of the various health issues on their male population'. This is an important point as it indicates that there are national and regional variations to be considered as well as those related directly to the issue of 'being male' or individual cultural beliefs. The environment is one such variable which could have an impact on men's health, as is evident when considering the rate of suicide in men living in Finland – 4 per cent of all male deaths as opposed to 0.6 per cent in Greece (White and Cash, 2003). This link between suicide and seasonal variations has been reported in many international studies and Bjorksten *et al.* (2005) found that most suicides in West Greenland were men. They considered a link to the long periods of daily sunlight in the summer months which affected mood and violent tendencies, which manifested in the way the men committed suicide.

Men's health and health care has in the past reflected the gender variations in life expectancy, with more focus on women rather than men. However, this is now changing and, in the UK, organizations such as the Men's Health Forum have made a significant step towards having the health needs of men of all cultures taken seriously by the Department of Health.

White (2001), who is also the world's first professor of men's health, made the following key points in relation to men's response to illness:

1. Men do not manage their health well and solutions need to be found to redress the current inequality in health.

2. Most men do not see their bodies as having problems and may need to be persuaded to visit the doctor when something does go wrong.

3. Health services are perceived as being less accessible to men and simply visiting the health centre may involve negotiating time off work.

4. By making services more male-friendly and accessible, men are more likely to seek advice and take an active role in managing their health.

(White, 2001, p. 18)

Reflective exercise

From your experience how true are these statements in 2009? Consider what additional health services are available for men specifically where you live and the kinds of information available. Discuss and share your findings with colleagues.

An excellent article to obtain some up-to-date information on the above points is that by the Men's Health Forum in the UK (see website at the end of this chapter), which is a policy briefing paper prepared for National Men's Health Week 2009. In this paper they offer numerous facts and figures with regard to men's health problems, men's use of services, why men do not seek help and where services for men are up to in terms of additional provision for men. These are considered briefly (in the report) in relation to men generally.

MEN'S HEALTH PROBLEMS AND SEEKING HELP

There are many health problems that both men and women experience but for men their incidence may be higher or the outcome very different. Men also respond to illness differently.

Sun and Liu (2007) discuss problems that Chinese men experience in relation to sexual health. In particular, they discuss the issue of erectile dysfunction and the fact that although it is common, it is under-treated. They note that for Chinese men to ask for medical help is to 'lose face' or 'being undignified', especially as the issue of sex for many Chinese people generally is 'considered dirty or abusive and the majority of ordinary people are unable to express their own sexual feelings or evaluate their sexual behaviours'.

They also note that many men with this health issue suffer from additional problems, such as diabetes or heart problems, which are associated with erectile dysfunction. Another major male health problem in China, as in other countries, is prostate cancer which 'is the fourth most common cancer in men in the world' (Sun and Liu, 2007).

Halbert *et al.* (2009) explored the reactions of African-American and white men to being told they had prostate cancer, and in particular whether their cultural beliefs and values made a difference. They did not find any significant difference between the two groups in terms of these issues but concluded that their coping mechanisms for the stress associated with the diagnosis were more likely to be related to their being men generally. Cultural differences in men of different ethnic origin were also the focus of a study by Hjelm *et al.* (2005) where they considered beliefs about health and diabetes in Sweden. The participants were mainly Arab, former Yugoslavian and Swedish men and all had a diagnosis of diabetes. Beliefs about health were found to vary and were clearly linked to issues of men's role in the family, as discussed earlier. For example:

> Swedish men stated the importance of a healthy lifestyle, with what they considered to be healthy food (low in fat and rich in fibre) and exercise. Non-Swedish men talked about the importance of employment to avoid mental strain: "having a job is very important. It affects your general well-being. It affects the relationship between man and woman". They described their frustration about being unemployed and not being able to have the "natural" role of breadwinner; this often led to conflicts within the family and thus increased blood sugar levels.
>
> *(Hjelm* et al., *2005, p. 51)*

Health problems experienced in the UK by men from different cultural backgrounds can be seen in Box 8.2.

Box 8.2 Men's Health Forum (accessed September 28, 2009)

The 1999 Health Survey for England found that:

- Higher rates of ischaemic heart disease (angina and heart attack) were reported by Indian, Bangladeshi and Irish men and higher rates of stroke by black Caribbean, Bangladeshi and Indian men (all compared with the general population).
- Higher rates of diabetes were reported by men from all the minority ethnic groups.
- Men from the South Asian and Chinese communities were less likely to be obese while Irish men were more likely to be obese.
- Bangladeshi men were nearly twice as likely to smoke as men in the general population; smoking rates were also higher among Irish and black Caribbean men. Chinese men were less likely to smoke than men in general.
- All minority ethnic groups consumed less alcohol than the general population except for Irish men.

Hjelm *et al.* (2005) also reported on men's beliefs about illness and how some of them even saw it as 'the will of God' (Arab men). Issues around sexual function were also considered, with the younger men of all cultures concerned about their sexual capability.

It is important for nurses and health professionals to take account of these views in order to help men manage their diabetes.

Case study

A 45-year-old Muslim man, married with three children, has diagnosed diabetes. He has been taking insulin for 20 years. He has come for a reassessment of his health needs and a note from his GP to the diabetes specialist nurse states that he has been to see the GP with regard to some erectile dysfunction problems.

Reflective exercise

You meet the man for the first time at the Diabetes Clinic where you are undertaking a 2-day clinical placement experience. What would be the key questions the nurse would ask him during the initial assessment of his needs for long-term care?

Using an assessment tool such as that based on Roper, Logan and Tierney's model of care (Holland *et al.*, 2008) may be helpful in terms of gaining an holistic picture of his healthcare needs. In particular would be the activities of living related to sexuality and eating and drinking. Use the other chapters in this book to assist in this exercise as well as the information in this chapter. An excellent website to help you is that of Diabetes UK at http://www.diabetes.org.uk/Guide-to-diabetes/Living_with_diabetes/Sex-and-diabetes/

You could make this kind of learning exercise part of a wider project during your course of study, such as developing a teaching/information package for men of different cultures who have diabetes – explaining about their illness, their future health behaviours, what they can do during periods of fasting during Ramadan and how to manage any additional health problems that may arise, such as impotency.

1. In many countries the life expectancy of men is lower than that of women and reasons for this vary.
2. The specific health needs of men are becoming more important on the health care agenda in different countries of the world.
3. Men respond to ill-health differently to women.

MEN'S HEALTH-RISK BEHAVIOURS AND THE USE OF HEALTH SERVICES

Galdas *et al.* (2005) in an extensive literature review on men and health help-seeking behaviour found that there was much inconsistency in the international evidence and that there was more than the issue of gender in why men do not seek help if ill. These other issues were: 'occupation, socioeconomic status and age'. They believed, however, that if nurses were to play a significant part in addressing the reasons men did not seek help, it was important that their practice should be 'informed by an understanding of men's beliefs, values and reactions to health services and ill-health'.

The attitudes of men towards health do, according to Peate (2004), have an effect on nursing care. In particular is the need for nurses and other healthcare professionals to understand the risk-taking behaviours associated with men's health problems in order to be able to offer advice on discharge home from hospital, or as part of health-promotion activities generally. These were linked to 'traditional masculine norms' and included:

- increased alcohol consumption;
- increased sexual risk-taking;
- a need to deal with problems alone;
- a reluctance to access health services.

(Nuttall, 2008, p. 540)

However, some of these do not apply to all cultural groups. Substance abuse in the form of increased alcohol consumption is one such health-risk behaviour that the majority of religious Muslim men would not consider. A study by Bradby (2007) explored how young British Asians (men and women) experience identity and substance abuse. In relation to drinking and identity she notes that:

Respectable Asian women did not drink, as a woman thought to be a drinker was dishonoured and her morality called into question. Taking alcohol would amount to forfeiting one's claim to being Muslim: for non-Muslim men, however, there was greater leeway to experiment with alcohol without jeopardizing a religious or ethnic identity. Providing Sikh and Hindu men did not indulge in the regular, sustained drinking associated with the ethnic majority, occasional and discreet celebratory drinks supported a worldly, manly image. Teetotal Sikh men demonstrated their religious devotion and a principled masculine strength.

(Bradby, 2007, p. 663)

It is interesting to note that smoking as a risk-taking behaviour elicited a very different response and that smoking was more tolerated by Asian groups in her study. She notes that:

> **"Smoking is bad, but at least it's not drink" was the Muslims' explanation of their elders' tolerance of cigarettes and non-Muslims said "Muslims smoke because they can't drink" ... Adult Muslim men hid their drinking but not their smoking because "smoking is not intoxicating" "it doesn't do anything to your mind ... you're still in control" so you do not lose sight of God's laws. However, a religious obligation to guard one's health and to steward one's finances was acknowledged to mean that ideally Muslims should avoid cigarettes as well as alcohol.**

> *(Bradby, 2007, p. 664)*

There are many other health problems that affect men specifically, in particular testicular cancer. It is noted, however, that this type of cancer is more common in white men rather than African-Caribbean or Asian men (Cancer Information+: see the website list at the end of this chapter). Regardless of the nature of health problems affecting men in particular (i.e. gender specific), most other health problems are non-gender specific but when affecting men they need to be addressed as such. A recent report by the European Men's Health Forum (Wilkins and Savoye, 2009), which considered men's health in 11 countries, highlighted this issue of men's health as related to male-specific actions and used this definition for a men's health issue:

> **A male health issue is one that arises from physiological, psychological, social, cultural or environmental factors that have a specific impact on boys or men and/or necessitates male-specific actions to achieve improvements in health or well-being at either individual or population level.**

> *(Wilkins and Savoye, 2009, p. 9)*

This makes an important distinction for those creating health policies but also for nurses and other health professionals who need to consider its meaning when developing any local services or care practices. The report states that it is about ensuring that services will need to be male-specific and not part of a wider 'men and women approach'. The definition above is clear about the fact that men's health is not just about the biological differences but also cultural and social differences, taking account of various health beliefs and the issues of masculinity that were discussed earlier in the chapter (Wilkins and Savoye, 2009). This is highlighted very well in Peate and Richens' (2006) paper on being a male refugee or asylum seeker (see Chapter 11), not only who have to contend with a new culture but also the impact of why they have arrived in another country. This is often as a result of war or persecution and may also have resulted in their losing their families. If one considers that in most societies the man is seen as the provider for the family, the possible traumatic loss of their family structure could lead to feelings of isolation and psychological stress. This is not to belittle similar events for women, but using the definition for male health issue it is clear that for health professionals in contact with men who are in these circumstances, a male-specific action would be essential to their self-respect and self-esteem.

CONCLUSION

Being a man in any society is influenced by cultural and religious beliefs but also, and most importantly, the way in which men relate to each other and to women generally. In this chapter we have tried to establish the basic principles and current evidence in relation to men's health in a multicultural society but realize that we could have written a whole book on this subject alone. The work being undertaken by the Men's Health Forum in the UK and Europe has begun to raise the agenda of men's health internationally. It is clear, however, that although there is more nursing and health-professional care practice evidence in relation to men and men's health generally, how to engage with the cultural aspects of men's health care in practice is not as evident. This is an area for further development if men's health is to achieve the importance it deserves at the point of contact with healthcare services.

> ## CHAPTER SUMMARY
>
> 1. The role of men in any society has an effect on their health behaviour and that of their families.
> 2. Men's health is influenced not only by their biological and physiological attributes but also their cultural background and religious beliefs.
> 3. Men are less likely than women to seek help in relation to their health and some groups such as asylum seekers and refugees are particularly at risk of not doing so.

FURTHER READING

Wilkins D and Savoye E (2009) *Men's health around the world: a review of policy and progress in 11 countries.* European Men's Health Forum, Brussels.

Wilkins D, Payne S, Granville G and Branney PL (2008) *The gender and access to health services study.* Men's Health Forum and University of Bristol, Department of Health, London: http://www.dh.gov.uk/en/Publicationsandstatistics/Publications/PublicationsPolicyAndGuidance/DH_092042 (accessed October 11 2009).

Harrison T and Dignan K (1999) *Men's health: An introduction for nurses and health professionals.* Churchill Livingstone, Edinburgh.

WEBSITES

http://afiyatrust.org.uk
    This is the website of the Afiya Trust which has as its aim 'Reducing inequalities in health and social care for racialized groups'.

http://www.cancerinfoplus.scot.nhs.uk
    Cancer Information+ website.

http://www.carersuk.org/Home

This website offers information for both carers and professionals with regard to support and training opportunities together with a range of resources.

http://www.emhf.org

This is the European Men's Health Forum website with a number of international focused reports and resources related to men's health and well-being.

http://www.equalityhumanrights.com/

This is the Commission for Equality and Human Rights website, which replaced some other organizations such as the Equal Opportunities Commission. There is useful information on men and caring roles and ethnicity.

http://www.in-practice.org/sexualhealth/index.php

This website offers an introduction to sexual health matters for nurses and healthcare workers, including a paper on ethnic and cultural differences in sexual health needs.

http://www.menshealthforum.org.uk

This website has factsheets and resources on all aspects of men's health.

http://www.nhscareers.nhs.uk/nursing.shtml#

The NHS Careers website. This has three life stories of men in nursing and reflects the drive to encourage more men to make nursing a career.

http://www.publications.parliament.uk/pa/cm200607/cmhansrd/cm070521/ text/70521w0023.htm#07052133000102

This is the Parliamentary website for the Hansard debate on men in nursing.

http://www.harpweb.org.uk/

This is the Health for Asylum Seekers and Refugees Portal and is a key resource site for healthcare professionals working with asylum seekers. This is an excellent site for men's health-related resources and information.

9 Child and family centred care: a cultural perspective

Christine Hogg

INTRODUCTION

From the day we are born, culture plays a part in our lives. Consider the following ritual in Islam:

> A Muslim welcomes a new baby into the ummah as soon as it is born, by whispering the call to prayer (the adhan, beginning 'Allahu Akbar!') into the baby's right ear, and the command to rise and worship (the iqamah) in its left ear, sometimes using a hollow reed or tube. Thus the word 'God' is the first word a baby hears.

(Maqsood, 1994, p. 173)

Cultural practices and cultural influences are already at work before a mother holds her baby. In Islam, it is decreed that the first sound children hear should be from a Muslim. This is in order that they should be introduced to the faith as soon as possible.

This chapter will consider the following issues:
• culture and the family;
• child-rearing practices across cultures;
• language and communication;
• patterns of illness and disease;
• good practices when caring for children.

In all societies, birth is accompanied by ritualistic practices that are influenced by culture. In the UK, most babies are born in hospital with the partner present as well as the midwife or doctor, who assists in the birth process. It is common practice for a woman to be discharged home (whatever her circumstances) soon after the birth. This may be within a matter of hours if she has had a normal delivery, and within a few more days if she has had a complicated birth with or without a Caesarean section. In her observations and study of a village in Iran, Kendall (1978) made the following observations of childbirth rituals:

> A woman in labour frequently cries that she is dying and she is urged to call upon Ali [Allah] for help. During delivery she kneels on a pile of old rags supported by female relatives on either

side ... When the baby comes out it is lifted to the rear of the kneeling mother, wrapped in old clean cloths and kept on the floor until the placenta is delivered.

(Kendall, 1978, p. 404)

Our introduction to the world is surrounded by customs and rituals. When a Hindu baby is born, a member of the family may write 'OM' (a mystical sound which represents the supreme spirit) on the baby's tongue with honey or ghee.

Cultural beliefs form the basis and foundations of people's lives. This premise is stressed by Dobson (1991), quoting Mead (1953):

Culture encompasses the overarching institutions in society and the small intimate habits of daily life, such as the way of preparing food or hushing a baby to sleep.

(Mead, 1953, p. 10)

Cultural practices and customs are subtle and are often taken for granted, and we may be unaware that they are unique to our culture. As Mead stresses, they are apparent in the small intimate habits, so simple but universal tasks such as hushing a baby to sleep may be undertaken in many different ways.

We assimilate cultural beliefs and attitudes as babies and children. Children are therefore continually learning and assimilating culture. The games they play, the food they eat, and the care and explanations that they are given when they are ill are all culturally determined. Cultural norms and values are a central part of a child's life, wherever they live. Thus, when a child is admitted to hospital, it may be the first time that they have encountered another culture, and they may therefore find the experience daunting and bewildering.

Children learn their beliefs about health and illness first from their family and later from their peers. Thus perceptions about health care should always be considered within the context of the family group. However, families do not live in isolation from external influences and sources of information. There are other significant influences, such as social and economic factors, that may play a large part in the development and health of a child, and it is imperative that these are borne in mind when we consider the health of the child as a whole.

CULTURE AND THE FAMILY

The family is a central issue when considering the health of a child, but even more so when the child is of a different culture from the majority population. Each of us has different ideas and beliefs about family life and family norms: for example, the size they should be, how to behave with other family members, and indeed what actually constitutes a family. In the UK in the twenty-first century the stereotype of a 'normal family' is a group of people 'tied with emotional bond, enjoying a high degree of domestic privacy occupied with the rearing of children' (Giddens, 1997).

This scenario is often reflected in advertisements on the television. In reality, the family may take on many different forms in our society, not least the single parent, black, gay or lesbian, extended, and so on (Schott and Henley, 1996).

The rights and responsibilities in families – who makes decisions and who undertakes certain roles (e.g. child-rearing) – will vary in different classes and cultures (Swanwick, 1996).

Mares *et al.* (1994) emphasize that the way in which the Western nuclear family is organized is only one of many possible ways. There is no such thing as a 'typical UK family', and all families are different. However, there are some common features to family life in the UK. These are also features of the nuclear family.

In the nuclear family, parents share responsibility for their children. In general, couples are financially and emotionally independent from their parents, although they may have frequent contact and live in close proximity to their extended family. In the nuclear family, home is regarded as a base and a place of independence. This reflects the Western notion of the value of the individual. For example, child-rearing practices in Western cultures encourage independence. Children are taught to 'think for themselves', and personal autonomy and independence are highly valued. These values also pervade our health belief systems. For example, we promote health education and encourage people to take responsibility for their own health.

Reflective exercise

1. Who are the members of your family?
2. Describe your family and the relationships you have with them.
3. How often do you have contact with them?
4. Who makes the decisions in your family, and why?

A study by Lau in 1984 explored the concept of family among 'Eastern' and 'Western' families. Her findings demonstrate that the indigenous white population in the UK values the individual as the most important unit, and that it rates self-sufficiency, personal autonomy and independence highly. A study by Stopes-Roe and Cochrane (1989) compared Asian people's attitudes to family values with those of indigenous white people in the UK. The study revealed that the Asian parents value conformity more and self-direction less than the white UK respondents. The conformist qualities included obedience and gender-appropriate behaviour.

Some minority communities (e.g. South Asian and traditional Chinese) find the pursuit of independence to be disrespectful and shocking. It may be misinterpreted as undesirable, selfish or a sign of coldness by the family, and a threat to traditional values and beliefs. Kakar (1982) explains the distinction between the Western concept of 'individual', meaning indivisible and pertaining to a person's homogeneous being, and the Eastern concept of 'dividual', where a person derives their own personal nature through interpersonal relationships and harmonious balance with the environment.

However, indigenous health workers may be tempted to encourage and praise people who appear to 'Westernize' themselves. We have remarked on the comment 'Oh, she's OK, she's learnt to be free, to stand up for herself, she's more like us'. However, culture is dynamic, it will change and people will become acculturated as they adapt (Helman, 2007). Yet, to expect people to become free and independent thinkers may cause great anguish not only among their elders but also among their peers and siblings. The quest for 'Western' independence may be interpreted as inhumane and as a rejection of family members and their values.

Young women in particular may find this conflict stressful. Feeling caught between two cultures, at home and at school, they may experience divided loyalties between the roles and behaviours that they are expected to assume. However, inter-generational conflict occurs in all cultures. It is normal for teenagers to rebel and establish their own identity, and occasionally to cast their parents in the role of villains and oppressors (this issue is discussed further in Chapter 6).

However, in some cultures people feel the pull and ties of the family more than in others. Strong family ties were evident in Gypsy (Roma) and Travelling families in a study by Parry *et al.* (2004). One woman noted 'we come from a big family community … and we're all very close'. Participants in this study placed great value on close family life and discussed how welcome children were. One respondent noted 'kids are everything to Travellers, that's why they get married … it's to have kids and rear up children'.

People may see themselves not as individuals, but as a component of a family. Consequently, decision-making may automatically be referred to another member of the family, and older members of the family may be consulted regularly, as the following Muslim man stated:

> **Even though my parents are back in Pakistan, we always ask them and discuss it with them if we are going to take a big step, or about the children. Like when we bought this house, or even you know about my daughter's school.**

> *(Mares et al., 1985, p. 83)*

In contrast to the nuclear family, some people may belong to a large family network – the extended family – where the welfare of one member is seen as dependent on the welfare of the whole family and all of its members. Families may live in large multi-generational homes or in close proximity to each other. Children may be raised by a number of female relatives, aunts, grandmothers and cousins. The roles of men and women are clearly defined, and they may lead separate lives, but above all else the support and centrality of the family are of greatest importance. People might also be conscious of the role they play in maintaining the good name and honour of the family. Marriage is often celebrated as a bond between two families. A couple remains part of a large family unit, both emotionally and physically, for all of their married life. The role of individuals within the family has implications for health care. For example, the care of a child in hospital may be undertaken solely by the mother, but any major decisions may be taken by the father, who may consult other male family members (e.g. his brother or father). The child and mother may not be consulted, which some healthcare professionals may find difficult to accept. The roles played by men and women may also be different, as they may have different responsibilities and areas of authority. In some communities, for example, women may take sole care of children and bring them up alone or with other female relatives. The worlds of men and women may be much more segregated and separate.

The Children's Act (Department of Health, 2004) in the UK stresses that help provided for the family should be appropriate to race, culture, religion and language and that regard and attention should be paid to the different racial groups to which the child and family belong.

The Act requires that those who work with children should consider fully the wishes of all children in the decisions that are made about their care. However, this may be in contrast to the perceptions of parents and families, who may regard their child as vulnerable and incapable of voicing their views and making decisions about their care. Yet, children's views about their health are influenced by their family and peers. Children's perspectives on health need to be considered within the context of the respective family groups (Fatchett, 1995).

Key points

1. The concept of family is culturally bound.
2. 'Western' family life may put emphasis on the value of the individual.
3. 'Eastern' family life may place the family at the centre of society at the expense of the individual.
4. In some cultures men and women may lead separate lives.

CHILD-REARING PRACTICES AND DAY-TO-DAY CARE OF INFANTS AND CHILDREN

In this section, consideration will be given to the day-to-day care of infants and children, and to the ways in which culture and health beliefs influence child-rearing practices. Weller (1993) states that:

> Beliefs about child-rearing are usually bound up with beliefs about life itself. These beliefs are culturally transmitted and culturally learned. They are also held without question.

> *(Weller, 1993, p. 40)*

Child-rearing is a universal occupation. However, the method of bringing up children will be dependent on the parents' values and the circumstances in which they live. Mares *et al.* (1985) emphasize that minority ethnic mothers in the UK are often aware that some health workers disapprove of and disagree with their ways of bringing up children. Naturally this will affect their confidence and self-esteem as parents, and it may also have a detrimental effect on the child. As one woman said:

> It's funny you know. Because you know they're watching you all the time, they don't really trust the way you are looking after your kids, you start to get really worried yourself. You start to think, well maybe they're right to be worried, maybe our way of bringing up kids is wrong, and maybe I am a no-good mother. It's funny what it does to you.

> *(Mares et al., 1985, p. 91)*

Raising children is a very personal and individual issue. The role of the nurse is therefore to support and help families in the way in which they wish to bring up children. Values and beliefs about child-rearing need to be respected and valued, not judged or criticized. Above all, they do not need to be changed or 'Westernized'.

Carrying and settling children and babies

As Mead (1953) indicates, it is the small, intimate habits of daily life that are beacons of our culture. One example is the way in which people carry babies and children. In the UK, Europe and North America, it is common to see babies and small children being pushed in a pram or carried in a sling. In South America, a mother may carry her child around all day on her back in a sling or papoose. Currer's research (1991) has explored the perspective of Pathan women and their beliefs about child-rearing. She argues that people in the Indian subcontinent believe that Western culture devalues and ignores children. An older man in Pakistan told her that he had been horrified, on a visit to the UK, to see a woman carrying a dog and pushing a baby in a pram. He stressed to her that in Pakistan babies were rarely left in cots with toys, instead they are stimulated, held and passed around. This practice was also described by Kendall (1978) in her study of an Iranian village:

> **After the first 10 days the mother alone cares for the baby. He sleeps on a quilt next to her and spends most of his waking hours in her arms. If she leaves the house for errands or visits she carries the baby, firmly swaddled in an upright position against one shoulder and under her chaddor ... Babies are swaddled to keep them warm, to keep them clean and because it helps their arms and legs to grow strong and straight.**
>
> *(Kendall, 1978, p. 405)*

The practice of keeping the baby with the mother at all times, and carrying on daily life alongside her is the norm in some cultures. Andrews (1995) stresses that from the moment of birth the Vietnamese mother has her infant with her constantly:

> **A mother carries the child with one arm, the child's leg straddling her hip, even during naps. If the mother is not holding the child and the child begins to cry, the mother picks up the child instantly ... "Bad mothers" are those who fail to attend to their babies' crying immediately.**
>
> *(Andrews, 1995, p. 137)*

However, in Western culture this approach may be interpreted as 'spoiling the child or fostering dependence'.

A study by Caudhill and Frost (1973) compared the settling practices of Japanese mothers with those of American mothers. It was noted that Japanese mothers spent a long time soothing and lulling their infants. In contrast, the American mothers spent time stimulating them with active chatting. The Japanese mothers viewed contented, quiet babies as the desired norm, whereas the American mothers considered open, expressive, assertive and self-directed children to be desirable.

These child-rearing practices may be a reflection of social and economic circumstances. When my first baby was born, I was aware that I was to return to work in a few months, so I made a conscious effort to ensure that the baby was ready to be with other caregivers. This practice was reinforced by the health visitor, who once reprimanded me for 'holding the baby too much'.

It is also interesting to consider babies and children with regard to sleeping arrangements. In some Eastern and African cultures, bed-sharing may be a common practice as parents may feel that they need to look after the child while sleeping or that the child may be seen as too young to sleep alone. However, in Western cultures bed-sharing may be frowned on as it may be seen as fostering dependence and linked to sudden infant death syndrome. Andrews and Boyle (2008) noted that in some cultures it is common for families to sleep in the same bed, and babies in particular are kept close to their mothers so that they can breastfeed on demand.

Hygiene practices

Good hygiene practices are essential for health and comfort, but are culturally influenced and often linked to health beliefs. Practices may therefore vary, but should not be interpreted as standards, so judgements must not be made.

Practices may vary both between different groups and over time. For example, my grandmother would bathe her children once a week in a bathtub in front of the coal fire. This was usually on Saturday night, prior to church on Sunday. However, in many cultures bathing is considered to be poor hygiene practice, as it is considered to be 'wallowing in one's own muck'. People in Scandinavia may prefer to take a sauna, and it is common to see saunas in nursing homes. Many cultures prefer to shower or use running water to wash, so that dirt can be carried away in the water flow.

Toileting practices may also differ. Hindus and Muslims may prefer to squat when excreting, and to wash in running water after using the toilet, instead of using toilet paper. The left hand only is used for this purpose. The right hand is kept pure for handling food and other clean things.

Feeding and nourishing babies and children

Food is an extremely important part of our culture, and is as important to children as it is to adults. The acquisition and preparation of food are universal occupations, but again these are culturally determined and influenced. We learn about food as children, and our choices and preferences for food may be formed in childhood. Food plays a large part in religious festivals and rituals, but it is also influenced by trends and fashions. For example, the feeding of babies and children has changed considerably in the last 100 years. In the early part of the twentieth century, breastfeeding was a working-class practice, mainly because it was cheap. Andersen (1997) points to records which demonstrate that solids were forbidden to children under the age of 1 year, and that meat and fish were not allowed until the child was 3 years old. It was not until relatively recently, in the 1960s and 1970s, that solids were recommended at an early age – that is, from around 4 months. However, in many developing countries babies may be weaned later than is current practice in the UK. Mares *et al.* (1985) stress that this is common practice in countries where malnutrition is frequent, as it generally increases the infant's chances of survival. Food is a very important issue in Gypsy (Roma) and Travelling families and is noted by Parry *et al.* (2004). One respondent noted 'travellers love fat children' and others mentioned the importance of giving children tonics to stimulate a good appetite. Food and being a good parent were closely associated.

During the Muslim holy month of Ramadan (or Ramzaan), young children are exempt from fasting. Children are usually encouraged to fast for a few days from the age of 7 years, and they may fast with their parents on Fridays and at weekends. Between the ages of 12 and 14 years they begin to fast for the whole month (Schott and Henley, 1996). People who are ill are exempted from fasting. However, this is an individual decision and many people prefer to fast for spiritual reasons.

In Judaism, most devout Jews adhere to the Jewish kashrut or dietary laws. As in Islam, they are part of a code of discipline. Jews may not eat pork, pork products or anything that contains or is made with these. Shellfish and any fish without fins are also prohibited. Jews may eat meat from other animals, but it must have been killed in a certain way – that is, kosher (meaning fit). Milk and meat may not be used together in cooking.

Hindus are not permitted to eat beef and beef products, as cows are considered to be sacred animals. Hindus believe that all of God's creatures are worthy of respect and compassion and thus

Hindus are encouraged to be vegetarians. Alcohol is generally forbidden, and fasting is commonly practised.

Sikh dietary restrictions are similar to those for Hindus. Few Sikhs eat beef or halal food, and alcohol is forbidden. Pork is generally avoided by both Hindus and Sikhs, as pigs are regarded as dirty scavenging animals.

In South-Asian cultures food may be eaten using the hands rather than cutlery. The right hand is considered to be clean and is used for eating purposes. The left hand is reserved for 'dirty' functions such as cleaning and washing the genital areas.

Reflective exercise

1. Think back to the last time you were ill. What did you eat? What were you advised to eat by your family or friends?
2. Do you eat different foods for different illnesses? Do you 'feed a cold and starve a fever' for example?
3. What did you eat as a child when you were ill?
4. If you are a parent, what do you give your children to eat when they are ill? Why?

A study by Chevannes (1995) explored children's views about health and illness. It emerged from the study that during illness, white children liked to eat foods such as mashed potatoes, ice cream, toast, eggs and soup. However, although African-Caribbean children also enjoyed these foods, they added a few that were specific to their ethnic group. They enjoyed plantain, pumpkin soup, chicken soup and soup with yam. Asian children mentioned soup, vermicelli, dhal, lentil curry, chapatti and hajmola tablets (unprescribed herbal medicine). They also described different drinks that they were given when ill. White and Asian children reported enjoying Lucozade and Ribena, whereas African-Caribbean children said they drank 'Andrews' (an antacid). Yet all of them drank tea when they were ill.

From this survey it is apparent that food preference is culturally determined and that food has properties for curing and helping illness. Food and nutrition are extremely important to all of us, but perhaps more so when we are ill. Understanding and respecting food and eating habits is important if we are to help children to feel comfortable and accepted. It is also vital to plan appropriate and adequate care.

Dressing babies and children

The clothes we wear and the way in which we present ourselves are all signs of our cultural orientation. Our style of dress is often related to our climatic conditions, but clothes also signify or preserve modesty.

1. Describe the clothes you are wearing today.
2. Which clothes shops do you buy from, and why?
3. Why have you chosen to wear these clothes?
4. What types of messages do they send out about you?
5. If a parent, how does your choice of clothes influence what your child wears?

In many cultures, strict attention is paid to female modesty (e.g. covering the limbs and hair). This may also be applicable to small children. Modesty is an extremely important issue for South Asian cultures. For example, Muslim girls may be encouraged to preserve their modesty at all times, and, therefore, parents do not like to see the child's body exposed. Instead, they may prefer to have just one part of the body exposed. In non-urgent examinations it may be preferable for Muslim girls to be examined by a woman. Nudity may be considered improper.

Modesty and the need for privacy was also indicated in the study by Parry *et al.* (2004). In this research, Gypsy (Roma) and Travelling families discussed their need for privacy and their embarrassment when receiving physical personal care or needing to undergo intimate examinations. Some people noted that this was linked to upbringing: 'it's our kind of shyness and embarrassment'. This may prove a difficult issue for young people in particular, who may avoid lessons about sexual health issues. In hospital care it may result in some children and young people being hesitant, shy or reluctant to discuss intimate issues in relation to health care. Some young women may prefer to avoid using ordinary day-to-day language such as 'periods' for menstruation and may resort to using euphemisms such as 'monthlies' or the 'curse'.

It is also customary for some children to wear adornments or religious symbols. Christian children may demonstrate their religion by wearing a cross or medallion bearing the picture of a saint. Muslim children may wear a chain or piece of string around the neck or wrist, bearing a pendant inscribed with verses from the Qur'an. Sikh children may wear a kara (a steel bracelet) and both boys and girls may have their hair held up on top of their head with a small handkerchief. The hair of Sikh boys must not be cut. Sikhs may also wear the kaccha (special shorts or underpants).

The way in which we present ourselves to the outside world provides messages about our identity. The above examples are externally worn symbols, and they may be used to signify good luck, good health or protection for children. It is important that they are valued and respected and not removed or thrown away. In pre-operative and post-operative care, for example, care must be taken to recognize and respect any religious objects that the patient is wearing.

Giving names

In nursing we have a professional and legal duty to address people correctly and to ensure that they receive the appropriate care. Schott and Henley (1996, p. 109) state that 'Names matter. Wilful or careless misuse of names is alienating and insulting and is unlikely to enable the development of good caring relationships'.

Names also play a major part in our social and cultural identity and heritage. Children are named in different ways in different cultures. For example, in African cultures personal names may have a meaning such as 'child of my dream', 'gift' or 'joy', and they do not denote gender differences. Some names are associated with days of the week. In Ghana, the name Kofi means male Friday, while Ama means female Saturday.

Hindu names may have three parts: a personal name and a complementary name (which are often used together), followed by a family name. The most common female complementary names are Behn, Kumari and Rani. The most common male complementary names are Kant, Kumar and Chand. Most women take their husband's family name when they marry.

In the South-Asian Muslim naming system, males may have two names – a religious name (e.g. Mohammed, Allah and Ullah) and a personal name, and they must be used together. Females may have a personal name followed by a title, such as Bibi, Begum, Bano or Khanum. Females do not traditionally take their husband's name, so a family might not share a common name. Sometimes babies are not given a name for some time after birth, as a member of the family may be given the honour of choosing the name. Baby girls are not usually given their title for some time and initially have only one name.

In Hinduism parents give their child's name from a priest on the 10th day. Naming systems in Sikhism are based on religious rules. This requires people not to use a family name but to use only a first name together with a male or female title. These are Kaur (meaning 'princess' for females) and Singh (meaning 'lion' for males).

It is important to note that people may change their names in order to 'fit in' with the UK system. It is also worth noting that some people might not know their date of birth or their age, as in some developing countries births may not be registered.

Reflective exercise

1. Tell someone your names and describe to them how you came to have these names.
2. Explain the meaning of your names.
3. How do you feel about your names? For example, what do they say about you?
4. Have you ever had your name changed, or do you get called by nicknames? If so, how do you feel about this?
5. Is there anything you would change about your name? If so, why?

Most of us have a story to tell about our name, and these stories are often deeply significant. For example, children may be taunted about their name, and many of us dislike our given name being mispronounced or misspelled.

Playing and developing

Play is essential for helping children to develop and to understand the world in which they live. In Western cultures, good-quality (and often expensive) toys are promoted as essential to child development. However, in some cultures, toys may be kept to a minimum. Currer's (1991) observations of Pathan family life demonstrate very different concepts of play. Among Pathan families, the notion of separate worlds is irrelevant, and childhood is viewed very differently. In some households, the children's world is integral to that of the family, and children may therefore spend more time alongside their mothers, grandmothers or siblings. Thus they may seem to lack separate play resources, but instead they spend more time engaged with the caregiver in everyday tasks:

> **In the homes I visited, young children looked after younger siblings rather than play with dolls, and helped with household tasks as soon as they were able.**
>
> *(Currer, 1991, p. 44).*

Currer (1991) notes that the children's social skills were very well developed. She argues that to judge these children as 'under-stimulated' because they lack separate facilities is wrong. The concepts of child development that are based on notions of individualism may therefore not fit notions of Asian family life and the values of the community that underpin it. In some communities parents may be reluctant to send their children to playgroups or nursery schools preferring to keep them at home, fearing that they are too young to go to 'school'.

People may value the opportunity to let their children run around in the open air as is common in rural communities, as illustrated by the following quote by an Afro-Caribbean woman:

> **The one thing I miss here is the space. Just the other day I was saying to the children "Are you going to pull our house apart?" They don't have enough room to play about. We children used to spend most of our time outside.**
>
> *(Mares* et al., *1985, p. 90)*

Parents may also be afraid to let their children play outside because of fear of racist attacks, the risk that they may fall on concrete areas, traffic hazards, litter, etc. Many parents fear for the safety of their children and may therefore be very protective and unwilling to let their children out alone. A study conducted in 1992 highlighted the issues in out-of-school play schemes for Asian children:

> **Making their way to and from the play projects was difficult for many children, especially on dark winter evenings. Some Asian children were physically harassed on the way to and from the play projects, and girls were sometimes sexually harassed as well.**
>
> *(Kapasi, 1992, p. 163)*

Child-rearing in a racist society

Black and minority ethnic children are often aware of negative attitudes at an early age. Even from the age of 2 or 3 years, children are able to distinguish between different racial groups. Children from black and minority ethnic groups may soon harbour the idea that white people are naturally superior or cleaner than them. It has been demonstrated that children may soon start to show an adherence to, or preference for, the dominant cultural group. There are documented cases of children trying to scrub or bleach their skin white because they wish to reject their black skin and identity (Milner, 1975).

Some children are subjected to racist attacks or remarks or negative attitudes at school. Parry *et al.* (2004) note that for Gypsy (Roma) and Travelling communities, children's education at school may suffer as families may move sites. Some people noted the difficulty in getting their children into a chosen faith school and many parents noted children being discriminated against or bullied in school. In a study by Williamson *et al.* (2009) direct prejudice was also noted by a female Traveller:

> When my little brother was ill, he was only three, and we were in a different place and the doctor refused to see him because he was a gypsy. So we then had to go to a different town, 20 or 30 miles to a different town, because there were no walk-in-centres at that time.

(Williamson et al.*, 2009, p. 39)*

Although many children have a strong sense of pride and self-esteem, some experience periods of self-rejection and self-dislike. They may be constantly aware of 'being different', and these negative messages may be reinforced by health workers. Some parents are bewildered and hurt when their children reject their culture in favour of the dominant white culture. This might take the form of rejecting food or being ashamed of the parents' language, style of dress, etc.

LANGUAGE AND COMMUNICATION

Language and communication are central issues with regard to caring for children and their families. The way we talk, the words we use, dialects and accents all convey messages and impressions about ourselves. Language is acquired as babies and children, and the influence of our parents is paramount in the early years. As children grow older, they are more likely to be influenced by the education system or peers.

Command of language and ease of expression are essential not only for safety and meeting basic human needs, but also for social fulfilment:

> An 11-year-old Somali girl, Fatima, had been on her own in hospital for over 1 week when she was interviewed. She lived with her mother, her 16-year-old brother and her grandmother, her father having been killed before their arrival in this country. A family member was visiting in the evenings but no one else was staying with her "because my mum and my grandma, they do not speak English". She was being cared for in an isolation cubicle, and busy hard-pressed staff generally only went in when medication or food was due, or if she called for something. The interpreter for the hospital's sizeable interpreting service had not been called to help this patient, despite the girl's limited knowledge of English, her age and the unfamiliarity of her environment. When the interpreter was called, her joy at speaking to somebody from her country in her own language was boundless.

(Slater, 1993, p. 9)

Children in particular are sensitive to language and communication problems. The inability to express oneself can be frightening and anxiety-provoking. Parents may be able to act as interpreters for children, but if the parents cannot speak English, other methods may have to be found. These might include interpreters, toys, books and picture boards. It is not acceptable to use siblings to translate except in emergencies.

Ways of communicating distress and pain may also vary across cultures. In cultures that value stoicism and fortitude, suffering silently when in pain may be viewed as appropriate and mature behaviour. This is particularly relevant to Anglo-Saxon cultures and is described as 'maintaining a stiff upper lip'. However, in some cultures (for example Jewish and Italian) it may be appropriate to display distress 'outwardly' that is by expressing pain and suffering verbally (Helman, 2007).

Even when people do speak a little English, they may experience problems in using healthcare services. For example, some parents may speak English well but do not understand the technical jargon/slang or dialect that is used in the hospital setting. They may experience humiliation in public situations where they do not understand others or are unable to make themselves understood. They may also be made to feel stupid and uneducated even though they have skills in other languages:

> Asian families from India and Pakistan, but Bengali-speaking families in particular, also stress language as the cause of the greatest difficulties when using health care.
>
> *(Slater, 1993, p. 9)*

(Children from refugee and asylum seeker families may find this to be of particular significance. This issue is explored in Chapter 11.) A Bengali woman in the same study commented on people who could not speak English:

> I don't think staff respect our people. Once there was a lady next to me who didn't speak English. The nurse was making fun of the mum, laughed at her for not being able to explain something.
>
> *(Slater, 1993, p. 10)*

This can lead to parents feeling invisible, and they may be reluctant to stay in hospital, for fear of being humiliated or judged. This is sometimes interpreted as an uncaring or disinterested attitude towards their children. Families need access to good interpreting and translating services that are sensitive to the needs of both children and their families.

Key points

1. Child-care practices are culture bound and may change over time.
2. Parents have a right to raise their children in the way that they feel is appropriate.
3. Children and their families may be particularly sensitive and vulnerable to criticisms about their lifestyle, so care must be taken to understand and acknowledge cultural differences.

PATTERNS OF ILLNESS AND DISEASE

There are important variations in the patterns of illness among different ethnic groups in the UK. Some conditions that affect specific minority ethnic groups are described here.

Sickle-cell anaemia

Sickle-cell anaemia is a genetic disorder of haemoglobin in the red blood cells. More than 12 500 people in the UK have sickle-cell anaemia. The majority of them are of African or Caribbean descent, although it also affects those from Asia, the Middle East and the eastern Mediterranean.

This type of anaemia is caused by an abnormality in the structure of the haemoglobin molecule in the red blood cells. The first symptoms usually appear after the age of 3–6 months, and include swelling of the hands and feet, and pain in the joints, abdomen and chest. Anaemia may be present, and the infant may be susceptible to bacterial infection. Sickle-cell crises are extremely painful. There is no cure for sickle-cell anaemia, and the aim of treatment is to reduce complications and manage pain. In children, the disorder can be fatal because of their susceptibility to infection (Ferguson, 1991; see website list at the end of this chapter).

Thalassaemia

Thalassaemia is an inherited disorder that affects the production of alpha- and beta-globin chains, which are an essential part of the structure of haemoglobin in the red blood cells. There are two main forms of thalassaemia – alpha-thalassaemia major and beta-thalassaemia major. Both disorders are potentially fatal.

In the UK the main groups at risk of inheriting thalassaemia are people from the Mediterranean, Cyprus, Italy, Spain and Portugal and individuals from the Indian subcontinent and the Far East. Thalassaemia usually becomes evident in children between the ages of 6 and 12 months. If the child becomes severely anaemic, they may die of cardiac failure or infection. They may require monthly transfusions or daily subcutaneous injections (Anionwu, 1993; see website list at the end of this chapter).

Rickets

There is a higher incidence of rickets in children from minority ethnic groups. Rickets is caused by a lack of vitamin D, which is normally obtained from the diet and by exposure to the sun. Children with this condition may become weak and irritable and may have bone abnormalities. Exposure to the sun is a contentious issue. Parents who live in inner-city areas may wish to keep their children indoors and protect them not only from the poor weather but also from racial harassment (Mares *et al.*, 1985; Ahmad, 1993; Smaje, 1995).

GOOD PRACTICES WHEN CARING FOR BABIES AND CHILDREN

Black children and families and those from ethnic minorities face many problems when they access healthcare services. Chevannes (1997) argues that nurses need to develop partnerships with families and acknowledge that family members provide care on an ongoing basis. For example:

> Nurses intervene during episodes of illness and surveillance, and this means that they have to negotiate their entry into family homes, to achieve a plan of care which is needs-based and to ensure quality for those receiving care.
>
> *(Chevannes, 1997, p. 162)*

Chevannes (1997) indicates that there are three stages of interaction necessary when working in partnership:

- family members should be encouraged to state the needs for caring as they see them;
- the patient and the carer, in conjunction with the nurse, should identify the types and patterns of caring that are desired in relation to the needs;
- the patient, carer and nurse should participate in devising and agreeing upon care plans.

She believes that:

> **There is a need for nurses to listen, hear and act on the views of different families and of family members – Indian or black Caribbean, an adult woman or a boy child – and to take into account the respective and diverse views in the care plan which is prepared and later agreed.**
>
> *(Chevannes, 1997, p. 163)*

Good practice in the care of sick children therefore centres on shared care between parents and health staff. Parents who are not from the same culture as the staff may feel reluctant to stay in hospital, as they may feel either that they are not welcome or that the hospital does not have adequate facilities related to their cultural or religious needs (e.g. somewhere to pray). Some parents are stigmatized as uncaring when they leave their children unaccompanied in hospital. However, it is important to remember that parents may have pressing commitments to other children or family members.

It is imperative, therefore, that parents and children are given adequate information about the services available as well as about the care of the child. This should include information not just about the diagnosis, treatment and prognosis of the child, but also about the routines involved and the facilities for the family.

Information-giving needs to take into consideration issues such as language and literacy skills. Families who are unable to read in their own language may find videos and posters useful. Children are also more receptive to visual information and this should be taken into account when giving them information about their care.

Play facilities in hospitals need to reflect the cultural and racial diversity of children and multicultural toys should be available. These could include signs and books in dual languages, jigsaw puzzles, black dolls, and toy fruits and vegetables that represent foods eaten by black and minority ethnic children. It may also be useful to provide toys that are appropriate to the traditions of the culture, such as domestic tools and utensils.

Nurses also need to familiarize themselves with the relevant customs and festivals of the local communities, such as Ramadan and Diwali (see Appendices). It might be useful, for example, to plan celebrations with children. Parents and siblings may also welcome facilities for prayer and worship.

Nurses should ensure that children and their families have appropriate washing and toilet facilities (e.g. showers, running water). For example, Muslims may prefer to wash before praying. If it is not possible to move the patient physically, they may appreciate having a bowl brought to them and the bed curtains being pulled round.

Many children from black and minority ethnic families eat British food or an amalgam of family and British food. However, in some families it is customary to eat British foods while adhering to religious or cultural rules. People may develop a taste for British type food but insist that it is cooked according to religious rules (e.g. no animal fats). However, it is important to show sensitivity in the way that food is handled and presented to children and their families. For example, it is important to separate food utensils when handling food, to ensure that prohibited foods are not mixed. It is also important to note that, in the absence of their parents, some children may request food that is prohibited. This may be because of the child's curiosity, a desire to be like other children or rebelliousness, but nurses should always be aware of the anxiety of the parents and respect their wishes as well as ensuring that the child receives adequate nutrition.

Visiting may cause staff tensions, and it should always be borne in mind that cultural expectations of care may differ between families. For example, it may be the norm for the close extended family to be present (especially the female family members) and for decisions to be made by the male family members. Female children in hospital may cause their parents a great deal of anxiety. Families may object to girls undressing in front of others, especially male staff. Care and sensitivity are paramount here. For example, it is practical only to expose the area that is to be examined. Some families may prefer their daughter to be cared for by a female doctor or nurse, and these wishes should be respected wherever possible. Consider the following Case Study.

Case study

Rachel is a 7-year-old girl admitted to the ward for myringotomy and insertion of grommets. She has glue ear. Rachel belongs to an Orthodox Jewish family and is accompanied to the ward by her father. Her mother is at home with their 6-month-old baby. She is admitted on Friday afternoon and is due to go to theatre on Saturday morning. Rachel's father is to be resident.

How would you ensure that Rachel's cultural and religious needs are met?

The following information would help you to make informed decisions when caring for Rachel (Schott and Henley, 1996).

- Giger and Davidhizar (1991) emphasize that Jewish parents, like many others, may be very protective of their children and vocal about their feelings and anxieties. This should not be misconstrued by nursing staff as the father and child being aggressive, 'difficult' or a 'problem patient'.
- Rachel will require a kosher diet, and care must be taken to ensure that the food is individually wrapped and not unwrapped until it is ready to eat. The family must unwrap the meal. Care must also be taken to ensure that milk and meat products are not mixed (e.g. do not offer milk to drink with a meat dish).
- Rachel's father may prefer to let her use her own plastic cup.
- Medication may be an issue. The family might not wish Rachel to take certain analgesics and other medicines unless they are kosher. These include Disprol and Calpol suspension. It may be necessary to consult the pharmacy department about this.

continued

Case study

- Rachel's father may consider some children's activities (e.g. watching videos) to be unsuitable for his daughter.
- The Jewish Sabbath (Shabbat) begins at sundown on Friday and finishes at nightfall on Saturday. It is a major festival and a day of rest. Orthodox Jews do not work, and they also avoid activities such as signing official documents on the Sabbath. This factor needs to be borne in mind when signing consent forms. However, this consideration may be waived if life or health is compromised.
- Modesty is very important in Jewish cultures, especially for females. The family may be protective of their daughter and wish to avoid any unnecessary exposure. This should be considered when examining Rachel, and it might be necessary to provide female staff.
- Rachel's father may wish to pray when he is staying in hospital, and a suitable room or a quiet area should be provided, if possible, on the ward. Alternatively, the curtains may be drawn round the bed area.
- Some Orthodox Jewish men avoid all contact with unrelated women and therefore may not shake hands or make eye contact.

CONCLUSION

Culture influences all aspects of a child's physical and psychosocial growth and development. For some children, admission to hospital may be the first time they encounter a new culture, particularly if they are under 5 years old. Hospitals can be frightening, stressful places for all of us, but these fears are compounded in children who may not understand the language or the customs and rituals of hospitals. However, children and families may face a host of problems when they access health services, and they may find that the services provided are either not sensitive to their needs, or that they do not understand what is happening to the family member. Research by Slater (1993) clearly indicated that some families from black and minority ethnic groups felt that healthcare staff disapproved of them, or else they did not feel respected and in some cases were humiliated. In some cases, the parents' knowledge of their child was ignored by staff who 'think that we don't know anything, we're not smart like them or we're stupid' (Slater, 1993). Services for children therefore need to take into account not only the individual needs and circumstances of the child, but also those of the family, and that often this needs to include the extended family. Caring for children from other cultures sometimes requires us to set aside our preconceived ideas about child-rearing and the norms and values with which we have grown up.

CHAPTER SUMMARY

1. Children need to be understood within the context of their families and their environments.
2. Beliefs about child care and child-rearing practices are valued and protected in every culture.
3. Children and their families are particularly vulnerable when they are receiving health care, and extra care and attention may be needed with regard to issues such as communication and provision of information.

FURTHER READING

Croot EJ, Grant G, Cooper CL, Mathers N (2008) Perceptions of the causes of childhood disability among Pakistani families living in the UK. *Health and Social Care in the Community* **16**(6), 606–13.

This qualitative research study explores the way that Pakistani parents account for and understand their child's disability. It is particularly interesting as it explores the relationship between religion, in particular Islam, and disability.

Quintana SM, Chao RK, Cross WE, Hughes D, Nelson-le Gall S, Aboud FE Conteras-Grau J, Hudley C, Liben LS, Vietze DL (2006) Race, ethnicity, and culture in child development: contemporary research and future directions. *Child Development* **77**(50), 1129–41.

This work is a comprehensive study of the complex issues in relation to child development and children's health.

Shah R (1994) Practice with attitude. Questions on cultural awareness training. *Child Health* **6**, 245–9.

There are some interesting questions and useful information included in this paper, which explores the issues related to the needs of Asian children with disabilities.

Syal M (1997) *Anita and me.* Harper Collins, London.

A very entertaining and funny novel, which depicts the life of Meena, the only daughter of a Punjabi family, as she is growing up in the Midlands in the 1960s.

Wilson P (2005) Jehovah's Witness children: when religion and the law collide. *Pediatric Nursing* **17**(3), 34–7.

This article examines the complex legal and ethical issues involved in making decisions when religious law is in conflict with civil law.

Purnell L (2009) *Guide to culturally competent health care*, 2nd edn. F A Davis & Co, Philadelphia.

Each chapter in this book has a section on family, pregnancy and childbearing practices which illustrate cultural practices in these aspects of life.

WEBSITES

http://www.forcedmigration.org/

This website is an on-line resource on human displacement and has a number of resources related to children and their experiences, including displacement after war or natural disasters. There are also links to other sites such as UNICEF on child related issues.

http://www.sicklecellsociety.org/

Sickle-Cell Anaemia. This website has a range of resources and information about sickle-cell anaemia.

http://www.ukts.org/

Thalassaemia. UK Thalassaemia Society. This website has a range of information about this disease including a set of standards for the clinical care of children and adults with thalassaemia.

10 Care of older people from black and minority ethnic groups

Christine Hogg

INTRODUCTION

We cannot control age – it is not a matter of choice. However, the way in which we grow old and the way we value age and older people are dependent on many factors including class, gender, status and the perceptions of those around us. Growing old can be difficult for anyone. Retirement may bring complex problems, including a decline in status, role loss and reduction in income. People may face loneliness, isolation and declining physical health. In addition to these problems, older people from black and minority ethnic groups may also face hostility and racism.

The chapter will discuss and examine the following issues in relation to older people from black and minority ethnic groups:

- patterns of migration;
- triple jeopardy theory;
- myths and stereotypes about older people;
- health beliefs and older people;
- health and illness patterns;
- providing services for older people.

PATTERNS OF MIGRATION

If when I first came here I had had five years with good money in my hand, then I could have gone back; then I could have done something for my home country. But at this age all I have is my home pension to live on. How can you go back? What are you going for?

We have done a lot for Britain. We bring life to them, no matter what they say. They have and we give them more. We give all our energy and our strength and all the riches that we can get. We give it to this country. We give them another culture and background that they didn't have before.

(Schweitzer, 1984, p. 35)

The experience of growing old is subject to many influences and differing life circumstances. Holmes and Holmes (1995) analysed the experience of growing old in many cultures, and discussed lifestyles on the Mediterranean island of Paros. The island is virtually crime free, the inhabitants fish, farm and provide a service to tourists, and they value physical work and mental activity. The diet consists of large quantities of fresh fruit and vegetables, fish, eggs and cheese. The study also cites work by Beaubier (1976), who claims that in a population of 2 703 there were at least five people over the age of 100 years. Holmes and Holmes (1995) provide photographic evidence of a sprightly man aged 105 years who still works on his land. It may be argued that the circumstances in which people find themselves directly affect the quality of their health, and this important issue is discussed throughout this chapter.

Western culture, in the so-called 'developed' world, is increasingly led and driven by younger people. As a society it is acceptable to try to look younger, and there is an increasing drive to undergo plastic surgery to help to capture the 'essence of youth'. Older people in modern Western society have a minority status of their own – they are often cast aside or marginalized in favour of younger generations. In pre-industrial societies, older people were valued for their experience and knowledge and were frequently used as a resource for the community. In industrial societies, however, old age is associated with loss of physical strength and consequently a diminished ability to contribute to the work-force (even though many of us are in employment that requires mental rather than physical stamina). Yet in some cultures old age is revered and respected, and in some cases it is even rewarded (Holmes and Holmes, 1995).

It is generally accepted that the NHS has been less than responsive to the needs of black and minority ethnic groups as well as those of older people, whose services are often described as marginalized or 'Cinderella' services. Henley and Schott (1999) have commented as follows:

> Health service culture tends to reflect society's prejudices. Professionals caring for older people often have low status and little recognition. Medical training focuses on acute illness and still pays little attention to the common disabilities of old age or to illness in relation to older people.

> *(Henley and Schott, 1999, p. 33)*

Services for older people tend to be perceived as less glamorous than the so-called 'high-tech' services. These problems are compounded for older people from black and minority ethnic groups.

Demography

The number of black and minority ethnic older people in the UK population compared with the number of white older people is still small but is growing. The 2001 Census (Office for National Statistics 2009 shows that, in general, minority ethnic populations have a younger age profile. The only exception to this is the white Irish groups who have the oldest age structure in the UK. Although this population is relatively small at the moment it is projected to grow significantly in the future as people who migrated to the UK in the 1960s and 1970s grow older. For example the young people who migrated to the UK from India and Pakistan in the 1970s will soon be able to retire.

The census also demonstrated that certain minority ethnic groups were more likely to be afflicted by limiting long-term illness. Bangladeshi, Pakistani, Indian and black Caribbean groups were found to be at risk of diabetes, coronary arteries disease, arthritis, stroke and respiratory disorders.

Migration

Most of those people who migrated to the UK in the 1950s and 1960s as adults (in their twenties and thirties) are now older people who did not intend to stay in this country. Migration from one culture to another can be a new stressful experience that involves major disruptions to an individual's life (Furnham and Bochner, 1986; Eisenbruch, 1988; Raleigh and Balarajan, 1992). For some people it can be both demoralizing and alienating.

On arrival in a new country, the migrant may experience isolation, bewilderment, helplessness and feelings of insecurity. They may have left behind family and friends, familiarity, routine and security. Immigration laws may mean that people experience the additional strain of waiting for their family to join them. Moreover, they may face language problems, which may in turn influence their chances of housing, employment, etc. The host population may be hostile, fearful or just indifferent (Mares *et al.*, 1985).

Reflective exercise

Imagine that you had a change in circumstances (redundancy, for example) and that you needed to find work overseas.
1. Where would you go and why?
2. What preparations would you make? For example how would you find out about language and cultural traditions?
3. Who would accompany you and why?
4. What would you take with you? Which possessions would you take and why?
5. How do you feel you might cope with a new lifestyle?

You may, for example, have considered contacting the embassy of the country you are about to emigrate to, in order to obtain a temporary work permit. If you have children, you may have sought information about children's schools or colleges.

Eisenbruch (1988) coined the term 'cultural bereavement' for those groups of people who have suffered a permanent and traumatic loss of their familiar land and culture. This sense of loss and stress is exacerbated if the migrant is a refugee or exile, and if they have had to leave their home country suddenly because of war or persecution:

> When I left Poland in 1939 it all happened so quickly, there was such a panic, that I hardly brought anything with me, just two suitcases. We were escaping from the Germans and the bombs, one didn't think ... I took my little girl to Romania and then to Yugoslavia where my sister was living. My husband was taken as a prisoner and spent the rest of the war in a POW camp. We arrived in Southampton, I still with my two suitcases, and were sent to an army camp near Leominster ... If the war had not happened I would of course have preferred to have stayed in my own country, and not be a burden to another country.
>
> *(Schweitzer, 1984, p. 61)*

The stress and pressures faced by many migrants may lead to higher rates of mental health problems. The effects of migration may last a lifetime, so these factors should be borne in mind when caring for older people. For example, they may always feel an 'outsider' in the host community, or the scars and negative experiences of their migration may be borne through life. There are several studies that have found high rates of mental illness among migrants. This issue was discussed in Chapter 6.

Migration to the UK has been evident for over 500 years, but mass migration only began after World War II. Migration results from 'push' and 'pull' factors. After World War II, the UK actively recruited labour from the Commonwealth countries to aid the reconstruction effort. This factor was a major 'pull', as many people left their homes believing that they would earn enough money to return home and live in comfort. The 'push' factors included political instability, poverty and oppression.

Patterns of Asian migration

The majority of migrants in the 1950s and 1960s were single men from rural areas who came to make up the shortfall of unskilled labour in areas of industrial decline. Others were forced to leave their homes because of displacement. For example, a large number of Pakistanis from Mirpur came to Britain in the early 1960s as a result of the construction of the Mangla dam. For some, migration may have represented a chance to strive for better employment and may therefore have been synonymous with increased family status at home.

British society in the post-war years was suffering austerity, and for most migrants their experience was a difficult one. British attitudes at the time were still influenced by ideas and beliefs founded in colonialism. Mistrust and elitist attitudes towards people from overseas still abounded, and many migrants were met with racist attitudes and a general coldness and reserve from British people. One man who came from Punjab in 1962 recounted his experience:

> Although I was educated (I had an MSc in Engineering) my friend had to bribe the seniors with a bottle of whisky to get me a job as a machinist ... I had four machines to run and got paid half the amount other machinists used to get who had only two machines to run.
>
> *(Schweitzer, 1984, p. 42)*

Robinson (1986) described the patterns of settlement for these migrant workers. The first groups began to settle in areas where there was a high demand for labour, in cities such as Birmingham and London and the textile towns of Lancashire and Yorkshire. These men acted as the bridgeheads, helping newly arrived migrants to settle, whether or not they were blood relatives. They often shared lodging houses and helped each other with language and bureaucracy problems. The myths about the British in South-East Asia still abounded. Britain had an image of being discriminatory and immoral, and therefore a dangerous place for women. However, in the 1960s and 1970s the wives and children and sometimes the parents of male migrants began to join the men. Housing provision was found mainly in run-down inner-city areas where homes were more affordable. By the 1980s and 1990s, family consolidation meant that UK-born Asians were creating their own families and identities here.

African-Caribbean migration

The pattern of African-Caribbean migration gradually developed in the post-war years. Migrants were actively recruited from Barbados and Jamaica by British Rail, London Transport and other large organizations. In the 1960s, the NHS began to recruit nurses and midwives. As British citizens they had the unrestricted right to come here to settle and work. In common with other migrants, they often arrived in their late twenties and thirties and were unable to pay enough National Insurance contributions for a full pension. They were also less likely to be able to gain promotions and more likely to be made redundant. Britain was perceived as the mother country, and in many cases young single women as well as men were recruited. Like many migrants, African-Caribbean people took the jobs that local people avoided, yet they faced a great deal of hostility and prejudice. The following comments were made by a woman from Jamaica:

> After the war, we were invited into this country by the Government. Enoch Powell was one of them that sanctioned for West Indians to come and help clean up this country after the war. Well, I was at home in Jamaica doing nothing at the time, so I decided to come, expecting a decent job and to be treated as an equal … What do I get? I go to Mile End Hospital and get a job there, and I was placed on the corridor with a bucket, a scrubbing brush and a mat to kneel on. I never do that type of work in all my life. I cried all night and I cried all day. Coming to this country was the hardest work I have ever done.

> *(Schweitzer, 1984, p. 31)*

Chain migration was also a feature, with the first migrants helping to find others accommodation and employment. Many people in all of these groups subscribed to the belief that their stay would only be temporary and that they would eventually return home. However, few of them actually did return. On revisiting their home country, they might find the reality to be different from the fantasy, or they might recognize that they have changed and become 'more British'.

An interview with a woman from Guyana illustrates this problem:

> Guyana is different now. I went home 11 years ago and it's not the British Guyana I used to know. I mean all the beauty has gone out of it. I planned to go home after retirement a few years ago. I kept ringing up me family and they say, 'You better stay where you are, the conditions here are terrible'.

> *(Schweitzer, 1984, p. 30)*

Key points

1. People who migrated to the UK in the 1950s and 1960s are now forming part of the older population.
2. Migration can be a difficult and alienating experience, and many older people may carry the scars from earlier years.
3. Patterns of migration and settlement may reflect social, political and economic pressures.

THE TRIPLE JEOPARDY THEORY

Researchers in the 1980s began to stress the notion of 'triple jeopardy' which black and minority ethnic older people often face (Norman, 1985). Older people in society are at risk by virtue of associated ill health and loss of role. These disadvantages are compounded by racism and discrimination, and may result in poor living conditions, low incomes and a sense of alienation ('not feeling as if I belong here'). Finally, older people may find it difficult or are reluctant to access health services, social services and housing provision, either because they believe that they do not deserve them or because they perceive those services as being for the white majority population. As Jones (1996) indicates:

> Whenever racism appears, and at whatever level, the effects are more accentuated when a person is older. The presence of one deepens the influence of the other; that is, prejudice and disempowerment due to bio-socio-economic deprivation associated with old age is further enhanced when race becomes a factor.

(Jones, 1996, p. 109)

Alternatively, there is the argument that 'age is a leveller', in that the differences between older people from differing groups decrease with age. For example, in old age there are many commonalities that transgress race and social class. The loss of paid work, declining health and increase in leisure time are all examples of common experiences. In other words, age tends to reduce the differences.

A consultation project with older people from minority ethnic groups carried out by Butt and O'Neill (2004) reported that language barriers in services caused problems. People reported that they often had problems explaining their symptoms of ill health and that as a result conditions could be misdiagnosed or diagnosis was late. Many older people felt that services saw communities as 'problems' rather than respecting different communities. Some people also preferred their own community voluntary groups after losing faith in mainstream services.

MYTHS AND STEREOTYPES ABOUT OLDER PEOPLE FROM BLACK AND MINORITY ETHNIC GROUPS

One of the prevalent myths about minority ethnic groups is that they 'look after their own'. This is a dangerous and misinformed stereotype that unfortunately pervades the health and social care system. It is often assumed that older black and Asian people live as part of extended families, and that their needs for care and support in old age are almost always met within the family and community. This notion is refuted by Fennell *et al.* (1988), who indicate that although many ethnic older people live in multi-generation homes, they may not be receiving adequate or appropriate care. Modern pressures and aspirations in family life may influence the ability to provide the expected level of support. For example, women traditionally provided unpaid care for older family members, but second and third generations of women may choose or be compelled (by financial pressures) to work outside the home. This may further increase the isolation that older people feel. Willis (2008), in her preliminary findings, challenges the idea that minority ethnic groups support each other and found that black Caribbean older people actually gave less support that their white counterparts. Butt and O'Neill (2004) also found that many people refuted the stereotype that black and minority ethnic groups might 'look after their own'. The participants in this study pointed out that family members often lived away or that intergenerational gaps and culture gaps may leave older people living alone and feeling isolated.

This stereotype has often been used to justify the poor provision of services for older people. A study in 1998 by the Social Services Inspectorate found that, although many services were making genuine attempts to provide relevant and appropriate levels of care, many staff still took the view that 'they look after their own'. As one white staff member said:

> I don't think the Asian community like us to be involved. They are very independent people and look after their old people. They usually have some family and feel reluctant to accept services from outside the family.

> *(Social Services Inspectorate, 1998, p. 41)*

The study identified a lack of empowerment for black and Asian older people, and low levels of expectations. Some older people reported feeling 'invisible' to service providers. Another common myth is that older people from black and minority ethnic communities are a homogeneous group with similar cultural beliefs and languages. For example, Robinson (1986) reported 17 different dialects in the Asian community in Blackburn. The term 'Asian' may be regarded as similar to the generalization 'European'. If we consider the needs (language, health beliefs, customs, religious beliefs, etc.) of an older person living in a residential home in Glasgow, they would not be considered similar to those of an older woman living in a remote village in Portugal. Although they may have commonalities (e.g. failing health, low income, isolation) they are likely to have had different life experiences, employment patterns, family systems, language, customs, etc. They live in different parts of Europe and may consider themselves to be completely different. One may be a regular attendee of the Church of Scotland, and the other may be a devout Catholic. Thus although they may be regarded as similar (older, Christian and European), they speak different languages, practise their faith in different ways and may have never visited each other's country.

Fennell *et al.* (1988) argue that health services still perceive minority ethnic groups as 'social problems'. For example, minority ethnic older people may still be perceived as 'immigrants', despite having lived in this country for most of their adult life. They are rarely included in UK social care and healthcare policies, despite their growing numbers. Discrimination, negative attitudes and stereotypes seem to pervade the system, as a student nurse described:

> I was on an elderly care ward where there were two old ladies in beds next to each other. One was a lady from Poland who had come over to this country after the war as a refugee. She didn't speak any English but would nod and smile at us. In the next bed there was an old lady from India. She had been in England for 26 years and her English was quite poor. However, I couldn't believe the attitude of the nurses. The Polish lady was the ward pet – the nurses would take time and trouble over her. They would say things like 'poor old thing – she's had such a bad life'. The Indian lady, however, was blamed for her inability to speak English – 'Just imagine! How many years has she lived here?' One of the nurses would get annoyed about the number of visitors she had. 'Can't they see they are making too much noise?' It struck me at

the time that they were being very unfair; I never said anything at the time because I was a student. But how can people be so prejudiced?

HEALTH BELIEFS AND OLDER PEOPLE

Culture and health beliefs are inextricably linked, and for older people there is often a greater reliance on traditional medicines and health practices (health beliefs are discussed in Chapters 2 and 3).

When older people become ill they may have special or different needs than other groups. Illness in older people tends to occur in multiple rather than single episodes. They might respond quite differently to medication, and might take longer to recover from health problems. Often physical illness may be linked to mental or emotional distress (e.g. depression) and poor social circumstances (e.g. poverty, poor housing and isolation).

In all cultures older people may have an ambivalent attitude towards modern medicines, often believing it to be suitable for treating acute conditions but not for strengthening the overall 'constitution'. They may be unfamiliar with modern healthcare practice and are suspicious of modern technology, and they may adhere to remedies or practices that they have grown up with and with which they are familiar.

Reflective exercise

1. Consider the health beliefs of older people from your own culture (e.g. your grandparents).
2. What are they?
3. How different are they from your own health beliefs?
4. Are your health beliefs different to those of your parents?

Older people from different cultures are often familiar with and favour alternative or traditional therapies. For example, many have grown up in communities where there are one or more alternatives to Western medicines. People from the Indian subcontinent may go to a vaid or hakim for treatment. The Chinese and Vietnamese may consult an acupuncturist or herbalist from their own community. Moreover, in rural communities access to modern or Western health care may necessitate a long or difficult journey to the nearest town or city. Modern medicine is not rejected, but people may find it more appropriate to consult several different practitioners. They may believe that there are several ways of obtaining treatment, and that these methods play complementary roles. In turn, the traditional healer may refer patients for more modern or conventional treatment.

The traditional practitioner may be attractive to older people because they spend more time with the patient and may also speak the same language or come from the same town or country of origin. The patient may therefore gain considerable psychological benefit from the consultation. Another attraction is that the patient feels a greater degree of control over their health.

Drugs in particular may cause problems for older people from other cultures, and unfamiliarity or language difficulties may be associated with non-compliance. Qureshi (1989) stressed that in Eastern cultures, rectal examination and rectal medication (e.g. suppositories and enemas) may be taboo and even cause deep offence and distress. This is because traditional cultures perceive rectal examination to be a form of punishment and insult.

In Western health care, great importance is attached to the rights, needs and perceptions of the patient as an individual. In the UK, for example, we place great emphasis on individual privacy and respect for confidentiality. Healthcare professionals in the UK are therefore extremely patient-centred. However, in Eastern cultures the person as a patient may be seen in the context of their family and care may be shared. An older person may be accompanied to hospital or to the GP by members of the family who expect to be told everything and may expect to be present at examinations. In Eastern cultures, illness is viewed as a crisis for the whole family, so the outcomes of care will affect all family members. In Western cultures, this approach to health care is sometimes interpreted as interfering or overprotective. Blakemore and Boneham (1994) indicate that in traditional rural or developing countries, provision for health care in hospital may be poor, so relatives are expected to provide care for the patient. For example, people from South-Asian cultures may believe that hospital care requires relatives to undertake the nursing care of a member of the family (e.g. washing and feeding). Indeed, to some people the notion of leaving a relative alone in hospital may seem neglectful or even abusive. However, visits to the ward by large family groups often cause great concern among healthcare staff, not least the nurses. This concern, in our experience, often leads to rigid and restrictive visiting rules on adult wards. In other parts of Europe hospitals are much more open to family members and there is no restriction on visiting:

> **I was in a bad car crash in Italy and spent five months in hospital, most of the time unable to move. I discovered that the family was supposed to feed the patient. I would literally have starved if my kind friends hadn't organised a rota of people to come and feed me every day.**
>
> *(English woman, Henley and Schott, 1999, p. 168)*

It is interesting to note that in other areas of health care in the UK, especially hospices and children's wards, restrictive visiting has been abolished and in children's services families are actively encouraged to stay with the child.

Key points

1. Older people from black and minority ethnic groups may face multiple hazards in health care owing to adverse factors such as racism and poor provision of services.
2. Myths and stereotypes about older people in this group may also jeopardize their access to the provision of care.
3. The health of the older person may be considered to be a family problem and not a problem for the individual.

HEALTH AND ILLNESS PATTERNS AMONG OLDER PEOPLE

The health of older black and minority ethnic people is intrinsically linked to historical and social factors that in turn have affected their economic and social position in society. There is an established association between ill health and poverty (Townsend and Davidson, 1982), and older minority ethnic individuals suffer particular disadvantages with regard to their health. Explanations for the excess morbidity include poverty, lifestyle and poor housing.

A report by The Joseph Rowntree Foundation (2004) found that some people who had migrated to the UK in the 1950s and 1960s and had worked in public services had not been properly advised on pensions and consequently found themselves in poverty in later life. Indeed, it was also found that benefit entitlement was poorly understood as information was not always available in appropriate languages.

However, health problems may arise in more subtle ways. Epidemiological studies show a number of trends that are worth noting. For example, osteomalacia is found in excess among older Asian women, and Calder *et al.* (1994) suggest that this may be caused by vitamin D deficiency. This may be due to deficiency in the diet or a lack of exposure to sunlight. Rates of hypertension are high in both the Asian and African-Caribbean populations, and there is a high mortality rate among African-Caribbean women (Smaje, 1995; Blakemore and Boneham, 1994; Ebrahim, 1996). Ischaemic heart disease is more common in Asian people, and older Asian people are at higher risk of heart attack compared with the national rate (Smaje, 1995). Both Asian and African-Caribbean populations have a higher prevalence of diabetes than the majority population. Ebrahim (1996) argues that rare or 'exotic' diseases are seldom encountered, but it may be difficult to diagnose heart failure, asthma or tuberculosis when there are communication problems. An earlier study undertaken by Ebrahim *et al.* (1991) found that a group of Gujarati elders in North London was more prone to diabetes, asthma, gastrointestinal bleeding, strokes and heart disease than white groups. However, in this study there were no significant differences in the problems found in old age (e.g. visual and hearing impairment, falls, urinary incontinence) between the Asian elders and the indigenous population. Around 50 per cent of the people in both groups experienced some type of visual impairment, and indeed more people from the indigenous groups admitted to being incontinent of urine. It is of significant interest that the Asian group reported higher levels of life satisfaction than the indigenous group. This may be related to the fact that South-Asian older people may have a more significant spiritual element to their lives. One person in the study commented that he felt that old age was a time of coming to terms with oneself and with God. However, one might argue that older South-Asian people might have come to expect less from life, given their life experiences. Ebrahim *et al.*'s study revealed that the Asian group had a higher rate of use of medication than the indigenous group. Other studies (e.g. Donaldson, 1986) have indicated that the number of consultations in general practice by people from ethnic minorities is high. Indeed, as Ghosh (1998) indicates, most people from minority ethnic groups believe that they are sicker than their white peers. It is difficult to know or understand why older minority ethnic patients visit their GP more often or receive more medication. One simple explanation may be that they have higher rates of morbidity than the indigenous groups. It may be that black and Asian people feel that they are not getting their needs met, or that their concerns are not being adequately addressed, so they are likely to revisit the GP for more or better advice.

When considering the health needs of black and minority ethnic older people, there may be a tendency to diagnose 'exotic' complaints that people bring back from travel abroad. However, this avoids the issue of disease patterns that have been influenced by living in the UK.

DEVELOPING SERVICES FOR OLDER BLACK AND MINORITY ETHNIC PATIENTS

Providing care for older people from black and minority ethnic groups is one of the most challenging issues for the nursing profession. The following principles and guidelines have been gleaned from the literature and represent guidelines for good practice.

Hilton (1996) cites examples of behaviour that may seem strange, and he offers alternative explanations (see Box 10.1).

Box 10.1 *Examples of behaviour and alternative explanations*

'He won't make a decision ...' – perhaps he needs to ask an authority figure in his community

'She is off her food ...' – perhaps she always washes her hands before eating; perhaps it is a fast day

'She has dementia and she is climbing all over the toilet ...' – perhaps she is trying to squat to use the toilet, the way she remembers from her own country

'She is terrified of physical investigations ...' – perhaps she has been tortured

'The family visit in a large group, they never look at the sign saying two visitors at each bed ...' – perhaps it is their custom to support the patient in this way, and the patient would be distressed by their absence

---

Above all, it is important not to treat older people as exotic specimens as Blakemore and Boneham (1994) indicate:

> When we reflect on the experience of a Jamaican widow or a Sikh grandfather going to a GP's surgery, or to a hospital for treatment, we should therefore remember it is not a matter of the older black patient bringing an "awkward" set of expectations or cultural attitudes with him or her. It would be more accurate to see the hospital or medical practitioner culture as exotic and "awkward", perhaps in the sense that it demands compliance to rules that are in part culturally defined and unlike the everyday rules of social behaviour. The relationship between patients and medical practitioners always involves some negotiation.
>
> *(Blakemore and Boneham, 1994, p. 105)*

Consider the following Case Study, which explores some of the issues already outlined.

Miss K is a 78-year-old Polish woman. Lately she has been getting quite forgetful and has been admitted to the ward with unstable diabetes and a chest infection. The warden (herself of Polish origin) says that she is a very private person who has few friends. According to the district nurses, Miss K's flat is quite chaotic, and there are complaints that she is hoarding things 'again'. Miss K is admitted to the ward today. She speaks little English, she is very tearful, speaking in her own language and is clinging on to her handbag, which contains all her medication.

What actions should the nurse take on the basis of this limited information?

The following nursing actions were taken:

- The nurse who was caring for Miss K interpreted her behaviour as resulting from fear and thought that she was frightened, bewildered and perhaps disorientated. From this point the nurse used her interpersonal skills to help the patient to feel at ease. She approached Miss K in a quiet but firm manner, talking to her slowly and calmly. She used plenty of non-verbal techniques, gentle touch and good eye contact. She made a conscious effort to avoid appearing hostile. She did not attempt to take Miss K's handbag away from her, and instead sat with her at the bedside and allowed her to cry, providing her with tissues and a cup of tea.

- The nurse also made sure that Miss K knew her name and knew how to call her with the call bell. She did this by introducing herself. This ensured that Miss K felt established and accepted. It also meant that she did not feel as lost and isolated in the hospital.

- The nurse then contacted the Polish interpreting service in the hospital. However, the person concerned was on holiday. The nurse then made enquiries and found a nurse who spoke Polish as her mother tongue. The Polish-speaking nurse was enlisted to orientate Miss K to the ward, bathrooms, etc.

- The nurse asked the Polish-speaking nurse's permission to write down some key words that would be useful when communicating with Miss K. Key words (e.g. pain, sugar, urine, bathroom, toilet, hungry, feeling ill, nurse, doctor) were written in Polish and, together with a signboard, were used when she was communicating with Miss K. Once she was able to make herself understood, the nurses began to notice a discernible difference in Miss K's mood.

- The nurse then carried out procedures with Miss K, using a few key words in Polish and the rest in English, quietly and gently. The nurse was aware that even though she might not respond in English, she might be able to understand it when being spoken to rather than speaking it herself. The nurse decided that it was better to continue to speak and explain even though Miss K did not understand everything that was being said to her, as this was preferable to caring for her in silence, which could possibly seem quite threatening.

continued

- The nurse then contacted the warden of the flats for some information and assistance. It became apparent that Miss K arrived as a young woman in the UK in 1946 as a refugee from Poland. Her family had been killed during the war, and she had spent some time in a concentration camp. The hardships and the trauma of this period had made her reclusive and anxious. Throughout her adult life she was inclined to hoard and treasure her possessions. It was felt that this was a direct result of living her life in a concentration camp where she had been stripped of possessions. The warden said that like many people who had experienced life in a concentration camp and as a refugee, she had a fear of destitution and poverty. She still experienced nightmares and had a deep mistrust of hospitals, as she had been physically assaulted by nursing staff while in the concentration camp hospital. Lately she had become even more reclusive and had forgotten to take her medication. She settled in a town in the North of England in a small community of Polish people so that she could be with others from her country. Miss K worked for some time as a cleaner and now lives in a housing association scheme that is warden controlled.

- The nurse asked if the warden could arrange for some of Miss K's personal belongings to be brought in for her. The next day the neighbour brought in her nightwear and a few personal items, including some prayer books, some holy water and a crucifix. She also brought a Polish newspaper. Miss K seemed to be comforted by these items.

Bearing these factors in mind, the nurse planned Miss K's care. As her religion was very important to her, she arranged for the local Polish-speaking priest to visit Miss K (this was done by contacting the chaplain at the hospital).

At handover, the nurse informed all of the other staff about Miss K's individual circumstances and the care and sensitivity that she would need. She also made the other nurses aware of the language resources. The next day the nurse bought a Polish–English dictionary with ward funds. This would be kept on the ward for future reference.

Miss K gradually became less anxious and her diabetes and general health improved. She formed a good relationship with the nursing staff, who were able to understand her in the context of her life experiences. Although communication was difficult at times, Miss K felt accepted and was more confident about trying to make herself understood. Miss K was discharged the following week. The nursing team commented that she seemed to be a different person from the frightened, tense individual who had been admitted to the ward the week before.

CONCLUSION

Blakemore and Boneham (1993, p. 139) comment that 'The trees of the world's rainforests are strong, mature and diverse, but growing on thin soils, they are extremely vulnerable to exploitation and destruction'. They believe that this image illustrates the position of black and minority ethnic older people in today's society in the UK. Many people are extremely resourceful and robust and have sometimes battled against extreme adversity in life. However, they may be vulnerable, and this vulnerability is perhaps heightened when they come into contact with health services. There are many health problems that are similar to those of the indigenous population (e.g. cardiovascular problems, diabetes, etc.) but older people from black and minority ethnic groups are often overlooked when services are planned. Unfortunately, the belief that the extended family is capable of coping with any disease or disability continues to discriminate against older people.

The diverse nature of the minority ethnic communities (e.g. the so-called 'Asian community') needs to be recognized and taken into consideration when planning and delivering services. Nurses in particular need to ensure that care assessment and planning take into account the context of the patient's life.

CHAPTER SUMMARY

1. Older people from black and minority ethnic groups need to be considered in the context of their individual life history and social circumstances.
2. There are some common myths and stereotypes about this group of people that may lead to poor service provision.
3. Older black and minority ethnic people may experience health problems in common with all older people, but these issues may be exacerbated by the effects of racism (e.g. poverty, poor housing).

FURTHER READING

Blakemore K (1997) From minorities to majorities: perspectives on culture, ethnicity and ageing in British gerontology. In: Jamieson A, Harper S and Victor C (eds), *Critical approaches to ageing and later life.* Open University Press, Milton Keynes, 27–38.

This is a stimulating and interesting chapter that considers the importance of including cultural issues in gerontology. There are some complex issues debated in the paper, which includes a comprehensive reading list.

Mold F, Fitzpatrick JM, Roberts J (2005) Caring for minority ethnic older people in nursing care homes. *British Journal of Nursing* **14**, 601–6.

This article discusses the issues in relation to caring for older people in nursing homes. It provides a useful framework and some key strategies.

Ndoro R and Marimirofa M (2004) West African older people in the UK with dementia. *Mental Health Practice* **7**, 30–2.

The mental health of older people from minority ethnic groups is often overlooked. The authors of this article consider the issues of dementia within a West African family and provide some practical insights.

Standing Nursing and Midwifery Advisory Committee (SNMAC) (2001) *Caring for older people: a nursing priority – integrating knowledge, practice and values.* Department of Health, London.

This is a report on caring for older people inclusive of all cultures. It offers a wide range of recommendations for the future care of older people, including the educational needs of nurses and adopting culturally sensitive practice.

Wambu O (ed.) (1998) *Empire Windrush – fifty years of writing about Black Britain.* Victor Gollancz, London.

This anthology of African-Caribbean and Asian writings charts the experiences of the first waves of migrants to the UK. Within the text there are essays, poetry and fiction which tackle issues such as racism and identity.

WEBSITES

http://www.advisorybodies.doh.gov.uk/snmac/caringforolderpeople.pdf
This is a direct link to the DoH report: *Caring for older people: a nursing priority.* The focus was on the standards of nursing care given to older people in acute hospitals.

http://www.ageconcern.org.uk/AgeConcern/black_minority_ethnic_links.asp
This links directly to the Age Concern webpage for black and minority ethnic elders.

http://www.jrf.org.uk/publications black-and-minority-ethnic-older-peoples-views-research-findings
This website links directly to a report on black and minority ethnic people's views about research findings and their involvement, as well as how it can bring about change in their lives.

http://www.scie.org.uk/publications/guides/guide03/minority/index.asp
Social Care Institute for Excellence (SCIE): this website links directly to a report on assessing the mental health needs of older people in black and minority ethnic communities.

11 Caring for the health needs of migrants, refugees and asylum seekers

Christine Hogg

INTRODUCTION

Migrants, refugees and asylum seekers are not a new or recent phenomenon. In the twenty-first century, war, persecution, political unrest, hunger, conflict, adverse economic conditions and social upheaval have led to significant demographic changes and the migration of populations. However, some health professionals may feel ill-equipped to deal with the complex medical and social needs of asylum seekers and refugees. Refugees and asylum seekers are often considered a single homogeneous population but the two groups have different needs and risk factors. There is also much diversity within groups as people originate from different parts of the world and have differing experiences and backgrounds.

> **This chapter will discuss the following issues:**
>
> * migration and health;
> * the universal legal definitions of refugee and asylum seeker status;
> * the healthcare needs of refugees and asylums seekers, focusing on mental health, children and young people's health, the effects of torture and women's health.

MIGRATION AND HEALTH

Migration

The UK has a long history of having received migrants, refugees and asylum seekers. For example, in post-war Britain, the UK drew from the Indian subcontinent and the Caribbean in order to help rebuild the economy.

Migration is often described as being caused by two factors: the 'push' factor (conditions that force people to leave their country such as oppression, violence, civil war, etc.) or 'pull' factors (the promise of better prospects, employment opportunities, etc.). In recent years the 'pull' factors in Western Europe – demand for labour, good economic conditions and opportunities – has attracted migrants from other parts of Europe, in particular former Eastern block countries. Citizens of the UK are also migrating to countries such as Australia, New Zealand and North America, 'pulled' by favourable economic conditions and the promise of better pay and conditions. It is estimated that 427 000 people emigrated from the UK in 2008 (Office for National Statistics, 2009). However, even when the 'pull' factors are high and seemingly beneficial, migration can be a stressful experience and migrants can still experience a period of adjustment. This period of adjustment occurs when a migrant needs to find out about the new culture they are entering. This means learning a new language, new customs and social norms, and encountering new foods and new laws. This is known as 'acculturation' and is a process of adaptation, which, depending on the individual, may take time.

Some migrants choose to lose their own cultural identity, preferring to fully embrace the cultural norms and values of the host country. This process is known as assimilation. Assimilation may also depend on factors such as the ability to speak the new language, social and economic well-being and gender. So, for example, older women may have considerably more difficulties than younger men in gaining employment. Others, however, prefer to remain apart, retaining the practices and values of their culture. Many people find a middle way. The process and experiences of living and adjusting to a new culture is individual. However, migration is a stressful and challenging time as people adjust to new lifestyles and new communities. Migrants often leave behind family and friends and their grief and sense of detachment may surprise them, as may the feeling of being an 'outsider'. Some may experience bouts of acute homesickness and isolation and expectations of the better life they expected might not be met.

Reflective exercise

Think of a time when you were a stranger somewhere. You may have been on holiday or working in an unfamiliar town or country.

1. What was it like? Describe you feelings.
2. How did your behaviour change as a result of being a stranger?

Refugees and asylum seekers

I had no husband left, no children, no friends, no roof over my head, no past, in short. I never imagined that when I left Rwanda, I would feel abruptly and profoundly torn apart. Especially as the bodies of my husband and children lay in common graves, in this country which never wanted us. As far I was concerned, I had nothing left to do on that soil, which swallowed up my family in an ocean of torture, humiliation, suffering unmatched – perpetrated by our brothers the Rwandans. I thought myself disgusted with my own country.

('The Road to Refuge', BBC)

Since 1945, civil war, unrest and violations of human rights in some countries has led to large numbers of people seeking refuge in other countries or people being internally displaced in their own country. Refugees may flee war, political oppression, violence or sexual or physical abuse.

The 1951 Refugee Convention was established after the Second World War to ensure that atrocities such as the Holocaust were never allowed to happen again. The UK is one of 142 countries that signed up to it. The United Nations High Commission on Refugees (UNHCR) uses the words of Euripides (431 BC) to describe the plight of being a refugee: 'There is no greater sorrow on earth than the loss of one's native land'. Asylum is a human right and is recognized by the 1951 United Nations Convention. Under the convention, countries are obliged to consider the application of anyone who claims refugee status and grant that person refuge on the basis of evidence.

Under the 1951 United Nations Convention, a refugee is a person who:

> **… owing to a well founded fear of being persecuted for reasons of race, religion, nationality, membership in a particular social group or political opinion, is outside the country of his nationality, and is unable to or, owing to such fear is unwilling to avail himself of the protection of that country.**

(Convention Relating to the Status of Refugees, United Nations, 1951)

A refugee therefore is a person whose asylum application has been successful. An asylum seeker is someone who has submitted an application for protection under the Geneva Convention and is awaiting a decision from the UK Home Office. An asylum seeker may describe himself or herself as a refugee, but they are classified as an asylum seeker while they are awaiting a decision on their application for refugee status.

The number of refugees in the worldwide population is difficult to measure but estimates are around 9.4 million (United Nations High Commissioner for Refugees, 2006). Most of these remain in developing countries. In the UK the number of applications for asylum in 2008 was 25 930. This figure has reduced significantly from its highest point in 2002 (84 130) (The Home Office) following increased restrictions. The most common nationalities of applicants were Afghan, Iranian, Chinese, Iraqi and Eritrean. Contrary to widespread beliefs and misconceptions, the UK received a lower number of applications than other European Union (EU) states. Sweden, for example, received 16 per cent of the total number of applications. Quickfall (2004) notes that Glasgow City Council has actively welcomed asylum applicants because Scotland has a declining population.

The number of asylum seekers is low and generally they are concentrated in particular parts of certain cities. In 2007, 80 per cent were under the age of 35 years only 4 per cent were 50 years and older, and 70 per cent of asylum seekers were male (The Home Office). In terms of health care this is perhaps a positive in that younger populations may be healthier. However, the majority of refugees throughout the world are women and many refugee families in the UK are without a parent.

The image of asylum seekers and refugees

The terms asylum seeker and refugee are often used in association with negative perceptions and with derogatory terms such as 'bogus', for example 'bogus asylum seekers' and 'scrounger'. The Refugee Council note that reporting in the media is often factually incorrect and unbalanced. A headline such as 'Britain is the Asylum Capital of the World' (*The Express* 23/3/05) is refuted as the UK is home to just 3 per cent of 9.2 million refugees worldwide. The UK might be a desirable destination for refugees and asylum seekers as people may have friends or family here, and English is widely spoken throughout the world. Indeed, the UK was 16th in the league table of industrialized countries for the number of asylum seekers per head of population. By contrast, Pakistan has 2.4 million Afghan refugees who fled the Taliban regime. Statistics show that two-thirds of refugees are living in developing countries, often in refugee camps (http://www.unhcr.org). Asylum seekers may sometimes be described as 'over-running' a country and are likely to be viewed with suspicion or as 'cheating the system'. Conversely, the term refugee tends to evoke sympathy.

In the UK, refugees and asylum seekers have perhaps always been viewed with suspicion. Prior to the Second World War, Jewish refugees fleeing racial oppression in Nazi Germany faced suspicion and prejudice in the UK:

> The way stateless Jews from Germany are pouring in from every port of this country is becoming an outrage: the number of aliens entering the country through back door – a problem to which the *Daily Mail* has repeatedly pointed …

(Karp, 2002)

Box 11.1 *Facts about asylum seekers and refugees*

- The top 10 refugee-producing countries in 2006 all have poor human rights records or are places where war or conflict is ongoing.
- There is no such thing as an 'illegal' or bogus asylum seeker as under international law, anyone has the right to apply for asylum in the UK and remain here until the authorities have assessed their claim.
- Despite the labels 'scrounger' or 'bogus' being attached to asylum seekers, they do not come to the UK to collect benefits. Evidence shows that many do not know about the UK asylum or benefits systems before arriving.
- Most asylum seekers live in poverty and experience poor health and hunger. They cannot jump the queue for local housing and cannot choose where they live. Indeed, accommodation allocated to them is nearly all 'hard to let' properties.
- About 83 per cent of female refugees and asylum seekers say they do not go out at night because they fear abuse and harassment (see Refugee Council website in list at the end of this chapter).
- The vast majority of refugees are law-abiding citizens and are no more likely to commit crime than anyone else.
- Many refugees have academic or teaching qualifications. It is estimated that there are more than 1500 refugee teachers in England.
- Asylum-seeking children contribute very positively to schools around the country.

Source: The Refugee Council (www.refugeecouncil.org.uk)

Misconceptions are highlighted in a story told by a colleague working in local authority housing:

> I was contacted one day by a senior healthcare professional who said that he had had a number of people in his practice complaining that some Muslim asylum seekers resident in a house in the area were deliberately stirring up feelings by their display of a picture of Osama Bin Laden in their front window. It was felt by many passers by that this was upsetting and was creating racial tensions in the area. On investigation the housing worker found that the house was inhabited by a group of Portuguese migrant workers employed in the local canning factory and that the picture was actually Jesus Christ. They had put this in the window as they couldn't afford curtains at the time.

1. To claim asylum is a human right.
2. The number of people seeking asylum in the UK has fallen in recent years.
3. The average age of the refugee and asylum seeker population is generally lower than that of the indigenous population.

HEALTH CARE FOR REFUGEES AND ASYLUM SEEKERS

The healthcare status of migrants is generally lower than the indigenous populations but for refugees this may be compounded because of previous experiences. Refugees by definition are people who have been forced or 'pushed' out of their home country. They may have experienced political oppression, torture, violence, social injustices and economic hardships prior to seeking refuge elsewhere. They may have experienced or witnessed intimidation, violence or rape and may well be scarred both emotionally and physically by their experiences.

The decision to leave may have been sudden and secretive so they may not have had time to sort their affairs or say farewells. They may have also been living in refugee camps, which can be hostile and frightening places. The process of flight itself may have been lengthy, dangerous and traumatic. On arrival in the host country people may feel a sense of immediate relief that they are in a safe haven while at the same time they are faced with difficult bureaucratic processes, language problems and the uncertainty of the application decision process. They are likely to be short of money, living in an unfamiliar country where the climate is often colder than their home country.

Reflective exercise

Consider this scenario: you are woken up in the middle of the night to be told that you and your family must escape now as your life is in danger. You have 10 minutes to pack your bags.

1. What would you take with you?
2. What has led to you making that decision?
3. How do you think you would feel?

Legal entitlements to health care

A person who has formally applied for asylum in the UK is entitled to NHS treatment without charge for as long as their application (including appeals) is under consideration. They are entitled to register with a GP and are deemed to be 'ordinary residents'. However, for some, accessing care may be a bewildering and confusing process. A young woman from a refugee community notes:

> Like here it is small and slow and if you don't have an appointment … the doctor is always busy and there are so many people all the time … you can't find somewhere to sit … In the surgery … a lot of people just sitting and a long time to wait … That's if you don't have an appointment …

(Williamson et al., 2009, p. 37)

Healthcare issues for refugees and asylum seekers

Although refugees and asylum seekers are not a homogeneous group, studies demonstrate that, in general, their health is poorer as a result of the process of migration (Carbello, 2007). They suffer poorer health in their country of settlement mainly as a result of adverse effects of poverty, poor housing, etc. These patterns are similar to the general health and well-being of minority ethnic groups.

Consider the following Case Study to explore some of the health issues faced by both of these groups.

Case study

Marika and Bernard have been married for 15 years. They arrived in the UK with their children a year ago, coming from a refugee camp in Malawi. The couple have three children aged 13 years, 7 years and 14 months old. They are finding it difficult to adjust to life in Britain. They live in local authority housing and receive income support and child benefit. Marika finds it difficult to cope in winter – the children struggle to wake up in the morning and they can't afford new clothes for winter. Bernard can't speak English so finds it difficult to communicate and is unable to help the children with their homework. One of the children is showing aggressive behaviour at school and there have been reports from school that he is bullying other children. Marika is tired much of the time, she complains of terrible headaches and seems hostile and angry to people trying to help her.

In Malawi the family experienced various kinds of trauma, as they had been separated while fleeing the war. They had been united in the camp but Marika and Bernard found out that their son, aged 7, had been recruited into the army as a child soldier.

The family avoids discussing issues from the past and say that they are happy to be in the UK. However the health visitor notices that Marika is neglecting herself and that Bernard seems to be away from the home. She advises Marika to see the GP but she refuses saying that she will be 'OK'.

The following information may help the reader to gain more understanding of the complex issues that impact on this family's health and well-being.

Refugees come from a variety of backgrounds and often show great resilience in their capacity to survive. Their experiences are likely to be diverse and their health status may be dependent on varying factors such as their prior experiences or the healthcare provision in their home country. For example, for some refugees and asylum seekers their home country may not have had good immunization programmes and this might make them susceptible to communicable diseases in the UK. Common communicable diseases are tuberculosis (TB), hepatitis A, B and C, HIV/AIDS and parasitic infections (British Medical Association, 2002). Some refugees might not understand the role of the GP or may have differing experiences of healthcare provision, so, for example, might expect a hospital referral or may be accustomed only to dealing with medical staff and may not be used to receiving help or advice from other healthcare professionals, such as nurses.

Some refugees may suffer from the adverse consequences of living in camps for extended periods. For example TB can spread rapidly through cramped and squalid living conditions in refugee camps. Women in particular may have been subject to sexual violence and abuse in refugee camps (Kelly and Stevenson, 2006).

Burnett and Peel (2001) estimate that as many as 20 per cent of asylum seekers and refugees have severe health problems. They may be placed in low quality temporary accommodation or inadequate or poor housing conditions and are likely to suffer adverse health consequences such as respiratory problems, dermatology problems and infections. Poverty has a negative effect on physical and mental health and thus good living conditions may be central to maintaining good health.

Torture

It is estimated that between 5 per cent and 30 per cent of asylum seekers have been tortured (British Medical Association, 2001). Torture is defined as 'the intentional infliction of severe pain or suffering, whether physical or mental, upon a person in the custody or under control of the accused' (Article 7.2(e) (excerpt of the Rome Statute of the International Criminal Court; cited in Burnett, 2002). Methods of torture commonly experienced are beating, slapping, kicking, burning or electric shocks. Women and some men may have been subjected to rape or other forms of sexual violence. The perpetrators of torture may be the military, police, government agencies or even health workers. The physical effects of war and torture may include:

- fractures and crushed bones;
- wounds and burns which may become infected;
- keloid scars;
- head injuries which may result in epilepsy, poor memory and concentration;
- ear damage – slapping round the ears is common during interrogation, resulting in otitis media;
- eye damage from detention in dark rooms;
- land mine injuries;
- partial loss of vision;
- dental problems caused by torture (British Medical Association, 2002; Burnett, 2002).

Schott and Henley (1996) note that in some countries doctors are involved in carrying out torture and thus medical instruments that are normally considered benign (for example syringes and oxygen masks) may be associated with methods of torture and may re-awaken terrors. People who have been tortured may not want to disclose or discuss their experiences, fearing shame or believing that they should and could be allowed to forget their experiences. However, during physical examinations they may become extremely anxious; they may feel frightened about being touched and may not cooperate with some medical and nursing procedures. They may be distrustful of healthcare workers and avoid seeking help as a result.

Patel (2009) states that therapeutic approaches to torture should:

> ... not aim narrowly to 'fix' symptoms but serve a significant function in bearing witness to atrocity, in offering humanity, compassion and honest communication ... Experiences of powerlessness, hopelessness and worthlessness need to be acknowledged and explored.

(Patel, 2009, p. 131)

Key points

1. Refugees and asylum seekers are likely to have been through adverse experiences that may negatively affect their health.
2. They are entitled to receive NHS treatment and care in the UK.
3. They may be vulnerable to health problems related to poverty and poor housing.

MENTAL HEALTH ISSUES

Bhugra and Jones (2001) argue that, as a group, migrants are more vulnerable to mental health problems. Thompson (2001) notes that the incidence of mental health problems in refugees is five times higher than the general population. Refugees and asylum seekers commonly experience mental health problems that often are related to their past experiences. Some might show signs of anxiety, depression, guilt or shame as a result of their previous traumas such as rape, torture or oppression.

There is no doubt that refugees and asylum seekers are vulnerable to emotional health problems either owing to their past experiences or to their current experiences (e.g. living in poor housing, attempting to adapt to new circumstances or being the victims of racism). Carey Wood *et al.* (1995) note that two-thirds of respondents said they had experienced some form of anxiety or depression. Burnett and Peel (2001) note that refugees and asylum seekers in primary care often show signs of panic attacks, agoraphobia, disturbed sleep patterns, poor memory or concentration. The stress of uncertainty about asylum claims can cause heart disease, increased susceptibility to infection, cancer and gastrointestinal difficulties (British Medical Association, 2002). In a study by Williamson *et al.* (2009) young people noted that money or lack of financial security causes stress for some parents.

> Well if you don't have money sometimes it can cause most parents depression and stress and that affects other people who are living in the family because when the parents don't have money and they've got stress they take it out on their kids ...

(Williamson et al., 2009, p. 27)

Others may be experiencing the negative effects of family breakdown such as grief, isolation and homesickness. Families may suffer separation during civil or national unrest. It is not uncommon for one adult to flee with the possibility that partners or children may follow later.

McColl *et al.* (2008) argue that the psychological health of asylum seekers in the UK is affected by the 'seven Ds:

1. **Discrimination:** being stigmatized by the host countries. This could be through the media or political processes.
2. **Detention:** there is evidence that the health of people held in detention centres worsens as access to health care may be impaired (Fazel and Silvoe, 2006).
3. **Dispersal:** asylum seekers generally have no choice in where they are sent and they may be moved many times. They may be cut off from social networks.
4. **Destitution:** asylum seekers receive benefits that amount to 70 per cent of the lowest level of income support.
5. **Denial of health care:** asylum seekers and refugees are entitled to free access to primary health services in the UK, although failed asylum seekers are no longer eligible for free secondary health care except in cases that are deemed life threatening.
6. **Delayed decision:** there is evidence that the length of the asylum process adversely affects health (Steel *et al.*, 2006).
7. **Denial of the right to work:** asylum seekers are prevented from undertaking work. Lack of work can inhibit social integration and increase poverty.

The majority of asylum seekers and refugees have no mental illness and are able to use their own coping strategies and resources to survive adverse circumstances. However, there is evidence that refugees and asylum seekers are more likely to suffer depression, anxiety and post-traumatic stress disorder (PTSD) than the general population (Burnett and Peel, 2001; Fazel *et al.*, 2005).

The traumatic experiences that some refugees and asylum seekers may have experienced might lead to people behaving in ways that may be described in Western frameworks as PTSD. The symptoms of PTSD include:

- anxiety;
- irritability;
- reliving the experiences in flashbacks or nightmares;
- avoidance of reminders of events/increased nervous system arousal (e.g. hypervigilance, jumpiness, excessive anger, sleep problems);
- low mood;
- frequent crying;
- headaches, palpations and sweating.

The use of the term PTSD is perhaps controversial. It is a 'Western' concept and healthcare workers should exercise caution before labelling people. However, the effects of trauma may be hidden as this health visitor describes:

> I had one refugee family from [country]. The children were on the register for child abuse ... she (the mother) always appeared very depressed. And we could never get to the bottom of this. And she would just say she was fine, she was fine. Things were happening at school and they were really concerned and I would see them at home again ... Eventually it all came out that her father was murdered in front of her when the country was in upheaval and there was a coup and the country was in anarchy. She was very traumatized. Her husband then left her

> with all the children. She has no other relatives or children around ... She is actually suffering from post traumatic stress, you know, and it has been quite some time before we actually found out that her father had been executed in front of her.
>
> *(Drennan and Joseph, 2005, p. 160)*

It is important therefore to be cautious about labelling people with a psychiatric disorder as this may compound the sense of shame, fear and isolation they may be experiencing. Furthermore, being diagnosed with a mental health problem may carry taboo or stigma and this may further alienate people. However, if the person continues to express or show signs of psychological difficulties, help from mental health services may be required.

Burnett (2002) notes that symptoms that may require specialist help include:

- consistent failure to perform basic tasks;
- frequently expressed suicidal ideas or plans;
- social withdrawal and self-neglect;
- behaviour or talk that is abnormal within the person's culture;
- aggression.

McColl *et al.* (2008) argue that by focusing on PTSD as a disorder, health workers might neglect current adversities causing distress. There is some indication that post-migration stresses may affect an individual's emotional well-being (Iverson and Morken, 2004).

The treatment for PTSD (National Institute for Clinical Excellence, 2005) suggests cognitive behaviour therapy or eye-movement desensitization reprocessing (EMDR). Summerfield (2001) points out that some people may prefer problem-focused rather than emotion-focused psychological work.

Working with people in emotional distress

Understanding and helping people who have mental health problems is challenging and, to date, there is little concrete evidence to facilitate the process. However there are some general principles.

Understanding the challenges and experiences of being an asylum seeker and refugee may help the health worker to empathize with the person's present difficulties. This might include gaining an understanding of the geopolitical context of the person's country of origin. It may also be useful to consider the language, cultural norm and expectations of healthcare provision and the medico-legal issues involved in the person's background. Information about health care is accessible from the World Health Organization (WHO), and the BBC website provides up-to-date, essential information on the geopolitical context of nations. Other agencies such as Asylum Aid, Health for Asylum Seekers and Refugees Portal (HARP) and the Refugee Council provide up-to-date information, support and guidance (see the website list at end of this chapter).

It should be remembered that asylum seekers and refugees are not a homogeneous group so there is no one method or approach to working with them. Health workers need to approach people with the principles of cultural sensitivity and cultural competence (Papadopoulos, 2003). This embraces the notion of clients as partners in care and the creation of an environment in which ideas, information and issues are shared, understood and exchanged between the client and the professional.

Working with people who may be experiencing mental health problems

There are some general guidelines when working with people from refugee and asylum seeker groups who may be experiencing mental health problems.

Prior to the assessment process, the health worker should find out what language the person prefers to speak in and arrange interpreters accordingly. Care and sensitivity should be taken when arranging interviews as past adverse experiences may impede the process of assessment. For example, if a woman has suffered sexual violence she may feel more comfortable being interviewed by female staff and using a female interpreter. It is also important to remember that some people may express their distress through physical symptoms and that they may describe their problems as physical and not psychological. In some cultures mental health problems may be taboo or stigmatizing and thus people may prefer to express their distress through physical symptoms such as headaches, weakness or pain.

Some people may find that the process of being listened to is therapeutic in itself. Allowing a story to be told may be helpful and supportive. Burnett (2002) advised listening but not expecting too much in one session, with Burnett and Fassil (2003) citing a Glasgow GP who stated that:

> **The catharsis of being listened to for long enough and patiently enough can be all that is needed to restore health to nearly a normal level.**

> *(Burnett and Fassil, 2003, p. 36)*

However, it must not be assumed that people should be expected to talk in order to recover and, indeed, talking through a problem may not be considered appropriate or helpful. Others may be extremely suspicious or fearful of disclosing personal information believing it may lead to denial of refugee status. Tribe (2002) notes that the idea of talking to a psychiatrist who is a stranger may be alien, particularly as he or she may be associated with 'madness'.

Discussing distressing events may be indicated but this should be undertaken at a pace and at a time when people feel comfortable. Rather than directly questioning about experiences of torture and violence Burnet and Fassil (2003) suggest the following as a gentle indirect opener:

> **I know some people in your situation have experienced torture and violence. This is something I might be able to help you with. Has this ever happened to you?**

> *(Burnett and Fassil, 2003, p. 38)*

Weaver and Burns (2001) suggest that discussion of distressing events should be done in a safe environment without probing or pushing a refugee to disclose information about trauma. They advise the health worker to take cues from the client about whether or not talking about the trauma is therapeutic or retraumatizing. The worker should be prepared to stop the discussion if it seems to be harmful.

Counselling may also be an unfamiliar concept for some people who might not be accustomed to talking about themselves or discussing intimate issues outside the close family. Refugees from Mozambique describe 'forgetting' as their usual way of coping with difficulties and Ethiopians call this 'active forgetting' (Summerfield, 1996). Burnett and Fassil (2003) recommend building on people's strengths and giving them control. For example, assisting people in meetings to make decisions may help them to feel less powerless. They quote the stance of a psychologist in London who described the importance of 'being a witness' and of 'politicizing and not pathologizing anger'.

Mental health needs and emotional distress may not be addressed by talking therapies but instead some people may respond to activities or help that reduces their social isolation. Gorst-Unsworth and Goldberg (1998) in a study of 84 Iraqi refugees found that depression was more closely linked to poor social support than with a history of torture. In this group depression was found to be more common (44 per cent) than PTSD. Depression was linked to poor social support, separation from children, lack of political organizations in exile, few confidants and social activities. Mental well-being may benefit from improved housing, acceptance in communities and access to links and friendships with people from the host country and their own cultural groups. Practical help in finding employment or education may be as helpful in allowing people to gain improved self-esteem.

Working with asylum seekers and refugees and hearing stories of trauma and oppression may be painful and difficult for health workers, and support and supervision should be sought on a regular basis.

> ### Key points
>
> 1. When working with people who have experienced trauma, care must be taken as being diagnosed with a mental illness may be stigmatizing and may compound people's distress.
> 2. Mental well-being may be enhanced through helping people to feel more in control of their social and environmental situation.
> 3. Working with people who have experienced trauma may be overwhelming and distressing for the health professional and guidance and support is advisable.

WOMEN'S HEALTH

The majority of the world's refugees are women although the number of women reaching industrialized countries and obtaining asylum is lower. As a group, women refugees are highly vulnerable and are more likely to suffer deteriorating health. They are less likely to have English language skills or to be literate. Women with children may neglect their own health but may bring their children for health consultations (Burnett, 2002).

Sexual health issues

HIV/AIDS

Some asylum seekers and refugees come from countries where exposure to HIV/AIDS is greater. Women may have been placed at risk of HIV/AIDS in countries where sexual crime is perpetrated by the military who may have a higher incidence of HIV. Other women may have been forced into paid, unprotected sex in order to survive and may again be at risk of HIV. HIV/AIDS continues to carry a stigma and many people may fear that disclosure of their experiences may bring shame.

Alternatively, these experiences may evoke strong negative emotions in people who may wish to forget the incidents rather than repeat them. Other people may fear that a positive HIV test will lead to deportation from the UK.

Rape

Rape has been used through history as a weapon of warfare to degrade and humiliate a nation. Women are more likely to be the subject of sexual or physical violence and many have stories that go untold. In most countries sexual violence is a shameful and taboo subject, leaving many women to feel guilty. Some women may prefer to suffer in silence or in isolation, fearing rejection or hoping that the memories of atrocities may, in time, fade. Women may be shunned by their communities and families. They might also find intimate examinations and investigations such as cervical screening to be difficult. Women may express their distress through physical symptoms. For example, they may complain of frequent headaches, panic attacks or forgetfulness. For other women, unwanted pregnancy may occur from sexual violence and rape and although termination of pregnancy may be stigmatizing and unacceptable, it may be a choice for some women. Women in this situation may need to have female workers and access to as much relevant information as possible.

Pregnancy and childbirth

Women may be vulnerable to health problems during pregnancy and childbirth. Access to antenatal care might have been poor in their home country and they may have suffered poor nutrition at home, in refugee camps, in fleeing and in their current circumstances as poverty and poor housing conditions compromise their health status.

CHILDREN AND YOUNG PEOPLE'S HEALTH

> When you're a refugee your life is never complete. There is always part of your life that is missing, and that part is home.
>
> *(Burnett and Fassil, 2003, p.10)*

Children and young people claiming asylum are a particularly vulnerable group. Consider the following example:

> One family we had in here, a [ethnic group] but living in [country]. The child at that time when I met him was about 8 months old. The child was continually being brought to the clinic and to the GP's surgery, mainly for problems around eating ... This family had problems. They've been the victims of torture in [country] and also the father of the family had been beaten up over here in a racist incident as well ... I managed to work with the psychologist with that family around the eating problem ... and the child is no longer being presented and he is a different child now.
>
> *(Drennan and Joseph, 2005, p. 161)*

Refugee children are at risk of ill health. They may suffer from physical problems associated with their physical and social deprivation prior to entering the UK, for example, if they have been living in a country where healthcare resources are scarce. They may have endured difficult and traumatic experiences while in flight. For some children and young people the flight experience may have been bewildering or frightening.

Central to the health development and well-being of any child is the ability of parents, carers or guardians to meet the needs of the child. In some cases asylum-seeking and refugee parents may themselves struggle to cope and may have endured severe adverse experiences that might compromise their ability to care for their children. When caring for the health needs of any child it is necessary to see them in the context of their family life, structure and context, but this is even more important in refugees and asylum-seeking families.

Box 11.2 *Some questions that may be asked or considered when caring for the health needs of a child*

Who is in this family?

How is the family made up?

Who is missing from the family?

What recent experiences have affected this family?

What was the status of the family in their home country?

What are the relationships between family members like? (Parents to children, children to grandparents, siblings)

Is there extended family nearby or is the family alone?

What relationships/connections exist outside the home?

How does the family see itself (e.g. complete, normal, incomplete, fractured)?

What are the strengths of the family?

How have they coped in adversity?

What are the positions in the family? (e.g. who is seen as head, if any, of the household?)

Physical health issues for refugee and asylum-seeking children

Health for children may be compromised *in utero* if the mother has left a country where there is poor antenatal care or poor nutrition. Pregnant women may also have low expectations of antenatal healthcare provision, or may be fearful or mistrustful of health services. Some children are born in countries where prolonged war, conflict or famine has led to poor child health facilities, which may lead to poor screening facilities and poor immunization programmes. Thus, routine screening for health conditions such as phenylketonuria or congenital dislocation of the hip may not have been offered. (Detailed information about immunization programmes is available from the World Health Organization (WHO) – see list of websites at the end of this chapter.)

Children from refugee families are more likely to be living in substandard or crowded housing or detention facilities and therefore are more prone to having accidents in the home, such as burns and falls. They are also more likely to have road traffic accidents, particularly if they have been brought up in rural areas (Levenson and Sharma, 1999). Refugee children and young people may also suffer from under-nutrition, particularly if they have been living in adverse circumstances such as refugee camps.

Other issues to take into consideration when working with families/children and young people are whether or not the child/family understands the importance the health services attaches to confidentiality. This may be vital when people are coming from countries where health service workers are involved in the perpetration of oppression, torture or violence. Families may also need help to understand the function of health visitors, school nurses and other health service personnel who may be involved in their care as these roles may be unfamiliar.

Other specific health issues that may be noted with children and young people are female genital mutilation (FGM), tropical diseases and recurrent conditions such as malaria. It is also worth noting if the child or young person has any physical injuries resulting from war or torture. Some children and young people may even have been child soldiers.

School and school life may play an important role in the health and well-being of refugee children. It may represent an opportunity to belong and to become part of a community, to make friends and to learn. School may also represent a haven – a place of safety, security and stability for children and young people. School nurses can play an important role in helping children to access health care. However, school may also be a place where refugee children and young people are subjected to bullying and racial abuse. They may also find that they are behind in their schooling because their life has been disrupted by flight from war and conflict. Refugee children may also inevitably need to learn a new language and adapt to different ways of learning in school. Generally it takes 2 years to acquire the expression of language to the level of the indigenous population. Their parents may also struggle to support their children in homework if, for example, their English is poor. However, it is important to note that they are often very resilient and like many migrants are often determined and motivated to do well and succeed. Integration and inclusion in schooling is a lynchpin to the well-being of refugee and asylum-seeker children.

Child protection issues

Children and young people may be living in families where domestic violence occurs. This may be occurring between parents, and a partner's violent behaviour may be tolerated because of the violence he or she may have experienced. Children and young people may be witnesses to such violence and this may cause emotional distress. Mental illness may also be affecting a parent's ability to care for a child. Parents themselves may be suffering from mental health problems even if they have not experienced trauma. Thus their abilities to parent may be compromised. Physical punishments of children may be more acceptable and common in families and thus a distinction should be made between what constitutes discipline and physical abuse. It is important to note that parenting and child-rearing patterns differ throughout cultures. Parents need support but ultimately the welfare of the child is priority.

In some cases young people describe 'living between two cultures'. Often, they may assimilate and adapt to their new country more quickly than their parents. They may want to adopt the fashions, language and behaviours of their peers at school, but at home expectations about dress rules, for example, may be different. Young people may describe living a 'double life' and this can cause some emotional stress and confusion. Families that originate from countries where traditional gender roles are still important may feel that their offspring, in particular their teenage children, are rejecting their values and morals and conflict may occur. Young women and girls, in particular, may struggle with leading a 'double life'.

Unaccompanied minors

Lewis (2007) offers this insight into the experiences of children:

> Afghan children Ramazan and Abdul-Khaliq admit they are haunted by their journeys, especially in their nightmares. Ramazan lost his family as they crossed a border on foot; rushing through a rough mountain terrain in the dead of night with hundreds of other refugees, they became separated in the chaos. "I was shouting, calling their names", he said. Whenever I asked the smuggler [to help] he said be quiet, I will take you to your parents. I was crying. Some of them [fellow travellers or agents] were laughing. Others said: "don't worry, we will take you to your parents."

(Lewis, 2007, p. 1)

Unaccompanied children are defined as those young people under the age of 18 years without adult family members or guardians. They are a particularly vulnerable group. Under the age of 15 years they will usually be 'looked after' by the local authority in the UK. They are usually defined as 'in need' and services are provided under Section 20 of the Children's Act (Department of Health, 1989). They will be provided with foster care or residential home placement, an allocated social worker, a care plan, financial cash support and full leaving-care services. Those aged 17 and 18 years usually receive services under Section 17 of the Children Act (1989) and may be living in bed and breakfast accommodation or hostels.

Emotional health needs of children and young people

The process and experience of asylum-seeking and becoming a refugee may lead children and young people to experience a range of emotions and feelings. Many are likely to have experienced terror, shame, grief, fear, helplessness and enormous anger. Children, for example, may have experienced imprisonment, beatings, rape, mines, bombs or gunshots. They may have been tortured or have witnessed torture. They may have been forced into becoming child soldiers and may have inflicted violence on others. Some are likely to have experienced oppression in the form of persecution because of their family's religious or political beliefs for example. It is likely that they have experienced loss of friends, family or siblings. They may also have witnessed or experienced violence:

Case study

A 12-year-old boy was referred by the local secondary school because of repeated aggressive outbursts that led to his permanent exclusion. He came from Angola where at the age of 8 he had seen his parents killed because one of his brothers had defected from the army. He and another brother were able to flee via Congo and came to London where they lived together. On interview it was found that he was having flashbacks and nightmares of his parents' killing. (*From Hodes 2000, p. 64.*)

Children respond to such experiences in different ways, and they may feel under pressure to keep information secret. Children who have been separated from their families may face particular problems. Some feel that their parents have failed to protect them and may feel disconnected from their carers. Their emotional health may be compromised, which can result in problems arising in other areas – for example, they may refuse to go to school, or they may be disruptive in school and face exclusion. Other behaviours they may display are listed in Box 11.3.

> ### Box 11.3 Behaviours exhibited by children (Burnett and Fazil, 2003)
>
> - withdrawal, lack of energy and lethargy
> - aggression and poor temper-control
> - irritability
> - poor concentration
> - repetitive thoughts about traumatic events
> - poor appetite, over-eating, breathing difficulties, pains and dizziness
> - regression (e.g. bed-wetting)
> - failure to thrive
> - nightmares and disturbed sleep
> - nervousness and anxiety
> - difficulty in making relationships with other children and adults
> - lack of trust in adults
> - clinging, school refusal
> - hyperactivity and hyper alertness
> - impulsive behaviour
> - self harm
> - unexplained headaches, stomach aches or other body pains
> - memory impairment

Children and young people may also take on responsibilities at home caring for parents whose health and well-being may be compromised, or assuming other roles such as interpreting, if their language skills are better than their parents'. Children and young people may also be affected by their own parents' psychological state; adults may be preoccupied with the implications of their refugee status and the traumas they have suffered. Hence, parents may not be able to take care of their children's emotional well-being.

Children and young people may face the negative effects of the attitudes of the host country such as bullying at school or racism and hostility in the community. This may be especially difficult when their expectations of a country as a haven and a place of safety are dashed. Other factors such as poverty, unemployment, poor housing and loss of status may also undermine their sense of well-being.

Strategies for helping promote emotional well-being in children and young people

Very few children need psychiatric care but they may instead need strategies to help them develop a range of coping skills and to improve their resilience (see Box 11.4). Care should be taken in labelling children and young people with a mental health problem as this may be stigmatizing.

> **Box 11.4 Strategies to help children develop a range of coping skills**
>
> - The negative effects of emotional distress may be ameliorated by having a key adult (ideally a parent) to have a close relationship with. This may help them to maintain and preserve a sense of belonging.
> - Children and young people may need time and space to talk about their experiences. This may be facilitated by creative therapies such as art, music, drama and story-telling. However, they may not be able to articulate their stories as they might not have the language skills or vocabulary to describe their feelings. Also, they may live in families where it is not felt appropriate to express feelings, or parents and siblings may have experienced traumatic or difficult experiences. It may be beneficial to talk with a health worker in an environment where time is afforded and privacy is maintained.
> - It is worth remembering that some children and young people may have experienced trauma or unpleasant events at the hands of adults.
> - Children and young people may benefit from keeping links with their refugee community in order to develop and integrate their cultural identity. This might help them to feel connected and supported. It may help them come together in a group to discuss their situation among other peers who understand their stresses and issues. They may also benefit from being part of a local community, for example a youth group, football team, etc.

Some families may avoid formal therapy with health professionals if the interviews remind them of traumatic adverse past experiences, such as torture and interrogation; parents might not be able to listen to their children's stories as they may be too painful. Hodes (2000) notes that some research demonstrates that many refugees, having escaped and survived terrible circumstances, may want to look forward and not back. For parents this might be expressed as their high aspirations for their children, preferring them to go to school rather than clinic or therapy sessions. Support is important in helping to raise their self esteem and provide a sense of belonging. Helping to them to acquire a 'normal life' and a sense of security and safety may be fundamental to this. Healthcare professionals can advocate for children and young people but a holistic approach is necessary where professionals work together to assess needs (e.g. health education and community links).

CONCLUSION

Refugees and asylum seekers have experienced great difficulties but it should be remembered that despite adversities they may often show great resilience and courage. They are not a homogeneous group; they come from diverse countries and backgrounds and their individual experiences are unique. They may have specific health needs as well as communication difficulties. It is important for health workers to take into account their past experiences and the 'road' they have travelled. Evidence shows that for many people there is a need to feel accepted and part of the community, and to be given the opportunity to get on with their lives.

1. Women and children from refugee and asylum-seeker communities are particularly vulnerable.
2. Women may suffer multiple and complex health issues if they have been subjected to sexual violence.
3. Children's emotional and social well-being may be tied into family health issues but schooling is often central to children and young people's well-being.

FURTHER READING

Anonymous (2007) *From here to there: sixteen true tales of immigration to Britain.* Penguin Books, London.

This book is a collection of personal accounts of migration to Britain. The stories are moving and provide an insight into the trauma and difficulties of migration and 'finding a place called home'.

Morehead C (2006) *Human cargo – a journey among refugees.* Vintage Publications, London.

This book is a collection of essays in which the researcher has carefully documented the predicament of refugees and asylum seekers across the world. It is an interesting read with some alarming and harrowing stories of the plight and human cost of migration across the world.

Hosseini K (2003) *The kite runner.* Bloomsbury Publications, London.

This novel traces the story of Amir, a young Afghan boy, his life growing up in Kabul and his forced exile as a refugee to Pakistan.

Tremain R (2008) *The road home.* Chatto & Windus, London.

This novel traces the story of an East European migrant, Lev, to Britain and his struggle to find work and accommodation. It is an interesting account of an 'outsider's' view of the UK.

WEBSITES

http://www.amnesty.org/

Amnesty International provide information and campaigns to protect human rights on an international level.

http://www.asylumaid.org.uk

Asylum Aid is an independent, national charity. They work to secure protection for people seeking refuge in the UK from persecution and human rights abuses abroad.

http://www.asylumsupport.info

Asylum Support (ASAP) is a small national charity which aims to reduce destitution amongst asylum seekers by protecting their legal rights to food and shelter. ASAP specializes in asylum support law – that is, the law relating to asylum seekers' entitlement to housing and welfare support.

http://www.harp.org.uk

HARP (HARP Health for Asylum Seekers and Refugees Portal) website.

http://www.rcn.org.uk/development/practice/social_inclusion/ asylum_seekers_and_refugees

This links directly to the Royal College of Nursing (RCN) website which has a wealth of information with regard to asylum seekers and refugees and links to other relevant websites such as the Children's Society (Supporting refugee young carers and their families – a toolkit), which includes personal stories and some excellent information to help nurses and health professionals care for asylum seekers and refugees.

http://www.refugeecouncil.org.uk/

The Refugee Council. The aim of Refugee Council is to provide support and help to refugees and asylum seekers and to make information and advice available to them directly. The website provides some important information.

http://www.torturecare.org.uk/

Medical Foundation for the Care of Victims of Torture (MFCVT). The Foundation has branches in London Glasgow, Manchester, Newcastle and Birmingham. It provides services for survivors of torture, offering counselling, advice and various forms of therapy.

http://www.unhcr.org/

The United Nations High Commissioner for Refugees (UNHCR) is a humanitarian organization mandated by the United Nations to lead and coordinate international action for the worldwide protection of refugees. The website provides a huge amount of valuable information about the plight of refugees across the world.

http://www.who.int/en/

The WHO website contains a range of information about immunization programmes and other issues.

12 Death and bereavement: a cross-cultural perspective

Karen Holland

INTRODUCTION

Death, dying and grief are personal life experiences that become very public when they occur in a hospital setting. The beliefs, rituals and customs associated with death in different cultures are extremely varied. This includes the nurse's own professional culture where, for a student nurse, meeting death for the first time is part of their initiation into the profession. As our society becomes more multicultural, both nurses and healthcare professionals are exposed to a wider range of spiritual and religious beliefs, which in turn influence the need for care practices to become culturally orientated. This chapter explores the meaning of death and bereavement in different cultures; it also examines various practices that nurses should adopt when caring for those who are dying, their family and friends.

> **This chapter will focus on the following issues:**
>
> - the meaning of death;
>
> - the meaning of bereavement;
>
> - nursing practice and caring for the dying and bereaved, with particular emphasis on Jewish, Sikh and Muslim cultures.

The examples used in this chapter illustrate the main issues for nurses in practice with regard to dealing with death and bereavement experiences, and they are in no way intended to convey a 'recipe' approach to care of the dying. Recommendations for good practice are included.

THE MEANING OF DEATH

Given its simplest meaning, death is the stage when a person ceases to exist in their previous 'physical form' (i.e. biological death). Two other definitions of death have been identified by Sudnow (1967), namely 'clinical death' and 'social death', the former being 'the appearance of death signs upon examination' and the latter 'when the individual is treated essentially as a corpse although still clinically and biologically alive' (Bond and Bond, 1986). An example of social death can be seen in hospitals where patients are moved from the main ward area into side rooms if there is any possibility of them dying. Death can occur at any time and for many reasons (e.g. miscarriage, abortion, suicide, illness, accident or old age).

Determination of the precise point in time at which death occurs has become an important issue in today's technologically advanced society, especially when someone else can benefit through, for example, organ donation. An article written by the Muslim Law Council (1996) stated their view and ruling on organ transplantation, to the effect that they accepted 'brainstem death as constituting the end of life for the purpose of organ transplant', which they supported as a 'means of alleviating pain or saving life on the basis of the rules of Shariah'. This process can also be viewed as a form of 'social death' (e.g. when relatives are asked if the dying person is a donor and if not would they, as next of kin, consent to organ donation taking place).

However, some cultures and religions will not believe in or accept this 'biomedical' interpretation of death. It is important to remember this when an actual diagnosis of the point of death is made because this is of major significance for any associated rituals. Many cultures (e.g. Chinese) regard death as a transition for the person who dies, and such an event is a time for rituals to take place (Pattison, 2008). These are known as 'rites of passage', and they occur when a person moves from one social status to another (e.g. birth, marriage or death). These rituals ensure that those who are dying or bereaved know what is expected of them. The way in which individuals experience death will therefore have a major impact on how nurses and healthcare professionals support the patient's families and relatives, and also how they cope with their own feelings when someone they have been caring for dies.

The issue of euthanasia, or assisted death, is also important to consider given the way this is often highlighted in the media. Sheikh and Gatrad (2000, p. 98) make it clear that 'Islam views life as sacred and a "trust" from Allah' and therefore both suicide and euthanasia are prohibited. However, they point out that 'undue suffering has no place in Islam and if death is hastened in the process of giving adequate analgesia then this is allowed ... what is important is that the primary intent is not to hasten death'.

Purnell and Selekman (2008) point out the views of Jewish culture and religion, whereby active euthanasia is forbidden and is considered murder. However, they explain that 'passive euthanasia may be allowed, depending on its interpretation'. Anything that prevents someone dying 'naturally' or 'prolongs the dying process' is not acceptable and point out that 'therefore, anything that artificially prevents death (e.g. cardiopulmonary resuscitation) may be possibly withheld, depending on the wishes of the patient and his or her religious views'.

According to Skultans (1980), death itself creates change 'in terms of individual loss and social disruption for the wider group' and because of this any rituals associated with death are extremely elaborate. However, this practice of death rituals is kept to a minimum in most communities in the UK today. For example, in many English homes there is no longer a ritual public display of mourning after death, such as the wearing of black clothes and armbands, although in Ireland the custom of the wake, at which family and friends gather to pay their respects to someone who has recently died, still remains.

THE MEANING OF BEREAVEMENT

Bereavement is a term that is associated with dying and the events that follow death. Its meaning implies that those who experience this life event have suffered a loss and that something or someone has been taken away from them. Andrews (2008) points out that 'it is a sociologic term indicating the status and role of the survivors of a death' (i.e. they are the 'bereaved').

According to Cook and Philips (1988), bereavement can involve four phases, as described in Box 12.1.

Box 12.1 *Phases of bereavement (adapted from Cook and Phillips, 1988)*

- Shock, numbness and grieving (Phase 1)
- Manifestations of fear, guilt, anger and resentment (Phase 2)
- Disengagement, apathy and aimlessness (Phase 3)
- Gradual hope and a move in new directions (Phase 4)

A similar staged pattern was also identified by Kubler-Ross (1970) and consists of denial, anger, bargaining, depression and acceptance.

This model is very much a Western view of how people manage the grieving process or response to a loss (Andrews, 2008), but these types of models have also been applied to other situations where loss is experienced. Examples are loss of cultural identity and social structure experienced as a result of migration or loss of homeland as with refugees (Bhugra and Becker, 2005).

The way in which individuals cope with or manage bereavement varies according to the culture to which they belong, and even within cultures there are individual differences. For example, when a Hindu person dies, the older women may continue to mourn in the traditional manner by wailing loudly to show their grief and the whole family 'may wear white as a sign of mourning, usually for the first 10 days after the death' (Henley, 1983b). Colour is significant in many cultures during the bereavement period following a death. In the UK, for example, black is still seen as symbolic of death and many people retain the practice of only wearing black as a mark of respect at a funeral. Black armbands are also symbolic of the period of mourning after death as is a period of silence, as experienced at a number of public events such as a football match when someone who is well known in the sport has died.

'Grief' is an emotion that may follow bereavement, and individuals experience and show their grief in different ways according to the culture to which they belong (Andrews, 2008; Pattison, 2008). However, the concepts of 'dying' and 'grief' are Western cultural concepts and this needs to be remembered when coping with the death of someone whose cultural beliefs differ from our own.

Grief is also experienced in different ways both individually as well as culturally. This can either be a physical response such as fainting or insomnia to aggressive behaviour (Pattison, 2008). A sudden or unexpected death may trigger complete denial that the person has died. How the patient died is also important and being denied access to their loved ones, as in the case of a serious infectious illness for example, can cause long term concerns on the part of close family members. This would be particularly important for individuals from cultures where there are specific death rituals to be undertaken or where they believe the person should not die alone (Galanti, 2008).

In Muslim culture and religion, relatives and friends visit the recently bereaved family in their own home. The dead are expected to meet God and, hopefully, find eternal peace. However, any prolonged grieving is discouraged and considered wrong, although according to Rees (1990) any traditional patterns of mourning are expected to be followed. Mourning, according to Andrews

(2008) 'is the culturally patterned behavioural response to death' and each culture will have its own way of responding.

Bhugra and Becker (2005) offer a definition by Eisenbruch (1991) for the concept of cultural bereavement:

> **The experience of the uprooted person – or group – continues to live in the past, is visited by supernatural forces from the past whilst asleep or awake, suffers feelings of guilt over abandoning culture and homeland, feels pain if memories of the past begin to fade, but finds constant images of the past (including traumatic images) intruding into daily life, yearns to complete obligations to the dead, and feels stricken by anxieties, morbid thoughts, and anger that mar the ability to get on with daily life.**
>
> *(Bhugra and Becker, 2005, p. 19)*

Einsbruch (1991) developed a diagnostic interview for Southeast Asian refugees to help him understand their 'grief reaction, and start the process of healing' (Bhugra and Becker, 2005). For those working in mental health, understanding the cultural and social factors behind some of the manifestations of grief, such as anxiety and depression, should be an essential part of their work.

To attempt to classify people into the different 'stages' of grief could be viewed as a very ethnocentric approach, rather than a culturally sensitive way of dealing with the bereavement process. Understanding the nature of bereavement, grief and associated mourning in various cultures is an essential part of nursing and healthcare practice.

NURSING PRACTICE AND CARING FOR THE DYING AND BEREAVED

The beliefs, rituals and customs associated with death in different cultures are extremely varied, and this includes the nurse's own professional culture. De Santis (1994) found that the nurse–patient encounter can be viewed as an interaction of a minimum of three cultures:

- the culture which is founded on the nurse's professional knowledge;
- the culture which is based on the patient's own individual belief systems;
- the culture of the organization or situation in which the patient and nurse actually meet (e.g. the hospital or home; see Chapter 1).

Nursing culture

If we examine the professional culture of nurses in relation to death and dying, it becomes apparent that there are many rituals and customs associated with their own nursing practice. As mentioned above, for a student nurse, 'meeting death' for the first time is part of their 'initiation' into the world of nursing, and for the majority of them this encounter will take place in a hospital. Student nurses worry a great deal about this, and Kiger (1994) found that the main causes of concern are the expected additional difficulties of caring for dying patients. These include the pain of seeing them suffer, the shock of seeing a dead body, and the difficulty of dealing with bereaved relatives. However, after students have encountered death-related experiences their perceptions begin to change, and they speak of caring for and communicating with dying patients, coping with cardiac arrest situations, laying out a dead body, coping with the family of the dead person, and handling their own responses to death (Sewell, 2002).

Smith (1992) believes that 'death and dying in hospital can be considered the ultimate emotional labour' for nurses and although her findings mirror those of Kiger's (1994) study of students, she also found that there were 'clearly defined technical skills required in dealing with death situations, e.g. resuscitation during cardiac arrest and laying out the body when the patient was pronounced dead'. These essential skills are very much part of the student's training experience, and are taught by mentors who usually have more experience of death (Pattison, 2008). Death and dying are thought by some to represent the ultimate emotional labour, but all nurses find their own ways to cope with this experience.

Superstitions about death and the dead person still exist within nursing (e.g. unlucky rooms, or death comes in threes), and according to Wolf (1988) post-mortem care or 'laying out of the dead' can be regarded as a nursing ritual. Many will be familiar with the rituals identified by Chapman (1983) in relation to death in a hospital ward, and she recalls what happened when a patient died in the hospital where she was undertaking research observation:

> **First the dead patient was screened from sight. No mention of the death was made to the inhabitants or visitors to the ward. The laying out procedure began. Although the corpse should lie for an hour before 'last offices' are performed, this time was diminished by the nurses who were perhaps anxious to dispatch the body. The laying out procedure involved washing the corpse. This was done even though the now deceased patient had recently had a bath. The body was clothed in a white gown and labelled. It was then wrapped in a white sheet or shroud. The nurses wore gowns to do this even though this was not necessary as a prevention against infection ... Next all the curtains in the ward were drawn up to and slightly beyond the deceased person's bed. In this way no other patients were allowed to view the corpse or the mortuary trolley on which it was wheeled away. The trolley was disguised by a sheet. The corpse was not seen at all as there was a sunken container within the trolley to conceal it. The corpse was wheeled away, the curtains drawn back and normal ward life continued. The dead person when mentioned at all was spoken about in hushed whispers.**

> *(Chapman, 1983, p. 17)*

How can we explain the events in this scenario? It could be that because of the stressful nature of their work nurses find this a reassuring 'ritual' – a way to help them cope with the death of patients. However, Lawler (1991) believes that 'death and the dead body are a problem for nurses' from a Western culture, because death is seen as a very private experience and not a topic for general conversation. It has become a taboo subject. This could make it difficult for nurses who are not only expected to cope with the dying person and their family, but are also expected to undertake care which requires handling a dead body. This practice is known amongst nurses as 'last offices'. However, Lawler (1991) believes that this difficulty in coping is also very much dependent on how nurses themselves 'see death and what they believe takes place at death'. A study by Goopy (2006) of the way in which Italian nurses managed the death of a person in a modern Intensive Care Unit was reflective of Chapman's observations 20 years earlier. She stated that:

Italian nurses make the 'sign of the cross'; they visibly recite prayers over the body of the deceased; they openly cry over the body, and they open the windows of the room in which the patient has died to 'allow the soul to pass to heaven.'

(Goopy, 2006, p. 113)

A similar example to Chapman's observation can be seen in Box 12.2.

Box 12.2 Observation from Goopy's study (2006, p. 114)

The deceased now shrouded looks like an oversize baby who has been wrapped in swaddling – the shroud neatly and firmly folded around the body, with only his face visible. (The face is left uncovered by the shroud as the body is now to be transferred to the lower ground 'viewing room'.)

The nurses lift the body onto to the trolley and cover the shrouded body, including the face, with another sheet. (In this case the sheet that had been covering the patient earlier, as it has been inspected and deemed clean enough for this purpose.)

The body is wheeled outside the unit and the lift is called. On its arrival the trolley with the deceased is pushed inside and the nurse reaches in and presses the button for the lower floor. As the lift doors close and the body disappears the nurse scurries down the internal staircase which is located beside the lift. The body is pulled from the lift – the nurse will not enter the lift even now – at the lower floor and wheeled into the viewing room.

Both the nurses and nursing assistants later tell me that they will not under any circumstances get in a lift with a dead body ... 'we do not have to stay in the lift with the body. Shall we say we are afraid of him (the body)'.

Bryan (2007) asks the question 'Should ward nurses hide death from other patients?' and discusses how as in Chapman's observation, the 'body' is 'mysteriously concealed behind ward curtains or wheeled, disguised under sheets, along a hospital corridor'. She offers a case scenario of how the dying patient is hidden away from others and how nurses' managed it (Box 12.3).

Case study

The Hidden Dying Patient: Case Scenario (Bryan, 2007, p. 79)

Mrs Roberts, aged 83 years, was admitted from a nursing home to a general medical ward. On admission she was frail and breathless but conscious. She was diagnosed with pneumonia and treated with intravenous antibiotics. Her chest infection did not improve. Over the next 24 hours her condition deteriorated and she slipped into unconsciousness. Her family (a daughter in New Zealand and a grandson in Belfast) was informed and all active treatment withdrawn.

continued

Case study

The following evening, as the patients were settling down for the night, the nurse in charge pulled the curtains around Mrs Roberts's bed, believing her to be dying. Mrs Roberts died at 2.30 am. At 5 am the curtains were drawn around the beds of the other sleeping patients and Mrs Roberts's body was removed. When the patients were woken at 6 am for the drug round, Mrs Roberts's bed had been stripped and it was empty. At morning handover, the nurse in charge reported that she had not spoken to any of the patients about Mrs Roberts's death because they had not asked.

Reflective exercise

When you next experience caring for a dying patient and you are required to undertake 'last offices', think about the care that you gave prior to death.

1. How will the care that you are about to undertake be any different now that you have read how people may grieve or what they might believe about death?
2. Chapman's experience of death and associated practices in hospital occurred in 1983. From your own experiences, are these rituals still taking place? Goopy's (2006) example appears to imply this as does Bryan's (2007).
3. Consider the cultural and religious beliefs of patients in your care and find out what information is available in the organization you are learning or working in to help them with the end-of-life period as well as their relatives' subsequent bereavement. In addition, find information about how nurses and other healthcare workers will know how to manage this.

Patient culture

The cultural beliefs of an individual are those related to religion and spirituality, which many people view incorrectly as one and the same. However, individuals who have no religious affiliations may have spiritual beliefs that contribute to their health. Naryanasamy (1991) claims that the 'provision of spiritual care is less than ideal in practice', and that holistic care (meaning care of body, mind and spirit) is therefore not an achievable goal without this. For example, a patient may tell you, when asked for details of their religion, that they are not religious and they do not go to church. However, later they tell you that they go to the park every day and sit there thinking about their day and 'feeling very much in tune with the world'. This could imply a 'spiritual well-being' which can give the person an inner strength to cope with life events such as death without the need to believe in and pray to God. Naryanasamy and Owens (2001) carried out a study to explore 'how nurses respond to the spiritual needs of their patients' as well as their interventions. They found that there were many variations in how nurses offered spiritual care to patients and their families, ranging from the 'cultural interactionist approach' of accommodating religious needs, such as enabling a patient to pray to Mecca in the ward, to an evangelical approach where the nurse's own religious beliefs were shared by the patient and in some instances even imposing their own personal ideals to 'fulfil their own religious beliefs'.

Religious beliefs also have a major influence on caring for dying patients and their families, especially their attitudes to and beliefs about death itself. By looking at a variety of religions we can explore the care that should be given to a dying patient.

An elderly man named Jacob Levy is admitted to your ward from the Accident and Emergency department unconscious after being knocked down by a car. His relatives have yet to arrive and he is alone. His condition suddenly deteriorates, and although resuscitation measures are undertaken, he dies before his relatives arrive.

Points to consider

1. What knowledge of Jewish religion and culture would help you to prioritize the care of Mr Levy?
2. What physical care can be given once his death has been diagnosed?
3. What help will his family require once they arrive?

The information below will help you to make informed decisions.

The Jewish community considers itself both as a religion and an ethnic group. There are two main groups within their community, namely Orthodox Jews and Progressive Jews. Orthodox Jews pursue a traditional religious lifestyle, whereas Progressive Jews seek to make their religious beliefs and practices fit more into a modern way of life. When caring for a dying Jewish patient in hospital, the nurse needs to determine which group they belong to because this will affect the care given to the patient and their body after death. The normal practices carried out when a Jewish person dies may not be practical in a hospital or hospice (e.g. placing the body covered with a sheet on the floor, with the feet towards the door, and then placing a lighted candle by the head). Therefore Rabbi Julia Neuberger (1994) recommends that the guidelines issued by the Sexton's Office of the United Synagogue Burial Society in 1960 can be followed instead:

> Where it is not possible to obtain the services of a Jewish chaplain, it is permissible for hospital staff to carry out the following: close the eyes, tie up the jaw, keep arms and hands straight and by the side of the body. Any tubes or instruments in the body should be removed and the incision plugged. The corpse should then be wrapped in a plain sheet without religious emblems and placed in a mortuary or other special room for Jewish bodies.

(Neuberger, 1994, p. 14)

In deference to 'not touching the body', it may be advisable for a non-Jewish nurse to use disposable gloves. The burial and funeral normally take place within 24 hours of death, so the time for which the body of a Jewish person is left alone will be short. After the hospital staff have finished administering the initial care, a member of the Jewish community may watch over the body day and night. Neuberger (1994) states that this practice (known as shemira) is part of the belief that 'the body is the receptacle of the soul and the body is to be honoured, respected and guarded'. The family will normally make the funeral arrangements, but in exceptional cases if there is no family the solicitor or the hospital social worker may have to make the arrangements (Neuberger, 1994).

The family will probably want to know that their relative did not die on their own and that they were not left on their own after death. If the patient dies on the Sabbath (from sundown on Friday to sundown on Saturday) they must not be moved from the hospital because this is their day of rest.

Nurses need to be aware that Orthodox Jews do not allow post-mortem examinations and organ donations unless the post-mortem is for medical reasons. Progressive Jews may believe otherwise, so if a post-mortem is necessary the nurse needs to approach the subject with the family in a sensitive way. Being aware of the cultural and religious needs of Mr Levy and his family will ensure that the nurses can offer support and help which will be appreciated.

An expected death may be dealt with in a different way as indicated in the following Case Study.

Case study

Amarjit Singh is a 48-year-old man in the terminal stages of cancer and aware of his condition. He has been admitted to hospital from the care of his family so that his pain management can be reassessed. He is only able to undertake a minimal amount of personal care.

Points to consider
1. What knowledge of Sikh culture would help you undertake an assessment of Mr Singh's needs?
2. How will you involve the family in his care during his stay in hospital?
3. If you were to care for him in the community, how would you ensure that Mr Singh's family were given support from healthcare professionals?

The information below will help you to make informed decisions.

The Sikh religion has its roots in Hinduism, and as such Sikhs believe in only one God and pray in a Sikh temple (Gurdwara), which usually contains a prayer room in which the Sikh Holy Book (Gura Granth Sahib) is kept. There are no appointed priests in the Sikh Community, but 'holy men' are identified. As a Sikh, Mr Singh may wish to pray, and he may have brought a prayer book (gutka) with him. Nurses need to be aware that this must be treated with respect, and if they find that they have to move it for some reason, it should only be touched with a clean hand. Mr Singh's family will probably wish to stay with him in hospital at all times, and this needs to be allowed for as part of his care.

Friends and other members of the community will also wish to visit him, and if they have travelled some way to do so, the nurses caring for him need to balance the need to ensure that no offence is caused to him or his family with the needs of other patients in the ward (e.g. by allowing more visitors than is usual). This change from the norm could be incorporated into a Patient Information Booklet which acknowledges the spiritual and cultural needs of all patients and ensures that patients from different cultures are conversant with each other's beliefs and customs.

If Mr Singh is a formally baptized Sikh man (Amridharis), he will probably wear the five signs of Sikhisim. These are known as the 'five Ks' – Kesh (uncut hair), Kangha (a comb), Kara (a steel bangle), Kirpan (a symbolic dagger) and Kaccha (symbolic undershorts). Although many Sikhs no longer wear kirpan and kangha, most men and women have retained the kara and kaccha. It is important that nurses understand the significance of these for the patient and do not remove them unless the patient or his family give permission to do so. As Mr Singh is unable to take care of himself, the nurses need to ensure that they do not cause unnecessary embarrassment or distress when undertaking his personal care. If Mr Singh requires patient-controlled analgesia as part of his pain management, it will be important to ensure that the nurse or doctor use the right hand to insert the intravenous needle (the left hand is traditionally used for washing the body after using the lavatory, and the right hand for eating, drinking, shaking hands).

After his pain management is seen to be effective, Mr Singh will be discharged home to the care of his family, who will still require the support of a community healthcare team. Caring for Mr Singh during his stay in hospital will have been enhanced by an understanding of his individual and cultural needs, and will enable the nurses to ensure that information required by the community team following his discharge home will reflect this.

Telling someone that they are going to die requires special skills and although the doctor will inform individuals and families, it is very often the nurse who has to explain the actual meaning and implications of the situation for them. In some cultures, however, telling someone they are going to die, even though they have the right to know, may not be acceptable. Galanti (2008, p. 167) points out that 'in many Asian countries, including China and Japan, it is customary for the physician to reveal a cancer diagnosis only to the patient's family, and leave it up to the family whether or not to tell the patient'.

In the following Case Study, the family may want more information about the future care of their mother and how they could ensure that her needs will be met.

Case study

Mrs Nasreen Akhtar is a 68-year-old Muslim woman who has undergone major surgery for cancer of the colon. During the operation, metastases are discovered and only palliative surgery is undertaken. Mrs Akhtar's family were informed by the surgeon about the decision and she has yet to be told, as she was very ill following surgery, and had to be admitted to the intensive-care unit (ICU) for 24 hours. Her condition is critical.

Points to consider

1. What knowledge of Mrs Akhtar's culture would help you to communicate effectively with the relatives once they have been told of her critical status?
2. How will the nurses working in the ICU arrange for both the patient's and relatives' needs to be met in the first 24 hours after her surgery?
3. What specific cultural care needs will nurses have to accommodate following surgery?

The information below will help you to make informed decisions.

The ICU can be regarded as a subculture of its own where, because of its critical nature, the nurse's assessment of the patient may not immediately focus on the patient's cultural needs. However, it is essential that there is an awareness of Mrs Akhtar's cultural background so that she and her family can be cared for effectively. Many ICU settings have a small number of critically ill patients and, given that the space around each bed is limited, the opportunity for family involvement in care may be restricted.

The grief and anticipatory loss for the family have to be allowed for, but because of the clinical condition of the other patients in the ICU, the nurses will need to ensure that they adopt a sensitive and culturally aware approach to meeting their needs while ensuring that the needs of the other patients and their families are also met. For example, it may not be possible for more than one or two members of the family to be present at any one time within the ICU setting because of the intense activity that is normally taking place, and this could be even more problematic if Mrs Akhtar requires acute interventions and resuscitation.

Muslims are followers of the Islamic faith, and they believe in 'living their lives according to the will of Allah (God)' (Karmi, 1996). Their guiding rules are to be found in the Qur'an, which is their holy book. Karmi (1996) also states that there is great emphasis on 'modesty, social responsibility, health, cleanliness and the importance of family ties and children'. If one considers that modesty is important and that 'nakedness is considered shameful' (Karmi, 1996), then the type of care that Mrs Akhtar will receive in the ICU will be crucial to her general well-being and the experience of her family. She has undergone major surgery and will be receiving life-sustaining treatment which is potentially invasive. It will be important to both her and her family that her body is not exposed unnecessarily, and for the healthcare staff to acknowledge that being touched and examined by male nurses and doctors may be frightening and totally abhorrent to her.

Prayer is very important to Muslim families, and although women do not go to the Mosque for public prayer, they do undertake this at home. Mrs Akhtar will be unable to do this because of her illness, so it is important to her care that prayers are read to her by relatives, and that the Islamic call to prayer is whispered into her ear.

Good communication and continuous assessment are essential in all such situations, and nurses can enhance their care by talking to the family and the patient so as to provide individualized care.

Organization culture – hospital and community

All care that is given to the patient and their relatives will depend very much on the effectiveness of the hospital or community responding to the needs of a multicultural–multiracial community. If it is acknowledged that patients should all receive individualized care, then this will be apparent in different policies and procedures throughout the hospital or community service. Hospitals that acknowledge the cultural needs of patients are likely to have not only a chapel but also a mosque and a temple (or their equivalent) for prayer. It is also recommended that 'symbols of Christianity should be removed from chapels of rest when these are being used by non-Christians' (Black, 1991).

Care plans and other documentation, both in the hospital and in the community, should reflect an awareness of cultural differences. Many NHS trusts have produced guidelines on the spiritual and bereavement needs of different cultures, which have been developed through collaborative multi-profession and multicultural groups.

Reflective exercise

1. Think about your own working environment and use the recommendations below to assess your experience of providing care that is culturally aware. You may wish to discuss this with colleagues, which may not only lead to learning about other cultures and their needs, but may also enable you to understand why nurses' own beliefs about death and dying are so important to delivering culturally sensitive and competent care.

2. Using a nursing assessment tool that is familiar to you, consider how you would initially assess a person's needs with regards to the issue of death and dying. You may then wish to consider the following questions identified in Holland *et al.* (2008, p. 495) with regard to the 'Activity of Living: Dying'.

Factors and possible questions to consider during the assessment stage of care planning for the dying

- Physical:
    - Are there any confirmed diagnostic factors threatening the person's life?
    - What are the physical effects upon the person, family and friends?
    - Is the person aware of the diagnosis, stage and progress of the life-threatening disorder?
    - Is the possibility actual or potential?

- Psychological:
    - Is the person expressing a 'desire to know', anxiety or fear of dying?
    - Does the person desire that significant others 'know'?
    - What is the person's behaviour, mood, personality?
    - What is the person's understanding of their own dying/death?

- Sociocultural
    - What are the person's attitudes, beliefs and life experiences about death?
    - Does the person have specific cultural, religious, social or personal requests?
    - Who needs to be contacted on behalf of the person: family, partners, friends?

- Environmental:
    - Choice of environment to facilitate a peaceful death (i.e. hospice, home or hospital)?
    - What resources will be required to meet the needs of the person, family and carers?

- Politico-economic:
    - Are there any economic, legal, ethical, resource, social or domestic factors inhibiting a peaceful death?
    - What is the effect of the death and reduced life expectancy of the person on others?
    - Are there sufficient and appropriate support services within the hospital and the home for the dying and bereaved?
    - Does the person wish to donate any organs and do the family know?

Demonstrating evidence of good practice is becoming an essential part of a nurse's role, and one way to do this is by encouraging cultural awareness and effective communication between all healthcare workers and the wider cultural community. The following statements (recommendations) are examples of how this good practice could be developed.

1. There should be access to specific information on death and dying practices, including the contact numbers of local religious and spiritual leaders.
2. Leaflets and booklets which outline hospital or community protocols for the bereaved should be available for healthcare workers and patients and their families.
3. Booklets should be made available that explain the terminology used by nurses and others when caring for individuals from different cultures.
4. Integration of cultural issues into care assessments and care plan documentation should be mandatory.
5. Visiting times based on cultural practice should be encouraged and information made available about special occasions (e.g. festivals or fasting times).
6. A learning environment that encourages cultural and racial awareness across the healthcare professions should be a priority for all those involved in developing educational programmes.

CONCLUSION

It is very important that patients receive culturally sensitive care at all times during their stay in hospital, and it is essential to ensure that there is no prejudice shown through any stated rules of the organization or institution in which the dying patient may be cared for. As societies become more multicultural, nurses and healthcare professionals will be exposed to a wider range of spiritual and religious beliefs, which will influence the need to adopt care practices that are culturally orientated.

The meeting of three cultural realities (the nurse, the patient and the organization) requires that all those involved acknowledge the differences in the needs of the nurses, the patients and the organization (which arise from individual belief systems about death and dying in both Western and non-Western societies). However, nurses are in the very privileged position of being able to care for those who are dying and those who may be bereaved, and they can directly influence the type of care that is given. The UK Nursing and Midwifery Code (2008) clearly states that nurses must:

> **Make the care of people your first concern, treating them as individuals and respecting their dignity;**
> **Must demonstrate a personal and professional commitment to equality and diversity.**

The *Standards of proficiency for achieving registration* (Nursing and Midwifery Council, 2004) also state that the student must:

> **Respect the values, customs and beliefs of individuals and groups**
> **Provide care which demonstrates sensitivity to the diversity of patients and clients.**

FURTHER READING

Galanti G-A (2008) *Caring for patients from different cultures*, 4th edn. University of Pennsylvania Press, Philadelphia.

Kirkwood NA (2005) *A hospital handbook on multiculturalism and religion: practice guidelines for health care workers*, 2nd edn. Morehouse, London.

Parkes CM, Laungani P and Young B (eds) (1997) *Death and bereavement across cultures*. Butterworth–Heinemann, Oxford.

This book uses case studies to describe rituals and beliefs of many religions with regard to care of the dying and bereaved.

Valentine C (2008) *Bereavement narratives: continuing bonds in the 21st century*. Routledge, London.

This book explores the experience of bereavement in British society, based on the narratives of bereaved people and how people make sense of their experience of bereavement.

WEBSITES

http://www.ggalanti.com/

This website links to Galanti's book and has resources such as articles on a range of topics and links to further resources. Although mainly focused on a US healthcare context it has valuable application in other countries.

http://www.cancerresearchuk.org/

This is the Cancer Research UK website and has a number of useful resources, including an option to purchase a resource book and DVD-ROM for development of skills for responding to patient diversity in relation to cancer. Topics in this resource include language and communication and ethnic diversity and cancer.

http://www.york.ac.uk/healthsciences/equality/cultural.htm

This website at the University of York offers links to a large number of websites on the topic of equality and diversity. Examples of topics are: cultural safety, health promotion and beliefs and customs of different cultures in relation to death and dying and other aspects of living.

13 Cultural diversity and professional practice

Christine Hogg

INTRODUCTION

The need for care delivery based on cultural understanding and lack of prejudice has been highlighted in the previous chapters. We consider that healthcare professionals working in both hospital and community settings require additional skills and knowledge in order to be able to ensure both quality and equality of healthcare provision in a culturally diverse society. However, these same professionals also require an equal opportunity to contribute and participate in such health care.

In 1999, the Macpherson Inquiry into the death of a young black teenager, Stephen Lawrence, revealed the extent of institutional racism within the Police Service. In the wake of the Macpherson Inquiry, a dispute emerged at the Royal College of Nursing's (RCN) annual conference, when a resolution aimed at improving minority ethnic involvement was rejected. Such was the profound reaction and dismay that a nurse who worked only 2 miles (about 3.2 km) away from where Stephen Lawrence had died said: 'It was like a nightmare come true.' This dispute within the RCN revealed some interesting but worrying trends that prompted the RCN General Secretary Christine Hancock to comment: 'I do not believe that the RCN is any freer of institutional racism than any other big organization'.

Institutional racism may take the form of failure to recognize racial differences or a 'feeling that these differences are not significant or that attention to individualized care will transcend them' (Papadopoulos et al., 2004). However the Race Relations (Amendment) Act (2000) (Commission for Racial Equality, 2000) places a duty on all public authorities to tackle racism in service delivery. The Act stresses that employers can be held vicariously liable if their organization is found to be at fault and there is a positive duty on employers to take a proactive approach to racial equality.

We will explore and discuss some of the issues with regard to racial inequalities in the nursing and healthcare professions, and the ways in which the NHS and colleges of nursing are seeking to address them.

This chapter will focus specifically on the following issues:

- the history of black and minority ethnic nurses;
- equal opportunities within nursing;
- recruitment in the nursing profession;
- preparation and education of nurses to care for patients in a culturally diverse society.

THE HISTORY OF BLACK AND MINORITY ETHNIC NURSES IN THE NHS

Racism and discrimination in the nursing profession are not new issues. Mary Seacole, a black woman from Jamaica, was a contemporary of Florence Nightingale in the Crimean War. Her humanitarian work for the British Army led Queen Victoria to recognize and reward her, yet until recently she was relatively unknown, despite her contributions to nursing, which are comparable to those of Nightingale. Her reflections revealed possible racist attitudes and behaviours:

> 'Did these ladies shrink from accepting my aid because my blood flowed beneath a somewhat duskier skin?'

> *(Lee-Cunin, 1989, p. 1)*

Since the advent of the NHS in 1948, black people have played an essential part in its development and survival. In the 1960s and 1970s, the Department of Health actively recruited nurses from the former British colonies (Sen, 1970). This was largely to address the acute labour shortage in the NHS in post-war Britain when, to combat the crisis, the Government at the time exempted the NHS from the Immigration Acts of 1962 and 1965. These nurses were mainly recruited from the West Indies, Africa, Singapore, Malaysia, Ireland, Mauritius and the Philippines. Their numbers grew in the 1960s, peaked in the 1970s and then gradually declined. However, in the late 1990s the NHS once again began to recruit from overseas in order to meet staff shortages (Carlisle, 1996).

It soon became apparent that racism in the NHS was rife. Many of these migrant nurses' earliest experiences were primarily ones of hurt, loneliness and exploitation. Many described systematic discrimination both in and out of the workplace. For example, Sen (1970) reported that one student, when trying to hire a car, was told that 'cars couldn't be hired out to coloured people'. Training schools also demanded higher academic qualifications from overseas nurses wishing to train as State Registered Nurses (SRNs) than from the indigenous populations. Many nurses describe how they were coerced into taking the State Enrolled Nurse (SEN) training, a qualification that was held in lower regard. Many were not informed of the lower status of the SEN training, and were unaware that in many countries (outside the UK) it was of little value, so that returning home to nurse would be impossible. A nurse who was recruited from Barbados in 1968 describes how she was unaware of the different types of training:

> Within my first week ... I realised there was a major difference ... all the nurses doing the two-year courses were black.

> *(Hicks, 1982b, p. 789)*

Many nurses faced poor and exploitative working conditions. The pupil nurses (SEN trainees) were regarded as the 'workers' and were given the heavy and unpleasant jobs on the wards:

> Life during training was bedpans everlasting bedpans ... You rarely saw a white student in any of the geriatric wards ... If a new procedure was being shown in the wards, it was only to the student nurses who were mainly white.

> *(Hicks, 1982b, p. 789)*

Some nurses were also subject to racist abuse from patients. A patient told one black nurse to 'remove her black hands or she would be kicked' (Macmillan, 1996).

Racism also took the form of direct and indirect discrimination in the workplace, as illustrated in the following statement:

> After my third year I was put on the heaviest geriatric ward in the hospital. All my colleagues were put on the acute wards except for me. They tried to persuade me to apply to go on another ward.

(Lee-Cunin, 1989, p. 8)

Nurses were often made to conform to uniform standards despite their religious conventions and beliefs. Asian women were refused permission to wear trousers, despite their desire to preserve modesty (Mares *et al.*, 1985). Some nurses were also channelled to the less 'glamorous' areas of nursing, such as care of older people, those with mental health problems and those with learning disabilities. These accounts of prejudice and discrimination are both shocking and upsetting, yet there is evidence to suggest that racism and discrimination are still prevalent in the NHS today, (Sprinks, 2008, Allan *et al.*, 2004, Harrison, 2004).

In recent years a shortage of nurses in the NHS has again led to a drive to recruit nurses from overseas (Royal College of Nursing, 2002). This is at a time when the global labour market is becoming increasingly competitive, and international travel has become somewhat cheaper and more accessible. By the mid-1990s one in ten of annual new entrants to the UK nursing register was from non-UK sources. By 2001–2002 more overseas nurses were added to the register than there were UK registrants (Royal College of Nursing, 2003a).

In a study of ten organisations (five NHS and five private sector) the RCN found that internationally recruited nurses (IRNs) made up between 4 and 65 per cent of their total qualified nursing workforce (Royal College of Nursing, 2003b). A Mori Poll in 2002 found that 48 per cent of those interviewed felt that UK colleagues were treated better than they were and 33 per cent felt that UK colleagues did not respect their qualifications.

Alexis and Vydelingum (2004) interviewed 12 nurses who were recruited from overseas and explored their experiences of working in the NHS. The nurses came from the Philippines, South Africa, the Caribbean and sub-Saharan Africa. The findings show that these nurses were marginalized and felt excluded. They described a feeling of being thrown into a different world, and struggling to cope with communication issues, if, for example, English was their second language. Many participants felt that they had little hope of promotion and some had experienced bullying. They described what is was like:

> I felt as not belonging to this group. Out of place, lonely and at times wanting to go home. Kept asking myself why am I here?

(Alexis and Vydelingum, 2004, p. 17)

Allan *et al.*'s (2004) work investigated the experience of 69 IRNs. These nurses also found widespread racism and discrimination, with hostility originating from both colleagues and patients. The RCN (2005) has developed a good practice guide which suggests ethical and practical issues employers need to consider before recruiting nurses from overseas and suggests ways of helping IRNs to feel respected and understood. They suggest, for example, that it helps to provide adaptation courses, which explain common conditions that UK nurses deal with (for example heart disease) and the complexities of the patient pathway, for example the differences between primary and secondary care. Other issues that might be explored are language differences, explanations of local dialect phrases and idiosyncratic colloquialisms (Royal College of Nursing, 2005).

EQUAL OPPORTUNITIES IN NURSING

The first major study investigating nursing in a multi-ethnic NHS was undertaken in 1995 by the Policy Studies Institute (PSI) on behalf of the Department of Health (Beishon *et al.*, 1995). The research was commissioned in order to obtain a comprehensive picture of the experiences and working life of nurses. The study suggests that black and minority ethnic nurses continue to suffer racial discrimination and harassment. In this report, racial harassment by patients appears to be a regular feature of people's working lives in the NHS:

> **You try to be kind but you can feel it. You know when it's racial. If someone is in pain or they have got problems, there is a difference [between that and] when someone despises you because of your colour. They give you a cold look and you can't reach them.**

> *(Beishon* et al., *1995, p.129)*

Despite widespread evidence of harassment in all areas of nursing, these nurses were expected to get on with the job and not to make a fuss. The research criticizes managers and health service employment policies that do not identify racial harassment by patients as a problem. The report also suggests that racial harassment is under-reported because staff do not feel that they will be taken seriously. There appears to be a widespread lack of clarity with regard to policy enforcement.

In terms of equal opportunities, black staff fell behind in obtaining senior nurse posts. Once more they were more likely to be working in the less prestigious areas of nursing, such as mental health and learning disabilities. They were also more likely to be working full-time and doing other paid work on top of their nursing jobs.

In 2004 the Nursing Standard conducted a survey on diversity in the NHS with 814 nurses, 641 of whom were white (Harrison, 2004). The survey demonstrated that one-third of black or minority ethnic (BME) nurses thought the NHS to be institutionally racist. Many nurses from a BME background gave examples of racism and racist abuse. Some of the racism was not overt but was more subtle. One nurse stated 'Each time you are on duty, for whatever reason, nobody else but you will remain on the ward until the end of the shift. Others are told to go early, which is unfair'. In this survey only 15 per cent of white respondents agreed that BME staff should be given extra support to climb the management ladder in contrast to 73 per cent of BME staff.

The report also highlights the ethical issues raised when patients refuse to be treated by certain staff because of their race. In 2004 a nurse, Rosie Purves, won an employment tribunal and £20 000 in compensation when the Southampton University NHS Trust complied with a woman's request that she did not want her child to be cared for by a black nurse. In a poll in the *Nursing Standard* in 2008, of 211 respondents 9 per cent were from minority ethnic backgrounds and 8 per cent said they had been the victim of racism or discrimination (Sprinks, 2008). Older people tended to be the worst perpetrators – 'They say they don't want to be touched by "dirty hands"'. 67 per cent of nurses said they had received no training in culturally sensitive care since joining the present employer and 56 per cent had witnessed racist behaviour from patients and/or visitors.

Key points

1. In the NHS there is a long history of recruitment from overseas.
2. Many nurses recruited in the 1950s and 1960s experienced racist attitudes and behaviours.
3. The evidence suggests that racial harassment is a regular feature of some nurses' working lives in the NHS.
4. The evidence also suggests that equal opportunities for black and minority ethnic staff are lacking.

RECRUITMENT IN NURSING

In the late 1980s there was a fear in nursing that black nurses were becoming an 'endangered species' (Iganski *et al.*, 1998a). There was a belief that young people of minority ethnic descent were being deterred from choosing nursing as a career because of discrimination and harassment experienced by their parents. The under-representation of black nurses in the NHS raises some fundamental questions about the health service. For example, if minority ethnic groups are under-represented, then the NHS cannot claim to be a genuine equal opportunities employer. The lack of black and minority ethnic (BME) staff therefore not only reflects an inadequate equal opportunities policy, but it also seriously compromises standards and quality of care. It can be argued, for example, that the efficiency and credibility of the NHS are questionable if a proportion of the community does not have fair representation within the work-force.

Reflective exercise

1. Consider your working environment and the population you serve.
2. What proportion of the patients/clients is from black and minority ethnic groups?
3. What proportion of your team is from black and minority ethnic groups?
4. If a student nurse, how many of your colleagues are from black and minority ethnic groups?

In our experience there appears to be a common belief among nurses that young black and minority ethnic people do not apply for nursing training because it is considered to be a low-status job and therefore 'beneath' the aspirations of some cultural groups. Another reason often suggested is that nursing may be perceived as unattractive to some people because they may be expected to deal intimately with people of the opposite sex. To a great extent these beliefs and stereotypes about black and minority ethnic groups are misleading, and they often lead to an impasse or reluctance to find more proactive ways to recruit.

Similar findings are reflected in a study by Iganski *et al.* (1998a) and the following example from a manager:

> **They engaged somebody to undertake a project and it was quite extensive ... what they came back with was the perception of nursing that it wasn't the sort of right status for the people to want to come into and it was those sorts of attitudes that we were up against, and there was not a lot we could do to change that.**
>
> *(Iganski et al., 1998a, p. 336)*

Other studies offer a different perspective. Lee-Cunin (1989) questioned 27 Asian schoolgirls in Bradford about the responses of their parents to their possible entry into the nursing profession. This study provided some interesting insights. In total, 19 young women felt that their parents would approve, and only seven thought that they would not (one did not answer). One response was as follows:

> **My family and relatives were all for it. My parents said that it would be nice to have Asian nurses who spoke Asian languages to help out at hospitals and help out our own people. They thought of it as a good career, and still want me to continue, but have given me the decision to do as I wish.**
>
> *(Lee-Cunin, 1989, p. 35)*

However, one young woman stated that:

> **My family would not like the idea of me working with men [male nurses] ... They would say no, because you would have to look after men and give them a bed bath.**
>
> *(Lee-Cunin, 1989, p. 36)*

Baxter's (1988) research indicated that young Asian women were often steered away from nursing careers on the basis of stereotypes with regard to dress codes and uniforms. Instead, they were often directed into occupations that required higher academic qualifications. In contrast, African-Caribbean women were advised to undertake nursing on the basis of stereotypical assumptions that nursing would be an appropriate career for them. There is also some evidence to suggest that people from black and minority ethnic groups do not choose nursing as a career because of racism and harassment experienced by their parents as health service workers. This issue was raised in Lee-Cunin's (1989) study, as one SEN informed her:

> **I wouldn't get a job now. No one would take me. I have to stay in nursing. Soon they will have no young black nurses in my hospital. They are not taking them, anyway my kids are not going to go into that profession.**
>
> *(Lee-Cunin, 1989, p. 11)*

There is a suggestion in Baxter's research that young Asian women are discouraged from entering nursing because of the nature and intimacy of nursing work. A similar study undertaken by Daly *et al.* (2004) examined attitudes of young South-Asian students, parents of South-Asian students, career advisors and a small group of South-Asian nurse practitioners. This study found that very few young South-Asian women and even fewer young South-Asian men had ever considered a career in nursing. Many of the student participants were found to have a limited view of nursing. For example nursing was seen as a 'girly job' or 'boring, same routine every day'. Hospitals and the NHS were generally considered in a negative light. The report highlights the need for more South-Asian role models to be available and particularly more male role models, as well as portraying the NHS as a more stable environment. The parents viewed nursing as a good career but they unanimously responded that they would not encourage their children in such a choice. Some Muslim fathers expressed their concern in relation to their daughters and dress code and the prospect of them interacting with male patients.

Research by Iganski *et al.* (1998b) provides additional information that raises some serious questions about nurse recruitment. The main findings demonstrate that Asian applicants are consistently under-represented and are less likely to hold an offer of training. Applicants from black and African groups, on the other hand, are over-represented. This research also suggests that there may be other factors at work in the selection process which may have the effect, intentionally or otherwise, of discriminating against some applicants on the basis of their ethnic group. The study highlights that a higher proportion of applicants from black and minority ethnic groups are rejected without being interviewed.

In the study by Iganski *et al.* (1998b), only one institution had sought systematically to remove this scope by formulating a tightly structured interviewing instrument, and a few had ensured that teams were trained appropriately so that bias and prejudice were kept to a minimum. There is a common misconception that failure to recruit nurses from black and minority ethnic communities is 'their fault' – that is, they are culpable, either because they do not come forward (for whatever reason) or because they reject nursing. However, when the evidence is exposed it appears that subtle prejudices and biases are prevalent in the recruitment and application processes. As Hastings-Asatourian (1996) suggests, the 'single white female' preference is clearly discernible throughout the process, thus maintaining a work-force that is predominantly caucasian and female. However, equality of opportunity and recruitment of students from minority ethnic groups can only benefit health care if they are accompanied by effective preparation of all nurses to provide care that is culturally appropriate.

Key points

1. There is evidence to suggest that people from black and minority ethnic groups are grossly under-represented in the nursing profession.
2. The reasons for this failure to recruit include a poor image of nursing as a career, and parents' and teachers' fears of racism and harassment in the NHS.
3. Failure to recruit is also due to methods of selection and recruitment by colleges of nursing.

DEVELOPING THE WORKFORCE TO CREATE A CULTURALLY COMPETENT ENVIRONMENT

If the nursing profession is to address the needs of black and minority ethnic groups and the environment is to be inclusive in a meaningful and sensitive way, then nurse educators have a vital, if not pivotal role, to play in this process. It would therefore seem logical for the nursing curriculum in both pre- and post-registration courses to be proactive in addressing both cultural competence and dissemination of good practice.

Cultural competence is a complex issue and is defined by Papadopoulos as:

> **The capacity to provide effective health care taking into consideration people's cultural beliefs, behaviours and needs ... cultural competence is the synthesis of a lot of knowledge and skills which we acquire during our personal and professional lives and to which we are constantly adding.**

> *(Papadopoulos, 2003, p. 5)*

Being culturally competent is considered to be essential for providing care that is culturally appropriate. However, there is evidence to suggest that education programmes in nursing that are designed to prepare practitioners to meet the needs of patients from other cultures are all too often inadequate (Gerrish *et al.*, 1996b). McGee (1994) argues that one way to ensure this is for transcultural nursing to be regarded as an essential element in the nursing curriculum and that failure to include it might be considered a form of institutional racism in which one section of the population is seen as the 'norm' from which others differ.

McGee (1994) suggests educational strategies to achieve this end. She argues, for example, that in order to be competent in the delivery of transcultural care, students should be able to recognize their own values and be able to demonstrate openness to cultural differences. For example, students may be encouraged to examine their own culture by explaining a familiar tradition to a stranger or someone from outside their culture.

Reflective exercise

1. Identify one tradition from your own culture and describe it to a colleague.
2. Ask them to describe a similar tradition, and compare the two with regard to both similarities and differences.

Madeleine Leininger, an American nurse anthropologist who is generally viewed as the founder of the transcultural nursing movement, has been central to the development of education programmes in the USA that teach cultural competence through the theory of 'culture care diversity and universality' (Leininger, 1984). For example, there are postgraduate programmes that prepare nurses to work as the equivalent of specialist practitioners in a particular culture. These nurses learn about the specific customs, beliefs, ethno-history and health belief practices of a particular group, with a focus on the discipline of anthropology. They also have to work in the different communities (e.g. Mexican-Americans or Hmong), in order to gain practice experience of healthcare needs. Leininger's work is comprehensive and provides valuable and illuminating analyses of other cultures. However, it is not without its critics. As was seen in Chapter 5, Bruni (1988) criticizes transcultural theory and argues that it does not acknowledge culture as a dynamic phenomenon. She argues that culture is not static and that individuals do not fit into neat stereotypes. She cites the work of Bottomley (1981, p. 2), an Australian anthropologist, who argues that there is 'no Greek culture or Italian culture, but an enormous range of ideas and practices of regional variation':

> The problem of stereotyping cultures is compounded by the assumption that the country of origin of a person (or his or her parents) identifies the most significant dimension of his/her experience. Hence 'Maria' as the daughter of Greek parents is primarily perceived in terms of her 'Greekness'. Her position as a factory worker is considered to be of secondary importance.
>
> *(Bruni, 1988, p. 29)*

Bruni (1988) argues that people are individuals and need to be considered in the context of the rest of their lives. Stokes (1991), another critic of the 'specialist' approach to cultural care, argues that not only is it patronizing, but it also leads to care becoming fragmented as a result of cultural determinants in health care becoming 'someone else's job'. In other words, the nurse specialist may deter general nurses from addressing the cultural needs of the client group in their care. Leininger's position may lead to stereotyping or reinforcing the idea of 'otherness' and problems that are in themselves extremely ethnocentric, and which may even be deemed racist. It also assumes that all nurses who enter the programmes are from the same ethnic group. Furthermore, Littlewood (1988) argues that this approach may serve to perpetuate the distance between nurses and patients.

Other authors have attempted to suggest ways of introducing cultural competence into nursing education and practice (Papadopoulos *et al.*, 1998) and the American Nurses' Association (1986) has identified four approaches that educators might use to achieve cultural diversity in the content of the curriculum. They are:

- **the concept approach:** integration of cultural concepts throughout the entire nursing curriculum. For example, when teaching a subject such as pain management, cultural perspectives on pain may be considered as part of the session.

- **the unit approach:** inclusion of cultural aspects of nursing care in specific units. For example, students may be offered a module on 'Cultural Awareness in Nursing' as part of a diploma or degree programme.

- **the course approach:** offering of a specific course in which the emphasis is on the cultural aspects of nursing care. For example, students may be offered a Masters programme in transcultural nursing.

- **the multidisciplinary approach:** teaching of cultural content by the nursing faculty, anthropologists, medical sociologists and others involved in health care. For example, an anthropologist and a nurse may team up to teach the students 'rites of passage' as a theory. Following this, the students may then relate the topic to the practice of nursing.

McGee (1992) argues that perhaps the most useful approach is where culture is woven into every aspect of the curriculum. The advantage of this approach is that cultural issues are constantly referred to and, as a result, they become an integral part of nursing care. Nurses would than have a general awareness and integrate culture into their care delivery, almost at an unconscious level. This approach may also ensure that nurses view cultural aspects of care as part of day-to-day life and not as a 'problem' or as 'otherness'. The alternative unit or modular approach may encourage tokenism, especially if this is optional. The whole-course approach that Leininger advocates – that is, offering full modules or even short courses – may be useful and is certainly a possibility at post-registration level. However, Mattson (1987) argues that to leave transcultural issues until nurses qualify may be too late, and that bad habits and prejudices may be difficult to unlearn.

Abdullah (1995) suggests that any educational programme should have four goals:

1. to promote sensitivity to multicultural concepts;
2. to aid the development of knowledge of cultural differences;
3. to develop an organized plan to integrate the identified multicultural content into the nursing curricula;
4. to plan experiential opportunities that enable the learners to develop their caring approach.

Abdullah (1995) also stresses the need for learners to examine their own cultural biases and behaviours, as well as those of the client.

McGee (1992) argues that multicultural education should move away from 'transmissionist' styles. In these styles, the student accepts whatever the teacher says and is not encouraged to question or criticize. For example, the teacher may lecture or present information to the group on 'Islam' (facts and figures, religious rulings, etc.). Alternatively, transcultural nurse education may be more concerned with 'transformationist styles', which allow students to examine their own attitudes, beliefs, values and feelings. This demands that teaching and learning styles should be student-centred and flexible – an approach that demands reflexivity from both the student and the teacher (e.g. inviting people who are happy to talk about their culture). Duffy (2001) suggests that a transformative education of culture is of value. Tranformative cultural education 'begins with the assumption of shared power between members of equal but different cultures and acknowledges that co-learning and co-creating occur through interaction between individuals and groups'. Duffy stresses the value of the process of learning and that students should use 'their hearts and their heads' to develop inclusiveness. Students might be guided to learn and understand universal commonalities such as love and protection of family and friends rather than emphasizing difference and 'otherness'. This type of session has been used on a number of occasions within our own courses, where we have invited several people to discuss their experiences of 'being Muslim'. Students have benefited from the opportunity to ask questions and discuss their ideas and experiences from clinical practice. It is interesting to note that the speakers themselves have also commented positively on the sessions.

These approaches to transcultural nursing are varied, and each has its own particular value. However, they are reliant on teachers and educators themselves being prepared and willing to teach transcultural nursing. Although there is evidence that serious efforts are being made by some individuals and in certain institutions to address these issues (McGee, 1992; Papadopoulos *et al.*, 1994), it is also clear that preparation is still often inadequate. This factor was highlighted by Gerrish *et al.* (1996a) in a national survey to examine the ethnic-related content of curricula, together with teaching and learning methods. The responses to the survey revealed that there were serious shortfalls in teaching transcultural care nationally. For example, only 20 per cent of respondents felt that coursework prepared them to meet the healthcare needs of minority ethnic communities, and only one-quarter of programmes provided placements specifically intended to develop culturally sensitive care. Perhaps the most revealing finding of the study was that only 20 per cent of teaching staff had had extensive personal development to enable them to prepare students. Gerrish *et al.* (1996a) remarked that the responsibility for overseeing the preparation of students tended to rest with those educationalists that had a personal interest and commitment to the subject.

Gould-Stuart (1986) has described a programme conducted in a nursing home where many of the residents were Jewish and the staff came from a different cultural group. The aim was to modify the 'them and us' situation that had arisen between the staff and the residents. Gould-Stuart (1986) discussed a programme of seminars that explored aspects of ageing in relation to a range of different cultures, which prevented the staff from feeling that they were being policed or made to change their attitudes. The programme appears to have been successful because it did not rely on prescriptive approaches, but gave the staff the opportunity to explore and consider the issues at their own pace in a non-threatening manner. Baxter (1998) argues that although education and training in cultural issues is now taking place, albeit on an *ad hoc* basis, there is a pressing need to incorporate work that promotes racial equality in the profession. This notion is echoed by Alleyne *et al.* (1994), who argue that nurse education must challenge racism and avoid approaches that merely reify culture. Race and racism should become central issues to be examined and understood in the context of nursing. It is argued, for example, that the contribution of racism and social deprivation to producing and perpetuating healthcare inequalities is largely ignored by healthcare professionals. Alleyne *et al.* (1994) also stress that racism and discrimination affect every level of the healthcare service, including nurses and other healthcare workers, as well as clients. The failure of nurse educators to address racism and discrimination is perhaps due to one of three reasons:

1. a lack of knowledge, lack of training, and poor skills and knowledge development;
2. it can be argued that many teachers themselves hold racist and discriminatory views and they therefore do not challenge such views in the classroom;
3. they are not interested in the subject, avoid it (e.g. by dismissing it as 'political correctness gone mad') and/or do not feel that it merits attention (which is in itself a form of institutionalized racism).

However, from our personal experience (and from anecdotal reports heard while talking with other nurse teachers), combating racism and other discriminatory attitudes in the classroom can be both daunting and intimidating. Although we may be able to prevent nurses from expressing racist attitudes and beliefs in the classroom, we cannot be sure of their behaviours and practices outside it. Moreover, it is very difficult to change people's attitudes – which may often be the result of many years of socialization, prejudice and institutionalized racism. However, we would argue that failure to tackle racism is racist behaviour in itself. Sawley (2001) notes racist comments in the classroom and on placement areas. A lecturer from a minority ethnic group noted that in the past a group 'had refused to be taught by me because I am black', and six students had noted racist comments made by lecturers.

Baxter (1998) stresses the need for a race equality tutor. This may ensure a highly skilled, competent and knowledgeable teacher delivering high-quality and challenging information in the classroom. However, as Baxter (1998) herself indicates, this approach may have the effect of passing the problem on to other people instead. Finally, Baxter (1998) advocates the recognition of the contribution of black and minority ethnic student nurses and tutors. Tilki *et al.* (1994) also advocate this approach, stating that:

> Given the right environment, the adequately empowered nurse has the capacity to offer insights into his/her culture which can enable colleagues to appreciate some of the beliefs about health and illness that clients hold and value.

> *(Tilki et al., 1994, p. 1119)*

In a further study, Tilki *et al.* (2007) explored perceptions and experiences of classroom racism among nursing students and lecturers. The study exposed evidence of racism that was manifested in different ways. Many lecturers lacked confidence in tackling sensitive emotive issues and the study suggested that classroom management is needed to support lecturers to become culturally competent. However, we need to guard against assuming that every black and minority ethnic nurse is willing and prepared to act as a spokesperson for their cultural group, or on issues related to racial equality. Alleyne *et al.* (1994) conclude:

> Only when we begin to appreciate the depth and the relative imperviousness of our own ethnicity, and the extent of our own prejudices, can we begin to transcend our culture and appreciate that of our clients who belong to different ethnic groups.

> *(Alleyne et al., 1994, p. 1124)*

Key points

1. Nurse education can play a central part in improving the quality of culturally sensitive care.
2. There are several approaches to transcultural education programmes, each with its own merits.
3. Racism awareness training has a vital part to play in providing care that is both comprehensive and holistic.

CONCLUSION

> Racial discrimination is unlawful. It harms society as well as the individuals concerned, and is a waste of talent, resources and potential. An organization made up of diverse groups, with a wide range of abilities, experiences and skills, is more likely to be alive to new ideas and possibilities than a more homogeneous one.

> *(Mensah, 1996, p. 27)*

At the beginning of this chapter, reference was made to the 1999 Macpherson Inquiry and the Royal College of Nursing's concerns with regard to institutionalized racism in the NHS. Although this remains a volatile and contentious issue, the anecdotal and research-based evidence presented in this chapter clearly show the extent of the prejudice, misinformation and stereotypical attitudes that pervade the nursing profession. The damage and hurt experienced by many black and minority ethnic nurses working in the NHS must give all of us cause for concern. Overt and direct racism is offensive and unlawful, but of equal concern is the indirect racism that is experienced by many black and minority ethnic nurses. Racial discrimination is difficult to prove, and of course many people do not want to carry the label of troublemaker, so they bury the hurt and humiliation that they have experienced. However, as Mensah (1996) argues, all health service staff have a responsibility to combat discriminatory practices regardless of who they are and what position they hold. Furthermore, it can be argued that nurse education is not exempt from this responsibility, and many would argue that it holds the key to effective and positive change.

Clearly, therefore, when we begin to see racism and discrimination as a collective issue in the nursing profession, and not just as someone else's problem, then we may begin to effect change. It is easy to shift the blame and abdicate responsibility, and (equally damaging) to offer solutions that are patchy or piecemeal. If nursing is to offer care to patients that is both respectful and sensitive to cultural needs, it must tackle the inequalities and discrimination in its own profession, embrace cultural diversity and aim to open the doors for everyone.

CHAPTER SUMMARY

1. The evidence clearly demonstrates that racism and discrimination are prevalent in nursing and health care in the UK.
2. In general, nurses are not adequately prepared to care for patients in a culturally diverse society.
3. There is a strong argument that, unless we tackle racism, ethnocentric ideas and beliefs, all other strategies to provide care that is culturally sensitive will be futile.

FURTHER READING

Baxter C (1997) *Race equality in health care and education.* Ballière Tindall, London.
An extremely interesting and illuminating text, that is well written, easy to read, and provides much valuable information and research.

Hayes L, Quine S and Bush J (1994) Attitude change amongst nursing students towards Australian Aborigines. *International Journal of Nursing Studies* **31**, 67–76.
This paper discusses a workshop designed to improve the attitudes of nursing students towards Australian Aboriginals. The workshops were conducted by indigenous people and resulted in significant changes in students' attitudes. The tables provide interesting insights into stereotypical views about Aboriginal peoples.

Mayor V (1996) Investing in people: personal and professional development of black nurses. *Health Visitor* **69**, 20–3.

In this paper Mayor discusses her research, which investigates the career progression of black nurses in the UK. Some alarming and challenging narratives and statistics are presented concerning the overt and covert discrimination experienced by senior nurses working in the NHS.

Papadopoulos I (2003) The Papadopoulos, Tilki and Taylor model for the development of cultural competence in nursing. *Journal of Social and Environmental Issues* **4**, 5–7.

This model is useful in assisting practitioners to consider the different aspects of developing a model for cultural competence.

WEBSITES

http://www.dh.gov.uk/en/Publicationsandstatistics/Publications/ PublicationsPolicyAndGuidance/DH_066059

This web site links to the report 'Positive Steps – Supporting race equality in mental healthcare', Department of Health (2007).

http://www.harpweb.org.uk/index.php

This website links to Health for Asylum seekers and refugees and is a resource for health professionals involved in their care and well-being.

http://www.kwintessential.co.uk/cross-cultural/intercultural-communication- translation-news/category/cultural-diversity/

This website is for intercultural communication and translation news and reports on cultural news items world-wide.

Appendix 1

CHRISTIANITY – BELIEFS AND PRACTICES

Christians believe in one God and are followers of Jesus, whom they believe is the son of God. Jesus was crucified by the Romans for his beliefs, and his life is marked by the following festivals of Christianity:

- Christmas Day – his birth;
- Lent – which lasts for 40 days (from Ash Wednesday to Good Friday) and marks his 40 days in the desert. This is a time for Christians to reflect on their lives;
- Good Friday – marks the end of Lent and the day when Christ was crucified;
- Easter Day – celebrates his resurrection;
- Whitsun – is celebrated 50 days after Easter (Pentecost). This is an important festival for many Christians; it celebrates the descent of the Holy Spirit to Jesus' apostles after his death (Schott and Henley, 1996).

Christians believe in an afterlife and in heaven (where 'good' Christians are believed to go after death) and hell (where the Devil exists and where 'evil' people go).

The different denominations and groups include the following:

- Anglican/Church of England;
- Roman Catholic;
- Methodist;
- Pentecostal;
- Seventh Day Adventists;
- Baptists.

Implications of Christian beliefs for nursing and healthcare

Christians in hospital may wish to read the Bible, pray and receive holy communion. The hospital chaplain will be able to support their individual needs. Holy Communion may be taken at the bedside if necessary. If their illness permits, patients may visit the hospital chapel for prayers and religious services. For Seventh Day Adventists the Sabbath day is a Saturday.

Most Christians have been baptized (when they commit themselves to God). Some parents of very sick children and babies may request that they are baptized in hospital. The chaplain or priest can perform this ceremony. Schott and Henley (1996) point out that in an emergency anyone can undertake this ceremony, but preferably someone who has also been baptized.

Roman Catholic priests may undertake to anoint the sick and say prayers. This is a particularly important service for those who are dying.

There are no special death rituals unless these are specifically requested; neither are there any objections to post-mortem or transplant of organs on religious grounds.

Appendix 2

BUDDHISM – BELIEFS AND PRACTICES

Buddhism can be regarded as both a way of life and a religion. It is the main religion in Bhutan, Nepal and Tibet. There are two main schools of Buddhism, namely Thervada or 'Teaching of the Elders' and Mahyar or the 'Greater Way'. One branch of Mahyar Buddhism is Zen Buddhism; Tibetan Buddhism is another. Buddhists acknowledge no single God as creator. Instead, Buddhism acknowledges many Gods, but 'these are all seen as lesser beings than Buddha himself' (Neuberger, 1994). Buddhists believe in rebirth, which is influenced by past and present lives. Adhering to Buddhist teaching in each life enables the person to learn from past existences and to continue to strive for perfection or nirvana.

To achieve this perfect state of existence, Buddhists must follow a path (the Eightfold Path) which encompasses Buddha's Four Truths. According to Neuberger (1994), these noble truths are as follows:

- suffering is strongly linked to our existence as human beings;
- suffering itself is caused by our craving for pleasure, which then prevents us from gaining knowledge and insight;
- human beings will only eliminate suffering by removing wrong desires and selfishness;
- the way to remove this suffering is to keep to the Eightfold path to enlightenment.

The Eightfold Path (Sampson, 1982; Neuberger, 1994):

1. The Buddhist aims to gain a complete understanding of life.
2. The Buddhist aims to have the right outlook and motives.
3. The Buddhist aims to have the 'right' speech (i.e. not lie or gossip).
4. The Buddhist aims to carry out perfect conduct, which involves being and doing good and not doing evil. This is linked to not taking a life. He or she must not be dishonest or deceitful.
5. The Buddhist must earn his or her own living in accordance with Buddhist teaching – known as the 'right livelihood'.
6. The Buddhist has to practise 'the right effort' (i.e. developing self-discipline).
7. The Buddhist has to develop 'right-mindedness', which is achieved through meditation.
8. The Buddhist aims to practise 'perfect meditation' leading to complete enlightenment.

A ritual which symbolizes entry into the Buddhist faith is an affirmation of faith in three Treasures (Jewels), namely the Buddha (historical Buddha and spiritual ideal of enlightenment), the Dharma (teaching and practices lead to enlightenment) and the Sangha (the spiritual community, i.e. people who practise the Dharma).

Implications of Buddhist beliefs for nursing and health care

Time and space for meditation may be required. Some Buddhists may follow strict rules of hygiene, requiring them to wash before meditation and after defecation and urination. Many Buddhists are vegetarians. Their philosophy of life and rebirth is that imminent death will require that they are in a clear and conscious mind. This may affect the taking of pain-relieving drugs which cloud the mind. Sensitivity and reassurance about the influence of any medication must therefore be shown. Buddhists are usually cremated. There are no special rituals other than specific cultural ones as appropriate.

Appendix 3

HINDUISM – BELIEFS AND PRACTICES

Hinduism is a religion and way of life. A central element in Hinduism is the Supreme Spirit from which the whole universe stems. Everything that happens in the world is categorized as being creative, preserving or destructive, and this is symbolized by the three main Hindu Gods:

- Brahma – the Creator, who symbolizes creative power;
- Vishnu – the Preserver, who preserves and maintains what has been created;
- Shiva – the Destroyer, who brings all things to an end (Henley, 1983b).

Hindus believe that all living things are reincarnated. This cycle of life is called Sansar. The source of all things (atman) is reborn in another body. Karma is related to the belief that nothing takes place without a reason which is linked to one's responsibility for determining one's actions. Good karma is achieved by following a religious life and doing good to others. The ultimate aim is to be released from this cycle of reincarnation (earthly existence) and reunited with the Supreme Spirit. This is called Moksha.

Duty or Dharma is a very important aspect of Hindu religion, as is purity.

All aspects of bodily functions and emissions are considered impure and therefore polluting. A Hindu's body must be cleansed before worship, especially if they have had contact with impure things. Running water is a purifying agent and Hindus will wish to wash or shower frequently, especially before prayer.

The Hindu Holy Book is known as the Bhagvad Gita. A mala (string of beads) may be used during prayer, and must only be touched with clean hands. A Hindu temple is known as a Mandir, and shoes are removed and women must wear a head covering before entering it. There is no segregation of the sexes in the congregation. These temples have a resident Brahmin (the highest Hindu caste), known as a pandit. Visiting priests and teachers are known as swamis.

Henley (1983b) states that it is 'illegal in India to discriminate on the grounds of caste'. However, it remains important in traditional aspects of Hindu life, such as marriage arrangements. The caste system is based on four main classes which are linked to key roles in Hindu society:

- Brahmins – mainly the priests;
- Kshatriyas – those who defend and govern;

- Vaishyas – those who produce goods and food (e.g. farmers and tradesmen);
- Shudras – those who serve the other castes.

In addition, there is another class of people, namely the Outcastes or Untouchables. These have no caste and are viewed as those who undertake spiritually polluting jobs.

Implications of Hindu beliefs for nursing and health care

Modesty is very important to both men and women. Women must cover their legs, breasts and upper arms, and they would prefer to be examined by a female doctor. They usually wear a sari and the midriff is very often left bare. Some Hindu women may wear a shalwar kameez both during the day and at night. Women wear jewellery in the form of bracelets and a brooch known as a mangal sutra, which is strung on a necklace. These must not be removed unnecessarily. This could have implications for preoperative care, and nurses should ensure that removal is absolutely necessary before removing jewellery that has religious significance, or they should provide alternative arrangements that are culturally appropriate. Many women also wear a bindi – a small coloured dot in the middle of the forehead. Some married women also put red powder (sindur) in their hair parting to indicate their married status.

Men usually wear a kameez and pajamas (trousers with a drawstring) or a dhoti. This a cloth about 5–6 m long which is wrapped around the waist and drawn between the legs. Older men may also wear a long coat (achkan) or a shirt with a high collar and buttons down the front, known as a kurta. Men also wear 'a janeu or sacred thread worn over their right shoulder and round the body' (Henley, 1983b). This should never be removed. Some men may wear a bead necklace or other jewellery of religious significance.

Washing in running water is important to maintain purity. A special jug or bottle (and a water supply) can be provided for patients in hospital toilets and bathrooms. Toilet paper is not traditionally used, and Hindus use the left hand to wash themselves. The right hand is used for handling food and other clean objects. Hindus will wish to shower before prayer, and if this is not possible they must be assisted to wash with running water. Because of their beliefs about pollution, shoes must not be put in the bedside locker with clean things, because the feet are considered to be the dirtiest part of the body. The head is the most sacred part. During menstruation and 40 days after the birth of a child, women are considered to be unclean and polluting. They are not allowed to go to the temple, pray or touch any holy books at this time, and sexual intercourse is prohibited. Some women may not cook at this time.

Many Hindus are vegetarian. The cow is a sacred animal and the pig is considered unclean. Eggs are eaten by many Hindus. Because of their beliefs about pollution, some Hindus will not eat anything that has been prepared in hospital and their families will bring food prepared at home for them. They may refuse to eat or drink in hospital because they are unable to ascertain that the food or drink is not polluted in some way. Nurses will need to be particularly vigilant with regard to those patients where starvation and dehydration may hinder their progress and care.

Many Hindus will wish to die at home rather than in hospital. This must be considered sensitively, and it should be enabled to take place whenever possible. Hindus are cremated, usually within 24 hours of death. Young children and babies are usually buried. A period of mourning then takes place, and family members very often wear white for 10 days after as sign that they are in mourning.

The recording and acknowledgement of Hindu names are both important. Names will have three parts – a personal name, a middle name (which can only be used with the first name) and the surname (or family name): for example, man – Rajchand Patel, woman – Lalitakumari Sharma. It is important to record all of the names, given that certain family names are quite common (e.g. Patel).

Appendix 4

ISLAM – BELIEFS AND PRACTICES

Islam is the religion of Muslims. Makka (Mecca) in Saudi Arabia is considered to be the birthplace of the prophet Mohammed, and is a place of pilgrimage. Muslims face Makka during prayer (south-east in the UK). The prayer leader is called the Imam. They believe in one God (Allah) and the Qur'an (Koran) is their Holy Book. Islam is based on five Pillars (duties).

1. Declaration of faith (Shahadah);
2. Five daily prayers (Namaz);
3. Fasting during Ramadan (1 month of abstinence from food and drink from just before dawn until sunset);
4. The giving of alms (Zakat);
5. Hajj – pilgrimage to Makka at least once during the person's lifetime.

Washing rituals are an important aspect of Islamic prayer. Before prayer, the face, ears and forehead, the feet to the ankles and the hands to the elbows are washed. The nose is cleaned by sniffing up water, and the mouth is rinsed out. Private parts of the body are also washed after urination and defecation if this takes place before prayer. Exemptions from prayer are given to women during menstruation and up to 40 days after childbirth. The mentally ill are also exempt, as are the seriously ill. Friday is the Muslim holy day. Women do not generally attend the mosque for prayer, meetings and other functions, although there are some mosques which provide separate prayer rooms for women.

Ramadan is an important time for Muslims. Fasting is compulsory although there are some exceptions, including young children under 12 years, menstruating women and pregnant or breastfeeding women. Muslims who are ill are exempt, and diabetic Muslims may require readjustment of their insulin to fit in with their Ramadan meal patterns to avoid hypoglycaemic attacks. The zakat (2 per cent of their disposable income given to the needy each year) is collected during Ramadan. The Festival of Eid-ul-Fitr (Festival of Almsgiving) takes place after Ramadan ends.

Implications of Islamic beliefs for nursing and health care

Women may wear a shalwar kameez and a chuni or duppata (long scarf). They must be covered from head to foot, except for their hands and faces. They may wear glass or gold bangles, which must not be removed unless absolutely necessary, and only then with sensitivity and reassurance. Men may wear a kameez and pajamas. They also wear a head covering such as a brimless cloth hat or cap during prayer. Whenever possible, women patients need to see female doctors and men patients need to see male doctors.

The Muslim diet involves avoiding pork altogether, and all other meat must be halal. This means that it has been killed according to Islamic law, which involves cutting the throat of the animal so that it bleeds to death. Many hospitals now provide halal meat for patients. Alcohol is specifically forbidden in the Holy Qur'an.

If the patient is seriously ill or dying they may wish to sit or lie facing Makka, and their family may read the Holy Qur'an to them. At death the nurses can turn the patient on to their right side and position the bed so that it faces Makka. The body is not to be washed, and preferably it should not be touched by non-Muslims. Post-mortem examinations are usually forbidden unless there is a legal or medical need for them. Muslims are buried, not cremated, and this must take place as soon as possible after death.

Asian Muslim names do not have a shared family surname. Their own name comes first, followed by the father's or husband's name. Henley (1982) cites the following example:

- Husband: Mohammed Hafiz
- Wife: Jameela Khatoon
- Sons: Liaquat Ali, Mohammed Sharif
- Daughters: Shameena Bibi, Fatma Jan

For recording purposes this would need to be documented as Jameela Khatoon (wife of Mohammed Hafiz) or Mohammed Sharif (son of Mohammed Hafiz). The male and female naming systems are different. The calling name of a man is usually used by friends (e.g. Hafiz). If it is the second name, then it is usually preceded by a religious name (e.g. Mohammed). This must not be used or recorded as his first or personal name (Henley, 1982). Men may also have a hereditary name (e.g. Quereshi) which they may use as a surname. Muslim women also have two names. The first is their personal name (e.g. Amina) and the second can be either a name which is the same as the UK female title (i.e. Mrs) or another personal name (e.g. Begum). Henley (1982) recommends that the second female name be recorded as the woman's surname, but it is important to remember to record her husband's name if she is married (e.g. Amina Begum, wife of Mohammed Khalid).

Appendix 5

JUDAISM – BELIEFS AND PRACTICES

Judaism is the religion of Jewish people. Early stories are to be found in the Old Testament of the Hebrew Bible. Israel is considered to be a Jewish homeland. There are two main groups – Orthodox Jews and Progressive Jews. The Orthodox Jews follow a religious life which adheres to the traditional interpretation of God's will in the Torah or Pentateuch (handed to Moses by God on Mount Sinai). However, Progressive Jews follow a more modern interpretation of the Torah. Jews pray in the synagogue. They believe in one God, and that the Messiah has not yet come: they do not believe that Jesus was the Messiah. The Laws and the Prophets are written about in the Talmud.

They celebrate the Sabbath, which begins at sunset on Friday and lasts until sunset on Saturday. Work is prohibited during this period, including everyday tasks such as cooking or even switching on lights. Candles can be lit at the onset of the Sabbath. The Passover is celebrated in March/April, when only unleavened bread is eaten. Some Jewish men keep their heads covered at all times, and Orthodox Jewish women dress modestly (e.g. never with bare arms). Married women wear a wig or keep their hair covered at all times.

Jewish Festivals include:

- Yom Kippur (the Day of Atonement);
- Rosh Hashanah (Jewish New Year);
- Pesach (the Passover).

Implications of Jewish beliefs for nursing and health care

Jews believe in life after death, and dying patients should not be left alone. They may ask to see a rabbi, who will say a prayer with them. This is often the affirmation of faith or the Sheema. Orthodox Jews can only be buried, and the funeral normally takes place within 24 hours of death. This can sometimes be difficult if death takes place on the Sabbath. When a Jewish person dies, the mouth and eyes can be closed, usually by a son or closest relative. The arms can be placed by the sides of the body.

Orthodox Jews only eat kosher food, and pork and shellfish are normally forbidden. Meat and milk are not eaten together, nor must they be prepared together.

All male babies are circumcized on the eighth day after birth, and this ritual is performed by the mohel, who is a 'trained and registered circumciser' (Sampson, 1982). This is both a medical procedure and a religious ritual, and if the child is still in hospital and there are no medical reasons for not performing the circumcision, then the ceremony should be allowed to continue along with the celebrations (Purnell and Paulanka, 1998).

Orthodox male Jews wear a skullcap (yarmulke) and a prayer shawl (tallith) when praying.

Appendix 6

SIKHISM – BELIEFS AND PRACTICES

Sikhs believe in one God and in reincarnation. A Sikh temple is known as a Gurdwara, and the Sikh Holy Book is the Holy Granth Sahib. The Gurdwara also acts as a community centre for the local Sikh community. Sikhs who have been formally baptized are called Amridharis, and the ceremony is known as taking Amrit (a mixture of sugar and water which is blessed). As a mark of faith Sikhs wear what are known as the five 'K's.

1. Kesh – long hair. Men wear this in a bun (jura) under a turban. Women may wear plaits and cover their hair with a scarf (dupatta or chuni). Sikh boys will usually wear their hair in a bun on top of their head covered with a small white cloth (rumal) or a large square cloth (patka).

2. Kanga – small comb worn at all times.

3. Kara – steel bracelet worn on the right wrist.

4. Kaccha – special type of underwear (white shorts).

5. Kirpa – symbolic dagger/sword.

Women may wear the salwar (trousers) and kameez (shirt) with a long scarf (chuni). The salwar and kameez are worn day and night. They will also wear glass or gold wedding bangles which are never removed unless they are widowed (their removal symbolizes the loss of a husband).

Men may wear a kameez and pajama or kurta (a long shirt with a high collar and buttons all down the front).

Sikhs do not eat halal meat. This is because their meat has to have been killed with one stroke (jhatra or chakar). There is no specifically prohibited meat (Karmi, 1996). However, very few Sikhs eat beef because it is sacred in India and the pig is considered unclean. Many are vegetarian and do not eat fish or eggs.

Implications of Sikh beliefs for nursing and health care

The importance of the five 'K's will influence the care that Sikhs receive. The hair must not usually be shaved, but this may have to be undertaken in cases of serious head injury or surgery. This will cause a Sikh great distress, and they and their family will need much reassurance. The removal of the kanga, kara and kirpan will also upset a Sikh, and a full explanation must be given for this, together with possible solutions for keeping the items close by. The kaccha are never removed, and when changing one leg is usually left on whilst a new pair is put on the other. They may also be kept on in the shower. Men will also wish to keep their turban on when they are in hospital.

A dying Sikh may derive comfort from having passages read from the Granth Sahib. A member of the local gurdwara will undertake this. There are no specific last-office rites, but Sikhs are normally washed and laid out by their family. However, if nurses have to do this it is preferable only to close the eyes, straighten the limbs and wrap the body in a plain sheet with no religious emblems. Sikhs are cremated and not buried, usually within 24 hours of death. If a body has to be removed from a ward to the mortuary for viewing by relatives it is essential that all Christian religious emblems are removed from the room and replaced by the Khanda (religious symbol of Sikhs) on the altar.

Karmi (1996) states that 'most Sikhs will have three names: a first name, a religious title (Kaur meaning princess for women and Singh meaning lion for men) and a family name.' This last name is not often used by Sikhs because of its links with the hereditary caste system, which they reject. However, to avoid confusion some Sikhs in the UK have started to use this family name. Henley (1983a) provides examples of how this can be identified by nurses and others.

Non-hereditary family names (Henley, 1983a):

- Husband: Jaswinder Singh (lion)

- Wife: Kuldeep Kaur (princess)

- Sons: Amarjit Singh, Mohan Singh

- Daughter: Harbans Kaur, Satwant Kaur

Hereditary family names (Henley, 1983a)

- Husband: Rajinder Singh Grewal (family name)
- Wife: Swaran Kaur Grewal
- Son: Mohan Singh Grewal
- Daughter: Kamaljeet Kaur Grewal

The patient or family need to be asked how they wish to be addressed, and the correct names should be recorded in their case notes and nursing records.

References

Abdullah S N (1995) Towards an individualised client's care: implication for education. The transcultural approach. *Journal of Advanced Nursing* **22**, 715–20.

Afiya Trust for National Black Carers and Carers Network (2008) *Beyond care – putting black carers in the picture*. NBCCWN and Afiya Trust, London; http://www.afiyatrust.org.uk/.

Ahmad W I U (ed.) (1993) *'Race' and health in contemporary Britain*. Open University Press, Milton Keynes.

Alam M Y and Husband C (2006) *British-Pakistani men from Bradford: linking narratives to policy*. Joseph Rowntree Foundation, York.

Alexis O and Vydelingum V (2004) The lived experience of overseas black and minority ethnic nurses in the NHS in the south of England. *Diversity in Health and Social Care* **1**, 13–20.

Allan H T, Larsen J A, Bryan K and Smith P (2004) The social reproduction of institutional racism: internationally recruited nurses' experiences of British health services. *Diversity in Health and Social Care* **1**, 117–25.

Alleyne J, Papadopoulos I and Tilki M (1994) Antiracism within transcultural nurse education. *British Journal of Nursing* **3**, 635–7.

Alleyne S A, Cruickshank J K, Golding A N L and Morrison E Y St A (1989) Mortality from diabetes in Jamaica. *Bulletin of Pan American Health Organization* **23**, 306–15.

American Nurses' Association (1986) *Cultural diversity in the nursing curriculum: a guide for implementation*. American Nurses' Association, Kansas City.

Andersen S (1997) Changing practices in the weaning of babies in Britain. *Professional Care of Mother and Child* **7**, 59–60.

Andrews M M (1995) Transcultural perspectives in the nursing care of children and adolescents. In: Andrews M M and Boyle J S (eds), *Transcultural concepts in nursing care*, 2nd edn. J B Lippincott, Philadelphia, 123–79.

Andrews M M (2008) Religion, culture and nursing. In: Andrews M M and Boyle J S (eds), *Transcultural concepts in nursing care*, 5th edn. Wolters Kluwer/Lippincott Williams and Wilkins, Philadelphia, 355–407.

Andrews M M and Boyle J S (1995) *Transcultural concepts in nursing care*, 2nd edn. JB Lippincott, Philadelphia.

Anionwu E (1993) Sickle cell and thalassaemia: community experiences and official response. In: Ahmad W I U (ed.), *'Race' and health in contemporary Britain*. Open University Press, Milton Keynes, 76–95.

Atwal A and Caldwell K (2002) Do multidisciplinary integrated care pathways improve interprofessional collaboration? *Scandinavian Journal of Caring Science* **16**, 360–7.

Arber S and Gilbert N (1989) Men: the forgotten carers. *Sociology* **23**, 111–18.

Arets J and Morle K (1995) The nursing process: an introduction. In: Basford L and Slevin O (eds) *Theory and practice of nursing – an integrated approach to care*. Campion Press, Edinburgh, 303–17.

Atkin K and Rollings J (1993) *Community care in a multiracial Britain. A critical review of the literature.* HMSO, London.

Australian Nursing and Midwifery Council (2008) *Code of Professional Conduct for Nurses in Australia.* Australian Nursing and Midwifery Council (ANMC), Dickson ACT, Australia.

Bahl V (1996) Cancer and ethnic minorities: the Department of Health's perspective. *British Journal of Cancer* **74**(Suppl 29), S2–10.

Baxter C (1988) *The black nurse: an endangered species.* National Extension College for Training in Health and Race, Cambridge.

Baxter C (1997) *Race equality in health care and education.* Ballière Tindall/Royal College of Nursing, London.

Baxter C (1998) Developing an agenda for promoting race equality in the nurse curriculum. *Nursing Times Research* **3**, 339–47.

BBC *The road to refuge.* http://news.bbc.co.uk/hi/english/static/in_depth/world/2001/road_to_refuge/default.stm (accessed 10/10/09).

Beaubier J (1976) *High life expectancy on the island of Paros, Greece.* Philosophical Library, New York.

Beavan J (2006) Responding to the needs of black and ethnic minority elders. *Nursing and Residential Care* **8**, 312–14.

Beiser M (1990) Migration: opportunity or mental health risk? *Triangle, Sandoz Journal of Medical Science* **29**, 83–90.

Beishon S, Virdee S and Hagell A (1995) *Nursing in a multi-ethnic NHS.* Policy Studies Institute, London.

Belliappa J (1991) *Illness or distress? Alternative models of mental health.* Confederation of Indian Organisations, London.

Bennett M (1988) An Aboriginal model of care. *Nursing Times* **84**, 56–8.

Bhugra D and Ayonrinde O (2004) Depression in migrants and ethnic minorities. *Advances in Psychiatric Treatment* 10, 13–17.

Bhugra D and Becker M A (2005) Migration, cultural bereavement and cultural identity. *World Psychiatry* **4**, 18–24.

Bhugra D and Jones P (2001) Migration and mental illness. *Advances in Psychiatric Treatment* vol **76**, 216–23.

Bhui K and Bhugra D (2002) Mental illness in Black and Asian ethnic minorities: pathways to care and outcomes. *Advances in Psychiatric Treatment* **8**, 26–33.

Bjorksten K S, Bjerragaard P and Kripke D F (2005) Suicides in the midnight sun – a study of seasonality in suicides in West Greenland. *Psychiatry Research* **133**, 205–13.

Black J (1991) Death and bereavement: the customs of Hindus, Sikhs and Moslems. *Bereavement Care* **10**, 6–8.

Blakemore K and Boneham M (1993) *Age, race and ethnicity.* Open University Press, Buckingham.

Blanche H T and Parkes C M (1997) Christianity. In: Parkes C M, Laungani P and Young B (eds) *Death and bereavement across cultures.* Routledge, London, 131–46.

Bond J and Bond S (1986) *Sociology and health care.* Churchill Livingstone, Edinburgh.

Bottomley G (1981) *Social class and ethnicity. Chomi Report No. 348.* Clearing House of Migrant Issues, Melbourne.

Bowler I (1993) 'They're not the same as us': midwives' stereotypes of South Asian descent maternity patients. *Sociology of Health and Illness* **15**, 157–78.

Boyce K (1998) Asserting difference: psychiatric care in black and white. In: Barker P and Davidson B (eds) *Ethical strife.* Edward Arnold, London, 157–70.

Bradby H (2001) Communication, interpretation and translation. In: Culley L and Dyson S (eds) *Ethnicity and nursing practice.* Palgrave, Buckingham, 129–48.

Bradby H (2007) Watch out for the Aunties! Young British Asians' accounts of identity and substance use. *Sociology of Health and Illness* **29**, 656–72.

Brink P J (1984) Key issues in nursing and anthropology. *Advances in Medical Social Science* **2**, 107–46.

British Medical Association (1995) *Multicultural health care – current practice and future policy in medical education.* British Medical Association (BMA), London.

British Medical Association (2002) *Asylum seekers – meeting their health care needs.* British Medical Association (BMA), London

Brown K, Avis M and Hubbard M (2007) Health beliefs of Afro-Caribbean people with Type 2 diabetes: a qualitative study. *British Journal of General Practice* **57**, 461–9.

Bruni N (1988) A critical analysis of transcultural theory. *Australian Journal of Advanced Nursing* **5**, 27–32.

Bryan L (2007) Should ward nurses hide death from other patients? *End of Life Care* **1**, 79–86.

Buchan J, O'May F and McCann D (2008) *Older but wiser? Policy responses to an ageing nursing workforce.* RCN Scotland, Queen Margaret University, Edinburgh.

Burnard P and Gill P (2008) *Culture, communication and nursing.* Pearson Education, Harlow.

Burnett A (2002) *Guide to health workers providing care for asylum seekers and refugees.* Medical Foundation, London.

Burnett A and Fassil Y (2003) *Meeting the health needs of asylum seekers in the UK. An information pack for health workers.* NHS London Directorate of Health and Social Care, London.

Burnett A and Peel M (2001) Asylum seekers and refugees in Britain: health needs of asylum seekers and refugees. *British Medical Journal* **322**, 544–7.

Butt J and O'Neil A (2004) 'Let's move on'. Joseph Rowntree Foundation, York.

Calder S, Anderson G, Harper W and Gregg P (1994) Ethnic variation in epidemiology and rehabilitation of hip fracture. *British Medical Journal* **309**, 1124–5.

Carbello M (2007) *The challenge of migration and health.* International Centre for Migration and Health; http://www.icmh.ch/publications.htm (accessed 16/10/09).

Carers UK (2009) *Facts about carers, January 2009 policy briefing;* http://www.carersuk.org/Home (accessed 28/09/09).

Carey Wood J, Duke K and Karn V (1995) *The settlement of refugees in Britain. Home Office Research Study No 141.* HMSO, London.

Carlisle D (1996) A nurse in any language. *Nursing Times* **92**, 26–7.

Carson V B (1989) Spiritual dimensions of nursing practice. W B Saunders, Philadelphia.

Cashmore E E (1988) *Dictionary of race and ethnic relations*, 2nd edn. Routledge, London.

Caudhill W and Frost L A (1973) A comparison of maternal care and infant behaviour in Japanese-American, American and Japanese families. In Lebra W (ed.) *Youth socialisation and mental health*. University Press of Hawaii, Honolulu.

Chapman G E (1983) Ritual and rational action in hospitals. *Journal of Advanced Nursing* **8**, 13–20.

Chevannes M (1995) Children's views about health; assessing the implications for nurses. *British Journal of Nursing* **4**, 1073–80.

Chevannes M (1997) Nursing caring for families – issues in a multiracial society. *Journal of Clinical Nursing* **6**, 161–7.

Cochrane R and Bal S (1989) Mental health admission rates of immigrants to England: a comparison of 1971 and 1981. *Social Psychiatry and Psychiatric Epidemiology* **24**, 2–11.

Colliere M F (1986) Invisible care and invisible women as health care providers. *International Journal of Nursing Studies* **23**, 95–112.

Coid J W, Kahatan N and Gault S (2000) Ethnic differences in admissions to secure forensic psychiatry services. *British Journal of Psychiatry* **177**, 241–7.

Commission for Race Equality (2000) The Race Relations (Amendment) Act. Commission for Racial Equality, London.

Commission for Racial Equality (2004) *Gypsies and Travellers: a strategy for the CRE*. Commission for Racial Equality (CRE), London.

Community Practice (1993) Beliefs and customs of the Hindu, Jewish and Muslim communities. *Professional Nurse*, February, **8**, 333.

Cook B and Philips S G (1988) *Loss and bereavement*. Austin Cornish, London.

Cope R (1989) The compulsory detention of Afro-Caribbeans under the Mental Health Act. *New Community* **15**, 343–56.

Corsellis A and Crichton J (1994) Crossing the language and culture barrier. Why we need a training scheme for specialist skills. *Psychiatric Care* **November/ December**, 172–6.

Cortis J D (1993) Transcultural nursing: appropriateness for Britain. *Journal of Advances in Health and Nursing Care* **2**, 67–77.

Cox J L (1977) Aspects of transcultural psychiatry. *British Journal of Psychiatry* **130**, 211–21.

Culley L and Mayor V (2001) Ethnicity and nursing careers. In: Culley L and Dyson S (eds) *Ethnicity and nursing practice*. Palgrave, Basingstoke, 211–30.

Currer C (1991) Understanding the mother's viewpoint: the case of Pathan women in Britain. In: Wyke S and Hewison J (eds) *Child health matters*. Open University Press, Milton Keynes, 40–52.

D'Alessio V (1993) Culture clash. *Nursing Times* **89**, 16–17.

Daley A (2004) Caring for women who have undergone genital mutilation. *Nursing Times* **100**, 32; http://www.nursingtimes.net (accessed 16/08/09).

Daly W M, Swindlehurst L and Johal P (2003) Exploration into the recruitment of South Asian nurses. *British Journal of Nursing* **12**, 687–96.

Darvill A (2003) Testing the water – problem-based learning and the cultural dimension. *Nurse Education in Practice* **3**, 72–9.

Davies C (1995) *Gender and the professional predicament in nursing.* Open University Press, Buckingham.

Davis H and Choudhury P A (1988) Helping Bangladeshi families: Tower Hamlets parent–adviser scheme. *Mental Handicap* **16**, 48–51.

Department of Health (1989) *Children's Act.* The Stationary Office, London; http://www.dcsf.gov.uk/childrenactreport/.

Department of Health (1992) *The Patient's Charter.* HMSO, London.

Department of Health (1996) *The Patient's Charter and you.* HMSO, London.

Department of Health (1998) *NHS Hospital and Community Health Services non-medical staff results for England: non-medical work-force consensus.* Department of Health, London.

Department of Health (2001) *Safety First: 5 year report of the national inquiry into suicide and homicide by people with mental illness.* Department of Health, London.

Department of Health (2004) *The Children's Act.* Department of Health, London.

Department of Health (2005a) *Elimination of mixed-sex hospital accommodation.* Department of Health, London.

Department of Health (2005b) *Delivering race equality in mental health care: an action plan for reform inside and outside services and the government's response to the independent inquiry into the death of David Bennett.* Department of Health, London.

Department of Health (2007a) *Privacy and dignity – a report by the chief nursing officer into mixed sex accommodation in hospitals.* Department of Health, London.

Department of Health (2007b) *A practical guide to ethnic monitoring in health and social care.* Department of Health, London.

Department of Health (2008) *Confidence in caring – a framework for best practice.* Department of Health, London.

Department of Health (2009) *Religion or belief – a practical guide for the NHS.* Department of Health, London.

De Santis L (1994) Making anthropology clinically relevant to nursing care. *Journal of Advanced Nursing* **20**, 707–15.

Dobson S (1986) Cultural value awareness: glimpses into a Punjabi mother's world. *Health Visitor* **59**, 382–4.

Dobson S M (1991) Transcultural nursing. Scutari Press, London.

Donaldson L (1986) Health and social status of elderly Asians: a community survey. *British Medical Journal* **293**, 1079–82.

Doran T, Drever F and Whitehead M (2003) Health of young and elderly informal carers: analysis of UK census data. BMJ **327**, 1388.

Drennan V M and Joseph J (2005) Health visiting and refugee families: issues in professional practice. *Journal of Advanced Nursing* **49**, 155–63.

Duffin C (2009) Would an increased proportion of male nurses benefit the profession? *Nursing Standard* **23**, 12–13.

Duffy M E (2001) A critique of cultural education in nursing. *Journal of Advanced Nursing* **36**, 487–95.

Dyson S, Culley L, Norrie P and Genders N (2008) An exploration of the experiences of South Asian students on pre-registration programmes in a UK university. *Journal of Research in Nursing* **13**, 163–76.

Ebrahim S (1996) Ethnic elders. *British Medical Journal* **313**, 610–13.

Ebrahim S, Patel N, Coats S *et al.* (1991) Prevalence and severity of morbidity amongst Gujarati elders: a controlled comparison. *Family Practice* **8**, 57–62.

Erens B, Primatesta P and Prior G (2001) *Health Survey for England: the Health of Minority Ethnic Groups, 99, Volume 1: Findings.* The Stationery Office, London.

Eisenbruch M (1988) The mental health of refugee children and their cultural development. *International Migration Review* **22**, 282–300.

Eisenbruch M (1991) From post-traumatic stress disorder to cultural bereavement: diagnosis of South Asian refugees. *Social Science and Medicine* **33**, 673–80.

Eisenbruch M (2001) *National review of nursing education: multi-cultural nursing education.* Department of Education, Science and Training, Canberra, ACT, Australia; http://www.dest.gov.au (accessed 05/08/09).

Ellahi R and Hatfield C (1992) Research into the needs of Asian families caring for someone with a mental handicap. *Mental Handicap* **20**, 134–6.

English National Board (1990) *Regulations and guidelines for the approval of institutions and courses.* English National Board for Nursing, Midwifery and Health Visiting, London.

Entwistle M (2004) *Women only? An explanation of the place of men in nursing* (Thesis). Victoria University, Wellington, New Zealand; http://hdl.handle.net/10063/35

Evans J A (2002) Cautious caregivers: gender stereotypes and the sexualisation of men nurses' touch. *Journal of Advanced Nursing* **40**, 441–8.

Fatchett A (1995) *Childhood to adolescence: caring for health.* Baillière Tindall, London.

Fazel M and Silvoe D (2006) Detention of refugees. *British Medical Journal* **332**, 251–2.

Fazel M, Wheeler J and Danesh J (2005) Prevalence of serious mental disorder in 700 refugees resettled in western countries: a systematic review. *Lancet* **365**, 1309–14.

Fennell G, Phillipson C and Evers H (1988) *The sociology of old age.* Open University Press, Milton Keynes.

Fenton S and Sadiq-Sanster A (1996) Culture, relativism and the expression of mental distress: South Asian women in Britain. *Sociology of Health and Illness* **18**, 66–85.

Ferguson M (1991) Sickle-cell anaemia and its effect on the new parent. *Health Visitor* **64**, 73–6.

Fernando S (1986) Depression in ethnic minorities. In: Cox J L (ed.) *Transcultural Psychiatry.* Croom-Helm, London, 107–38.

Fernando S (1991) *Mental health, race and culture,* 1st edn. Macmillan Education, Basingstoke.

Fernando S (1992) Roots of racism in psychiatry. *Open Mind* **59**, 10–11.

Fernando S (2002) *Mental health, race and culture,* 2nd edn. Macmillan Education, Basingstoke.

Finn J and Lee M (1996) Transcultural nurses reflect on discoveries in China using Leininger's sunrise model. *Journal of Transcultural Nursing* **7**, 21–7.

Fleming E, Carter B and Pettigrew J (2008) The influence of culture on diabetes self-management: perspectives of Gujarati Muslim men who reside in Northwest England. *Journal of Nursing and Healthcare of Chronic Illness* in association with *Journal of Clinical Nursing*, **17**(5a), 51–9.

Furnham A and Bochner S (1986) *Culture shock: psychological reactions to unfamiliar environments.* Routledge, London.

Galanti G-A (2008) *Caring for patients from different cultures,*4th edn. University of Pennsylvania Press, Philadelphia.

Galdas P, Cheater F and Marshall P (2005) Men and health help-seeking behaviour: literature review. *Journal of Advanced Nursing* **49**, 616–23.

Gatrad A R (1994) Attitudes and beliefs of Muslim mothers towards pregnancy and infancy. *Archives of Disease in Childhood* **71**, 170–4.

Gebru K, Ahsberg E and Willman A (2007) Nursing and medical documentation on patients' cultural background. *Journal of Clinical Nursing* **16**, 2056–65.

Gebru K and Willman A (2003) A research-based didactic model for education to promote culturally competent nursing care in Sweden. *Journal of Transcultural Nursing* **14**, 55–61.

Gebru K and Willman A (2009) Education to promote culturally competent nursing care – a content analysis of student responses. *Nurse Education Today* (in press).

Gerrish K, Husband C and Mackenzie J (1996a) *An examination of the extent to which pre-registration programmes of nursing and midwifery education prepare practitioners to meet the health care needs of minority ethnic communities.* Research Highlights. English National Board, London.

Gerrish K, Husband C and Mackenzie J (1996b) *Nursing for a multi-ethnic society.* Open University Press, Buckingham.

Gervais M C and Jovchelovitch S (1998) *The health beliefs of the Chinese community in England: a qualitative research study.* Health Education Authority, London.

Ghosh P (1998) South Asian Elders – a group with special needs. *Geriatric Medicine* **January**, 11–13.

Giddens A (1997) *Sociology.* Polity Press, Oxford.

Giger J N and Davidhizar R E (1991) *Transcultural nursing.* Mosby Year-Book, St Louis.

Giger J N and Davidhizer R E (2004) *Transcultural nursing - assessment and intervention*, 4th edn. Mosby, St Louis.

Goopy S (2006) … that the social order prevails: death, ritual and the 'Roman' nurse. *Nursing Inquiry* **13**, 110–17.

Gould-Stuart J (1986) Bridging the cultural gap between residents and staff. *Geriatric Nursing* **November/ December**, 19–21.

Gorst-Unsworth C and Goldberg E (1998) Psychological sequelae of torture and organised violence suffered by refugees from Iraq. *British Journal of Psychiatry* **172**, 90–4.

Hagger V (1994) Cultural challenge. *Nursing Times* **90**, 70–2.

Halbert, C H, Wrenn G, Weather B, Delmoor E, Have T T and Coyne J C (2009) Sociocultural determinants of men's reactions to prostate cancer diagnosis. *Psycho-Oncology* (Early view on-line DOI:10.1002/pon.1574).

Hall E T (1966b) *The silent language.* Greenwood Press, Westport.

HARP Health for Asylum Seekers and Refugees Portal; http://www.harpweb.org.uk.

Harrison G, Owen D, Holton A *et al.* (1988) A prospective study of severe mental disorder in Afro-Caribbean patients. *Psychological Medicine* **18**, 643–57.

Harrison S (2004) Racism and the NHS. *Nursing Standard* **19**, 12–14.

Hastings-Asatourian B (1996) Single white female. An investigation into the recruitment and selection practices of a college of nursing. (Unpublished MSc thesis).

Healey M A and Aslam M (1990) *The Asian community medicines and traditions.* Silverlink Publishing, Huddersfield.

Health Education Authority (1998) *Sun knows how: the skin cancer fact file.* Health Education Authority, London.

Healthcare Commission (2008) *Count Me In (National census of inpatients in mental health and learning disability services in England and Wales).* Healthcare Commission (now Care Quality Commission), London.

Helman C (1994) *Culture, health and illness,* 3rd edn. Butterworth-Heinmann, Oxford.

Helman C (2007) *Culture, health and illness,* 5th edn. Hodder Arnold, London.

Hendry J (1999) *An introduction to social anthropology.* Macmillan Press, Basingstoke.

Hendry J and Martinez L (1991) Nursing in Japan. In: Holden P and Littlewood J (eds) *Anthropology and nursing.* Routledge, London, 56–66.

Henley A (1982) *Caring for Muslims and their families: religious aspects of care.* Department of Health and Social Security and King's Fund, London.

Henley A (1983a) *Caring for Sikhs and their families: religious aspects of care.* Department of Health and Social Security and Kings' Fund, London.

Henley A (1983b) *Caring for Hindus and their families: religious aspects of care.* Department of Health and Social Security and King's Fund, London.

Henley A and Schott J (1999) *Culture, religion and patient care in a multi-ethnic society. A handbook for professionals.* Age Concern Books, London.

Her Majesty's Stationery Office (2004) *Civil Partnership Act 2004.* HMSO, London; http://www.opsi.gov.uk/acts/acts2004/ukpga_20040033_en_1 (accessed 24/11/09).

Herberg P (1995) Theoretical foundations of transcultural nursing. In: Andrews M A and Boyle J S (eds) *Transcultural concepts in nursing care,* 2nd edn. J B Lippincott Co, Philadelphia, 3–47.

Heslop P (1991) A preventable tragedy. *Nursing Times* **87**, 36–9.

Hicks C (1982a) Racism in nursing. *Nursing Times* 5 May, 743–8.

Hicks C (1982b) Racism in nursing. *Nursing Times* 12 May, 789–92.

Hilton C (1996) Global perspectives: a sensitive view. *Elderly Care* **8**, 12–15.

Hjelm K, Bard K, Nyberg P and Apelqvist J (2003) Religious and cultural distance in beliefs about health and illness in women with diabetes mellitus of different origin living in Sweden. *International Journal of Nursing Studies* **40**, 627–43.

Hjelm K G, Bard K, Nyberg P and Apelqvist J (2005) Beliefs about health and diabetes in men of different ethnic origin. *Journal of Advanced Nursing* **50**, 47–9.

Hjelm K, Nyberg P, Isacsson A and Apelqvist J (1999) Beliefs about health and illness essential for self care practice: a comparison of migrant Yugoslavian and Swedish diabetic females. *Journal of Advanced Nursing* **30**, 1147–59.

Hodes M (2000) Psychologically distressed refugee children in the United Kingdom. *Child Psychology and Psychiatry Review* **5**, 57–68.

Hoga L A K, Alcantara A C and De Lima V M (2001) Adult male involvement in reproductive health: an ethnographic study in a community of Sao Paulo City, Brazil. *Journal of Transcultural Nursing* **12**, 107–14.

Holland C K (1993) An ethnographic study of nursing culture as an exploration of determining the existence of a system of ritual. *Journal of Advanced Nursing* **18**, 461–70.

Holland C K (1996) *Teaching and learning strategies handbook. Pre-registration Diploma in Nursing curriculum.* School of Nursing, University of Salford, Salford.

Holland K, Jenkins J, Solomon J and Whittam S (2008) *Applying the Roper, Logan and Tierney Model in practice*, 2nd edn. Churchill Livingstone, Edinburgh.

Holmes E R and Holmes L D (1995) *Other cultures, elder years.* Sage Publications, Thousand Oaks.

Iganski P, Mason D, Humphreys A and Watkins M (1998a). The 'black nurse': ever an endangered species? *Nursing Times Research* **3**, 325–38.

Iganski P, Spong A, Mason D, Humphries A and Watkins M (1998b) *Recruiting minority ethnic groups into nursing, midwifery and health visiting.* English National Board for Nursing, Midwifery and Health Visiting, London.

Inoue M, Chapman R and Wynaden (2006) Male nurses' experiences of providing intimate care for women clients. *Journal of Advanced Nursing* **55**, 559–567.

Iverson V C and Morken G (2004) Differences in acute psychiatric admission between asylum seekers and refugees. *Nordic Journal of Psychiatry* **58**, 465–70.

Izzidien S (2008) *'I can't tell people what is happening at home' – domestic abuse within South Asian communities: the specific needs of women, children and young people.* NSPCC, London.

Jackson L E (1993) Understanding, eliciting and negotiating client's multicultural health beliefs. *Nurse Practitioner* **18**, 30–43.

James J (1995) Ethnicity and transcultural care. In Basford L and Slevin O (eds) *Theory and practice of nursing.* Campion Press, Edinburgh, 611–30.

Jervis L L (2001) The pollution of incontinence and the dirty work of caregiving in a U.S. nursing home. *Medical Anthropology Quarterly* **15**, 84–99.

Jones H (1996) Gender, race and social responses to an ageing client. In: Wade L and Waters K (eds) *A textbook of gerontological nursing perspectives on practice.* Ballière Tindall, London, 108–34.

Jones L J (1994) *The social context of health and health work.* Macmillan Press Ltd, Basingstoke.

Joseph Rowntree Foundation (2001) *Perceptions and experiences of counselling services among Asian people.* http://www.jrf.org.uk/knowledge/findings/socialcare/341.asp (accessed 18/09/09).

Joseph Rowntree Foundation (2004) *Black and minority ethnic older people's views on research findings.* http://www.jrf.org.uk/knowledge/findings/socialcare/564.asp (accessed 23/09/08).

Kakar S (1982) Shamans, mystics and doctors: a psychological inquiry into India and its healing traditions. Unwin, London.

Kaminski (2006) *Nursing through the lens of culture: a multiple gaze.* University of British Columbia, Faculty of Education, Vancouver; http://visiblenurse.com/nurseculture.html.

Kapasi H (1992) Out-of-school play schemes and Asian children. *Professional Care of Mother and Child* **June**, 163–4.

Karmi G (1996) *The ethnic health handbook. A fact file for health care professionals.* Blackwell Science, Oxford.

Kaunonen M and Koivula M (2007) Cultural healthcare issues in Finland. In: Papadopoulos I (ed.) *Transcultural health and social care: development of culturally competent practitioners.* Churchill Livingstone, Edinburgh, 203–20.

Karp A (2002) We've been here before. *The Guardian*; 08/06/2002; http://www.guardian.co.uk/uk/2002/jun/08/immigration.immigrationandpublicservices.

Keats D M (1997) *Culture and the child. A guide for professionals in child care and development.* Wiley, Chichester.

Kelleher D and Cahill G (2004) The Irish in London: identity and health. In: Kelleher D and Leavey G (eds) *Identity and health.* Routledge, London.

Kelly N and Stevenson J (2006) *First do no harm: denying health care to people whose asylum claims have failed.* Refugee Council, London; http://www.refugeecouncil.org.uk/Resources/Refugee%20Council/downloads/researchreports/Healthaccessreport_jun06.pdf (accessed 16/10/09).

Kendall K (1978) Maternal and child nursing in an Iranian village. In: Leininger M (ed.), *Transcultural nursing. Concepts, theories and practices.* Wiley Medical Publications, New York, 399–416.

Keogh B and Gleeson M (2006) Caring for female patients: the experiences of male nurses. *British Journal of Nursing* **35**, 1171–5.

Kiger A M (1994) Student nurses' involvement with death: the image and the experience. *Journal of Advanced Nursing* **20**, 679–86.

King M and Bartlett A (2006) What same sex partnerships may mean for health. *Journal of Epidemiology and Community Health* **60**, 188–191.

Kleinman A (1986) Concepts and a model for the comparison of medical systems as cultural systems. In: Currer C and Stacey M (eds) *Concepts of health, illness and disease: A comparative perspective.* Berg Publishers, Oxford, 27–50.

Koffman J, Fulop N J and Pashley D (1997) Ethnicity and the use of acute inpatients beds: a one day survey in north and south Thames Regions. *British Journal of Psychiatry* **171**, 238–241.

Kubler-Ross E (1970) *On death and dying.* Tavistock, London.

Kuhn T (1970) *The structure of scientific revolutions*, 2nd edn. University of Chicago Press, Chicago.

Kulakac O, Ozkan I A, Sucu G and O'Lynn C (2009) Nursing: the lesser of two evils. *Nurse Education Today* **29**, 676–80.

Kuo C L and Kavanagh K H (1994) Chinese perspectives on culture and mental health. *Issues in Mental Health Nursing* **15**, 551–67.

Kyung-Rim S (1999) On surviving breast cancer and mastectomy. In: Madjar I and Walton J A (eds) *Nursing and the experience of illness – phenomenology in practice*. Routledge, London, 77–97.

La Fontaine J S C (1985) *Initiation*. Penguin Books, Harmondsworth.

Lau A (1984) Transcultural issues in family therapy. *Journal of Family Therapy* **6**, 99–112.

Lauder W, Roxburgh M, Holland K, Johnson M, Watson R, Porter M, Topping K and Behr A (2008) *Nursing and midwifery in Scotland, being fit for practice. The report of the evaluation of Fitness for Practice pre-registration nursing and midwifery curriculum project*. University of Dundee; http://www.nes.scot.nhs.uk.

La Var R (1998) Improving educational preparation for transcultural health care. *Nurse Education Today* **18**, 519–33.

Lawler J (1991) *Behind the screens. Nursing, somology and the problem of the body*. Churchill Livingstone, Melbourne.

Leach P (1989) *Baby and child – from birth to age five*. Penguin Books, Harmondsworth.

Leavey G (1999) Suicide and Irish migrants in Britain: identity and integration. *International Review of Psychiatry* **11**, 168–72.

Lee-Cunin M (1989) *Daughters of Seacole. A study of black nurses*. West Yorkshire Low Pay Unit, Batley.

Leininger M M (1978a) Changing foci in American nursing education: primary and transcultural nursing. *Journal of Advanced Nursing* **3**, 155–66.

Leininger M M (ed.) (1978b) *Transcultural concepts, theories and practices*. John Wiley and Sons, New York.

Leininger M M (1984) Transcultural nursing: an essential knowledge and practice field for today. *Canadian Nurse* December, **80**, 41–57.

Leininger M M (1985) Transcultural care diversity and universality: a theory of nursing. *Nursing and Health Care* **6**, 208–12.

Leininger M M (1989a) Transcultural nursing: quo vadis – (where goeth the field?). *Journal of Transcultural Nursing* **1**, 33–45.

Leininger M M (1989b) The transcultural nurse specialist: imperative in today's world. *Nursing and Health Care* **10**, 251–6.

Leininger M M (1990) The significance of cultural concepts in nursing. *Journal of Transcultural Nursing* **2**, 52–9.

Leininger M M (1991) *Cultural diversity and universality: a theory of nursing*. Nurses League for Nursing, New York.

Leininger M M (1994) Transcultural nursing education: a world-wide imperative. *Nursing and Health Care* **15**, 255–7.

Leininger M M (1998) Transcultural health care: a culturally competent approach. *Journal of Transcultural Nursing* **9**, 53–4.

Leininger M M (2002) Culture Care Theory: a major contribution to advance transcultural nursing knowledge and practices. *Journal of Transcultural Nursing* **3**, 189–92.

Levenson R and Sharma A (1999) *The health of refugee children – guidelines for paediatricians*. Royal College of Paediatrics and Child Health, London.

Lewis C (2007) Healthcare beliefs of Indian patients living with leg and foot ulcers. *British Journal of Nursing* **16**(11) S22–6.

Lewis G, Croft-Jeffreys C and David A (1990) Are British psychiatrists racists? *British Journal of Psychiatry* **157**, 410–15.

Lewis P (2007) The sorry plight of refugee children. *The Guardian* 24/04/07; http://www.guardian.co.uk/society/2007/may/24/asylum.immigrationasylumandrefugees1 (accessed on 11/10/09).

Lipowski Z J (1988) Somatization: the concept and its clinical application. *American Journal of Psychiatry* **145**, 1358–68.

Lipsedge M (1990) Cultural influences on psychiatry. *Current Opinion in Psychiatry* **3**, 252–8.

Littlewood J (1988) The patient's world. *Nursing Times* **84**, 29–30.

Littlewood J (1989) A model for nursing using anthropological literature. *International Journal of Nursing Studies* **26**, 221–9.

Littlewood R (1986) Ethnic minorities and the Mental Health Act. *Bulletin of the Royal College of Psychiatrists* **10**, 306–8.

Littlewood R and Cross S (1980) Ethnic minorities and psychiatric services. *Sociology of Health and Illness* **2**, 194–201.

Littlewood R and Lipsedge M (1988) Psychiatric illness among British Afro-Caribbeans. *British Medical Journal* **296**, 950–1.

Littlewood R and Lipsedge M (2001) *Aliens and alienists*, 2nd edn. Unwin Hyman, London.

Lloyd K (1993) Depression and anxiety among Afro-Caribbean general practice attenders in Britain. *International Journal of Social Psychiatry* **39**, 1–9.

London M (1986) Mental illness amongst immigrant minorities in the United Kingdom. *British Journal of Psychiatry* **149**, 265–73.

Loring M and Powell B (1988) Gender, race and DSM-III: a study of the objectivity of psychiatric diagnostic behaviour. *Journal of Health and Social Behaviour* **29**, 1–22.

Loughrey M (2008) Just how male are male nurses? *Journal of Clinical Nursing* **17**, 1327–34.

MacLachlan M (1997) *Culture and health*. John Wiley and Sons, Chichester.

Macmillan I (1996) Colour no bar. *Nursing Times* **92**, 30–1.

Macpherson W (Chair) (1999) *The Stephen Lawrence Inquiry. Report of an inquiry by Sir William Macpherson of Cluny*. The Stationery Office, London.

Manley K (1997) Knowledge for nursing practice. In: Perry A (ed.) *Nursing: a knowledge base for practice*. Edward Arnold, London, 301–33.

Maqsood R (1994) *Teach yourself Islam*. Hodder, London.

Mares P, Henley A and Baxter C (1985) *Health care in multiracial Britain*. Health Education Council, London.

Mares P, Henley A and Baxter C (1994) Different Family Systems. In: Geoff M and Moloney B (eds) *Child health – a reader*. Radcliffe Medical Press, Oxford, 73–84.

Market and Opinion Research International (MORI) (2002) *Internationally recruited nurses member study. A study of the Royal College of Nursing internationally recruited nurse members.* Mori, London.

Mattson S (1987) The need for cultural concepts in nursing curricula. *Journal of Nursing Education* **26**, 206–8.

McCalman J A (1990) *The forgotten people*. King's Fund, London.

McColl H, McKenzie K and Bhui K (2008) Mental health needs of asylum seekers and refugees. *Advances in Psychiatric Treatment* **14**, 452–9.

McDermott M Y and Ahsan M M (1993) *The Muslim guide*. The Islamic Foundation, Leicester.

McDonald M (1997) Reflecting on ritual: an anthropological approach to personal rituals and care among Gujarati women in east London. In: Brykszynska G (ed.) *Caring – the compassion and wisdom of nursing*. Edward Arnold, London, 131–54.

McGee P (1992) *Teaching transcultural care. A guide for teachers of nursing and health care*. Chapman and Hall, London.

McGee P (1994) Educational issues in transcultural nursing. *British Journal of Nursing* **3**, 1113–16.

McGovern D and Cope R (1987) The compulsory detention of males of different ethnic groups with special reference to offender patients. *British Journal of Psychiatry* **150**, 505–12.

Mead M (1953) *Cultural patterns and technical change*. World Federation for Mental Health, Paris.

Meetoo D and Meetoo L (2005) Explanatory models of diabetes among Asian and Caucasian participants. *British Journal of Nursing* **14**, 154–9.

Megson D (2007) Equality and diversity in the curriculum: exploring ethnic identity and appreciating cultural diversity in a group of nursing and social work students, Education in a Changing Environment Conference. University of Salford, Salford; http://www.ece.salford.ac.uk/proceedings/author2.php?id=129 (accessed 10/08/09).

Mensah J (1996) Everybody's problem. *Nursing Times* **92**, 26–7.

Men's Health Forum (2009) Challenges and choices – improving health services to save men's lives: a policy briefing paper for National Men's Health Week 2009, 1–6. Men's Health Forum, London; http://www.menshealthforum.org.uk (accessed 10/10/09).

Midwifery Council of New Zealand (2007) *Competencies for entry to the register of midwives*. Midwifery Council of New Zealand, Te Tatau o te Whare Kahu, Wellington.

Miller M N and Pumariega A J (2001) Culture and eating disorder: a historical and cross-cultural review. *Psychiatry: Interpersonal and Biological Processes* **64**, 93–110.

Milner D (1975) *Children and race*. Penguin, Harmondsworth.

Mizuno-Lewis S and McAllister M (2006) Taking leave from work: the impact of culture on Japanese female nurses. *Journal of Clinical Nursing* **17**, 274–81.

Momeni P, Jirwe M and Emami A (2008) Enabling nursing students to become culturally competent – a documentary analysis of curricula in all Swedish nursing programs. *Scandinavian Journal of Caring Sciences* **22**, 499–506.

Moodley P and Perkins R (1991) Routes to psychiatric in-patient care in an inner London borough. *Social Psychiatry and Epidemiology* **26**, 47–51.

Moodley P and Thornicroft G (1988) Ethnic group and compulsory detention. *Medical Science Law* **28**, 324–8.

Mootoo J S (2005) *A guide to spiritual awareness, Nursing Standard*. RCN Publishing, London.

Morris J and Worth J (2006) Managing diabetes during religious festivals. *Practice Nursing* **17**, 478–84.

Mufune P (2009) The male involvement programme and men's sexual health and reproductive health in Northern Namibia. Monograph 1. *Current Sociology* **57**, 231–48.

Mulhall A (1994) Anthropology: a model for nursing. *Nursing Standard* **8**, 35–8.

Mullany B C (2006) Barriers to and attitides towards promoting husbands' involvement in maternal health in Katmandu, Nepal. *Social Science and Medicine* **62**, 2798–809.

Muslim Law (Shariah) Council (1996) The Muslim Law (Shariah) Council and organ transplants. *Accident and Emergency Nursing* **4**, 73–5.

Nairn S, Hardy C, Parumal L and Williams G A (2004) Multicultural or anti-racist teaching in nurse education: a critical appraisal. *Nurse Education Today* **24**, 188–195.

Nandi P K (1977) Cultural constraints on professionalization: the case of nursing in India. *International Journal of Nursing Studies* **14**, 125–35.

Naryanasamy A (1991) *Spiritual care – a resource guide*. BKT Information Services and Quay Publishing Ltd, Nottingham.

Naryanasamy A and Owens J (2001) A critical incident study of nurses' responses to the spiritual needs of their patients. *Journal of Advanced Nursing* **33**, 446–55.

National Association of Health Authorities and Trusts (1996) *Spiritual care in the NHS – a guide for purchasers and providers*. National Association of Health Authorities and Trusts (NAHAT), Birmingham.

National Black Carers' Network (2004) *We care too. A good practice guide for people working with Black Carers*. National Black Carers' Network (NBCWN) in association with Afiya Trust, London.

National Institute for Clinical Excellence (2005) *CG26 Post-traumatic stress disorder (PTSD): full guideline, including appendices 1-13*. National Institute for Clinical Excellence (NICE), London.

National Institute for Mental Health in England (2004) *Inside outside: improving mental health services for black and minority ethnic communities in England*. National Institute for Mental Health in England (NIMHE), London.

National Nursing Research Unit (2009) *Who wants to be a nurse?* Policy+. (Issue 15). Kings College London.

Neuberger J (1994) *Caring for dying people of different faiths*, 2nd edn. Mosby, London.

Norfolk, Suffolk and Cambridgeshire Strategic Health Authority (2003) *Independent Inquiry into the death of David Bennett*. Norfolk, Suffolk and Cambridgeshire Strategic Health Authority, Cambridge.

Norman A (1985) *Triple jeopardy: growing older in a second homeland*. Centre for Policy on Ageing, London.

Nursing and Midwifery Council (2004) *Standards of proficiency for pre-registration nursing education*. Nursing and Midwifery Council (NMC), London.

Nursing and Midwifery Council (2008) *The Code – standards of conduct, performance and ethics for nurses and midwives.* Nursing and Midwifery Council (NMC), London.

Nursing and Midwifery Council (2009) *Standards of proficiency for pre-registration midwifery education.* Nursing and Midwifery Council (NMC), London.

Nursing Council of Australia (2008) *Australian Code of Professional Conduct.* Australian Nursing and Midwifery Council, Dickson, ACT.

Nursing Council of New Zealand (2005) *Guidelines for cultural safety, the Treaty of Waitangi and Maori Health in nursing education and practice.* Nursing Council of New Zealand (Te Kaunihera Tapuni o Ao tearoa), Wellington.

Nuttall D (2008) Public health and men: needs and strategies. *Nurse Prescribing* **6**, 538–42.

Office for National Statistics (2009) Migration statistics 2008; http://www.statistics.gov.uk/pdfdir/mignr1109.pdf (accessed 16/10/09).

Office of Population Censuses and Surveys (1991) *Census for Great Britain.* HMSO, London.

Ohnuki-Tierney E (1984) *Illness and culture in contemporary Japan. An anthropological view.* Cambridge University Press, Cambridge.

Okley J (1983) *The traveller–gypsies.* Cambridge University Press, Cambridge.

Papadopoulos I (2003) *The Papadopoulos, Tikki and Taylor model for the development of cultural competence in nursing. Journal of Health, Social and Environmental Issues* **4**, 5–7.

Papadopoulos I (ed.) (2006) *Transcultural health and social care: development of culturally competent practitioners.* Churchill Livingstone, Edinburgh.

Papadopoulos I, Alleyne J and Tilki M (1994) Promoting transcultural care in a college of health care studies. *British Journal of Nursing* **3**, 116–18.

Papadopoulos I, Tilki M and Lees S (2004) Promoting cultural competence in healthcare through a research-based intervention in the UK. *Diversity in Health and Social Care* **1**, 107–115.

Papadopoulos I, Tilki M and Taylor G (1998) *Transcultural care: a guide for health care professionals.* Quay Books, Dinton.

Parry G, Van Cleemput P, Peters J, Walters S, Thomas K and Cooper C (2004) *The health status of gypsies and travellers in England. Report for the Department of Health.* The University of Sheffield, Sheffield.

Parsons L, Macfarlane A and Golding J (1993) Pregnancy, birth and maternity care. In: Ahmad W I H (ed.) *'Race' and Health in Contemporary Britain.* Open University Press, Milton Keynes, 51–75.

Patel N (2009) Developing psychological services for refugee survivors of torture. In: Fernando S and Keating F (eds) *Mental health in a multi-ethnic society.* Routledge, London.

Pattison N (2008) Caring for patients after death. *Nursing Standard* **22**, 48–56.

Payne-Jackson A (1999) Biomedical and folk medical concepts of adult-onset diabetes in Jamaica: implications for treatment. *Health* **3**, 5–46.

Peate I (2004) Men's attitudes towards health and the implications for nursing care. *British Journal of Nursing* **13**, 540–5.

Peate I and Richens Y (2006) Being a male refugee or asylum seeker. *Practice Nursing* **17**, 602–4.

Penachio D L (2005) *Cultural competence: Caring for Muslim patients*. Modern medicine (May 6, 2005) http//:www.modernmedicine.com/modernmedicine/Young+Doctors/27+Resource+Center/3a+Practice + Management/3a+Patient+relations/Cultural/Competence-Caring-for-your-Muslim-patient/ ArtideStandard/Article/detail/158977 (Accessed 02/02/10).

Perry A (1997) *Nursing: a knowledge base for practice*, 2nd edn. Edward Arnold, London.

Perry F (1992) Black and white issues. *Nursing Times* **88**, 62–4.

Phoenix A and Woollett A (1991) Motherhood: social construction, politics and psychology. In: Phoenix A, Woollett A and Lloyd E (eds) *Motherhood: meanings, practices and ideologies*. Sage, London, 13–27.

Pierce M and Armstrong D (1996) Afro-Caribbean lay beliefs about diabetes: an exploratory study. In: Keller D and Hillier S (eds) *Researching cultural differences in health*. Routledge, London, 91–102.

Pilgrim D and Rogers A (1993) *A sociology of health and illness*. Open University Press, Buckingham.

Pillsbury B L K (1978) 'Doing the month': confinement and convalescence of Chinese women after childbirth. *Social Science and Medicine* **12**, 11–22.

Pinikahana J, Manias E and Happell B (2003) Transcultural nursing in Australian nursing curricula. *Nursing and Health Sciences* **5**, 149–54.

Polanyi M (1958) *Personal knowledge*. University of Chicago Press, Chicago.

Poonia K and Ward L (1990) Fair share of (The) care? *Community Care* **796**, 16–18.

Prior L, Chun P L and Huat S B (2000) Beliefs and accounts of illness. Views of Cantonese-speaking communities in England. *Sociology of Health and Illness* **22**, 815–39.

Purnell L D (2009) *Guide to culturally competent health care*, 2nd edn. F A Davies, Philadelphia.

Purnell L D and Paulanka B J (1998) *Transcultural health care*. F A Davis, Philadelphia.

Purnell L D and Paulanka B J (2008) *Transcultural health care – a culturally competent approach*. F A Davis, Philadelphia.

Purnell L D and Selekman J (2008) People of Jewish Heritage. In: Purnell L D and Paulanka B J (eds) *Transcultural health care – a culturally competent approach*. F A Davis, Philadelphia, 278–92.

Quickfall J (2004) Developing a model for culturally competent primary care nursing for asylum applicants and refugees in Scotland: a review of the literature. *Diversity in Health and Social Care* **1**, 53–64.

Qureshi B (1989) *Transcultural medicine*. Kluwer Academic Publications, Lancaster.

Race Relations (Amendment) Act (2000). Office of Public Sector Information, London.

Raleigh V and Balarajan R (1992) Suicide levels and trends among immigrants in England and Wales. *Health Trends* **24**, 91–4.

Rees D (1990) Terminal care and bereavement. In: McAvoy B R and Donaldson L J (eds) *Health care for Asians*. Oxford University Press, Oxford, 304–19.

Rickford F (1992) Culture shocks. *Social Work Today* **25 June**, 10.

Robertson S and Williamson P (2005) Men and health promotion in the UK: ten years further on? *Health Education Journal* **64**, 293–301.

Robinson V (1986) *Transient settlers and refugees: Asians in Britain*. Clarendon Press, Oxford.

Romem P and Anson O (2005) Israeli men in nursing: social and personal motives. *Journal of Nursing Management* **13**, 173–8.

Roper N, Logan W W and Tierney A J (1996) *The elements of nursing*, 4th edn. Churchill Livingstone, Edinburgh.

Rosenhan D L (1973) On being sane in insane places. *Science* **179**, 250–8.

Ross L J, Laston S L, Nahar K, Muna L, Nahar P and Pelto P J (1998) Women's health priorities: cultural perspectives on illness in rural Bangladesh. *Health* **12**, 91–110.

Royal College of Nursing (1994) Black and ethnic minority clients: meeting needs. *RCN Nursing Update* **7**, 3–13.

Royal College of Nursing (2002) *International Recruitment United Kingdom Case Study*. Royal College of Nursing, London; www.rcn.org.uk/rcnpublications.

Royal College of Nursing (2003a) *Here to stay? International nurses in the UK*. Royal College of Nursing, London; http://www.rcn.org.uk/rcnpublications.

Royal College of Nursing (2003b) *We Need Respect: experiences of internationally recruited nurses in the UK*. Royal College of Nursing, London; http://www.rcn.org.uk/rcnpublications.

Royal College of Nursing (2005) *Success with internationally recruited nurses*. Royal College of Nursing, London.

Royal College of Nursing (2006) *Female genital mutilation*. Royal College of Nursing, London.

Sainsbury Centre for Mental Health (2002) *Breaking the circles of fear. A review of the relationship between mental health services and African Caribbean communities*. The Sainsbury Centre for Mental Health (SCMH), London.

Sampson C (1982) *The neglected ethic. Religious and cultural factors in the care of patients*. McGraw-Hill, Maidenhead.

Sashidharan S P and Francis E (1993) Epidemiology, ethnicity and schizophrenia. In: Ahmad W I U (ed.) *'Race' and health in contemporary Britain*. Open University Press, Milton Keynes, 96–113.

Sawley L (2001) Perceptions of racism in the health services. *Nursing Standard* **15**, 33–5.

Schott J and Henley A (1996) *Culture, religion and childbearing in a multiracial society*. Butterworth–Heinmann, Oxford.

Schreiber R, Stern P N and Wilson C (1998) The contexts for managing depression and its stigma among black West Indian Canadian women. *Journal of Advanced Nursing* **27**, 510–17.

Schweitzer P (ed.) (1984) *A place to stay. Memories of pensioners from many lands*. Age Exchange, London.

Schytt E (2006) *Women's health after childbirth*. Karolinska Institute, Stockholm, Sweden.

Sen A (1970) *Problems of overseas students and nurses*. National Foundation of Education Research in England and Wales, Slough.

Serrant-Green L (2001) Transcultural nursing education: a view from within. *Nurse Education Today* **21**, 670–8.

Sewell P (2002) Respecting a patient's care needs after death. Nursing Times, http://www.nursingtimes.net (accessed 23/09/09).

Shaechter F (1965) Previous history of mental illness in female migrant patients admitted to a psychiatric hospital, Royal Park. *Medical Journal of Australia* **2**, 227–9.

Sheikh A and Gatrad A R (2000) *Caring for muslim patients.* Radcliff Medical Press, Abingdon.

Skultans V (1970) The symbolic significance of menstruation and the menopause. *MAN* **5**, 639–51.

Skultans V (1980) A dying ritual. *MIMS Magazine* 15 June, 43–7.

Slater M (1993) *Health for all our children – achieving appropriate health care for black and minority ethnic children and their families.* Action for Sick Children, London.

Smaje C (1995) *Health, race and ethnicity – make sense of the evidence.* King's Fund, London.

Smith P (1992) *The emotional labour of nursing.* Macmillan Press Ltd, London.

Smyke P (1991) *Women and health.* Zed Books, London.

Social Services Inspectorate (1998) *They look after their own don't they? Inspection of community care services and ethnic minority older people.* Department of Health, Wetherby.

Soh N L, Touyz S W and Surgenor L J (2006) Eating and body image disturbances across cultures: a review. *European Eating Disorders Review* **14**, 54–65.

Somjee G (1991) Social change in the nursing profession in India. In: Holden P and Littlewood J (eds) *Anthropology and nursing.* Routledge, London, 31–55.

South Australia Health (2008) *Aboriginal Nursing and Midwifery Strategy.* Nursing and Midwifery Office, SA Health, Adelaide.

Spector R E (1996) *Cultural diversity in health and illness.* Appleton and Lange, Stamford.

Spector R E (2009) *Cultural diversity in health and illness,* 7th edn. Pearson Education/Prentice Hall, Upper Saddle River.

Sprinks J (2008) Diversity Champions needed to tackle discrimination against NHS staff. *Nursing Standard* **23**, 12–13.

Sproston K and Nazroo J (eds) (2002) *Ethnic minority psychiatric illness in the community (EMPIRIC) – quantitative report.* The Stationery Office, London.

Standing H (1980) Beliefs about menstruation and pregnancy. *MIMS Magazine* **1**, 21–7.

Stead L and Huckle S (1997) Pathways in cardiology. In: Johnson S (ed.) *Pathways of care.* Blackwell Science, Oxford, 56–67.

Steel Z, Silvoe D, Brooks R *et al.* (2006) Impact of immigration detention and temporary protection on the mental health of refugees. *British Journal of Psychiatry* **1888**, 58–64.

Stokes G (1991) A transcultural nurse is about. *Senior Nurse* **11**, 40–2.

Stopes-Roe M and Cochrane R (1989) Traditionalism in the family: a comparison between Asian and British cultures and between generations. *Journal of Comparative Family Studies* **20**, 141–58.

Strange F (1996) Handover: an ethnographic study of ritual in nursing practice. *Intensive and Critical Care Nursing* **12**, 106–12.

Street A F (1992) *Inside nursing: A critical ethnography of clinical nursing practice.* State University of New York Press, New York.

Sudnow D (1967) *Passing on. The social organisation of dying.* Prentice-Hall, Upper Saddle River.

Summerfield D (1996) *The impact of war and atrocity on civilian populations: basic principles for NGO interventions and a critique of psychosexual trauma projects.* Relief and Rehabilitation Network Overseas Development Institute, London.

Summerfield D (2001) Asylum seekers, refugees and mental health services in the UK. *Psychiatric Bulletin* **25**, 161–3.

Sun Y and Liu Z (2007) Men's health in China. *Journal of Men's Health and Gender* **4**, 13–17.

Swanwick M (1996) Child-rearing across cultures. *Paediatric Nursing* **8**, 13–17.

Swartz L (2000) *Culture and mental health: A Southern African view.* Oxford Publications, Oxford.

The Home Office. http://www.ukba.homeoffice.gov.uk/sitecontent/newsarticles/2009/november/immigration-asylum-stats

Thomas L (1992) Racism and psychotherapy: working with racism in the consulting room – an analytical view. In: Karem J and Littlewood R (eds) *Intercultural therapy: themes, interpretations and practice.* Blackwell Scientific Publications, Oxford, 133–45.

Thompson A (2001) Refugees and mental health. *Diverse Minds Magazine* **9**, 6–7.

Thorne S (1993) Health belief systems in perspective. *Journal of Advanced Nursing* **18**, 931–41.

Tierney M J and Tierney L M (1994) Nursing in Japan. *Nursing Outlook* **42**, 210–13.

Tilki M (1994) Ethnic Irish older people. *British Journal of Nursing* **3**, 902–3.

Tilki M (2000) Mental health of Irish in England. *Diverse Minds* **5**, 9–10.

Tilki M, Dye K, Markey K, Scholefiled D, Davis C and Moore T (2007) Racism: the implications for nursing education. *Diversity in Health and Social Care* **4**, 303–12.

Tilki M, Papadopoulos I and Alleyne J (1994) Learning from colleagues of different cultures. *British Journal of Nursing* **3**, 1118–24.

Towers C (2009) *Recognising fathers: a national survey of fathers who have children with learning disabilities.* Foundation for People with Learning Disabilities, London.

Townsend P and Davidson N (1982) *Inequalities in health.* Penguin, Harmondsworth.

Trevelyan J (1994) A woman's lot. *Nursing Times* **90**, 48–50.

Tribe R (2002) Mental health of refugees and asylum seekers. *Advances in Psychiatric Treatment* **8**, 240–8.

Tribe R and Raval H (2002) *Working with interpreters in mental health.* Routledge, London.

Tuohy D, McCarthy J, Cassidy I and Graham M M (2008) Educational needs of nurses when nursing people of a different culture in Ireland. *International Nursing Review* **55**, 164–70.

Turan J M, Nalbant H, Bulut A and Sahip Y (2001) Including expectant fathers in antenatal education programmes in Istanbul, Turkey. *Reproductive Health Matters* **9**, 114–15.

Tylor E B (1871) *Primitive culture: researches into the development of mythology, philosophy, religion, language, art and customs.* Murray, London.

United Kingdom Central Council for Nursing, Midwifery and Health Visiting (UKCC) (1989) *The nurses, midwives and health visitors approval order 1989.* UKCC, London.

United Kingdom Central Council for Nursing, Midwifery and Health Visiting (UKCC) (1992) *Code of professional conduct for nurses, midwives and health visitors.* UKCC, London.

United Nations (1951) *Convention relating to the status of refugees.* United Nations Office of the High Commissioner for Human Rights, Geneva.

United Nations High Commissioner for Refugees (2006) *Refugees by numbers.* United Nations High Commissioner for Refugees (UNHCR), Geneva; http://www.unhcr.org (accessed 12/10/09).

Vernon D (1994) The health of traveller-gypsies. *British Journal of Nursing* **3**, 969–72.

Vivian C and Dundas L (2004) The crossroads of culture and health among the Roma (Gypsies). *Journal of Nursing Scholarship* **36**, 86–91.

Walker C (1987) How a survey led to providing more responsive help for Asian families. *Social Work Today* **19**, 12–13.

WaterAid (2009) *Is menstrual hygiene and management an issue for adolescent school girls? A WaterAid publication.* http://www.wateraid.org/uk/ (accessed 23/09/09).

Watkins M (1997) Nursing knowledge in practice. In: Perry A (ed.) *Nursing – a knowledge base for practice.* Edward Arnold, London, 1–32.

Weaver H N and Burns B J (2001) 'I shout with fear at night': understanding the traumatic experiences of refugees and asylum seekers. *Journal of Social Work* **1**, 147–64.

Webb-Johnson A (1992) *A cry for change – an Asian perspective on developing quality mental health care.* Confederation of Indian Organizations, London.

Weller B (1991) Nursing in a multicultural world. *Nursing Standard* **5**, 31–2.

Weller B (1993) Cultural aspects of family health nursing. *Professional Care of Mother and Child* **February**, 38–40.

White A (2001) How men respond to illness. *Men's Health Journal* **1**, 18–19.

White A (2006). Social and political aspects of men's health. *Health* **6**, 267–85.

White A and Cash K (2003) The state of men's health across Europe. *Men's Health Journal* **2**, 63–5.

Whittock M and Leonard L (2003) Stepping outside the stereotype. A pilot study of the motivations and experiences of males in the nursing profession. *Journal of Nursing Management* **11**, 242–9.

Wilkins H (1993) Transcultural nursing: a selective review of the literature, 1985–1991. *Journal of Advanced Nursing* **18**, 606–12.

Wilkins and Savoye (2009). *Men's health around the world: a review of policy and progress in 11 countries.* European Men's Health Forum, Brussels.

Williamson T, Ryan J, Hogg C, and Fallon D (2009) *'YOUNIQUE VOICES' A study of health and wellbeing: experiences, views and expectations of seldom heard and mariginalised groups in Rochdale Borough.* Final report. University of Salford, Salford.

Willis R (2008) Ethnicity and family support. *Working with Older People* **12**, 27–30.

Wolf Z R (1986) Nurses' work: the sacred and the profane. *Holistic Nursing Practice* **1**, 29–35.

Wolf Z R (1988) *Nurse's work: the sacred and the profane.* University of Pennsylvania Press, Philadelphia.

Wright C (1983) Language and communication problems in an Asian community. *Journal of Royal College of General Practitioners* **33**, 101–4.

Yazdani A (1998) *Young Asian women and self-harm.* Newham Inner City and Newham Asian Womens' Project, Newham, London.

Zaman S (2009) Ladies without lamps: nurses in Bangladesh. *Qualitative Health Research* **19**, 366–74.

Index

acculturation 133, 166
activities of living 73, 75
Afghan people 180
African culture 79, 139–40
African-American people/culture
    17, 20, 125
African-Caribbean people/culture
    child-rearing 141
    diabetes 13–14, 37–8, 73
    diet 37–8, 138
    folk models of illness 73
    mental health 81, 84, 85, 86, 109
    migration patterns 153–4
    nurses 10, 204
    older people 159
afterlife 213, 219
Afyia Trust 120
agoraphobia 82, 83
AIDS 176–7
alcohol intake 87, 126, 127
alternative and complementary
    therapies 29–30, 32–3, 37, 157
American culture 94, 136
    see also African-Americans;
        Vietnamese Americans
amok (syndrome) 82
anaemia, sickle-cell 144
Angolans 180
anorexia nervosa 83
antenatal care 178
anthropological nursing model 71–2
anti-discriminative practice 59
Arabic people/culture 90, 125, 126
Asian people/culture
    child-rearing 141
    diet 138
    families 133
    female stereotypes 110–11
    language barriers to health care
        143
    migration patterns 153
    and nursing as a career 204–5
    older people 155, 156–7, 159
    see also South Asian people/
        culture
assimilation 132, 166, 179
asthma 34
asylum seekers 128, 165, 166–84
    children and young people's health
        177–82
    health care 169–72
    image 167–8

mental health issues 172, 179, 181
mental/physical trauma 169, 170,
    171–6, 177, 179, 180
numbers 167
torture 171–2
women's health 176–7
Australian Aborigines 21, 62, 79, 90
Australian Code of Professional
    Conduct 2008 2
autotransfusion 45
Ayurvedic medicine 23–4

balance 22
Bangladeshi people/culture 50, 103,
    112–13, 120
baptism 213
bed-sharing 136
beliefs see cultural beliefs; health
    beliefs; illness beliefs; religious
    beliefs
Bengali people 39
Bennett, David 'Rocky' 85
bereavement
    cultural 152
    meaning of 186–8
    phases of 187
Bhagavad Gita 52, 55, 215
bias 7
biological variation 70
biomedicine
    and belief systems 40
    criticisms of 33–4, 41
    and death 186
    and folk models 73
    giving explanations of 40
    and health beliefs 18–19, 21, 29,
        33–4
    and the popular/lay health sector
        25, 34–5
    public dissatisfaction with 29–30
    superiority claims 33
    and superstition 35–6
biradari (relations) 100
black and ethnic minority people
    child and family centred care
        141–2, 147
    and mental health 80–1, 84–5, 86,
        90, 92
    nurses 200–6, 209–11
    older people 150–63
    and racism and child-rearing 141–2
    women 104

drawing 70
    religious beliefs about 45–6
blood products 45–6
blood transfusions 45–6
body, laying out 189–90, 192, 220
body products, as polluting 55
Brahma 52, 215
breast cancer 44
British Medical Association (BMA) 12
Buddha 214
Buddhism 66, 214–15
burial practices 46, 192

cancer
    breast 44
    prostate 125
    terminal 193–5
    testicular 128
Cantonese-speaking populations 17
care mismanagement 38
care plans 40
Care Programme Approach (CPA) 85
carers
    female 102–5, 120
    health 121
    male 120–1
    young 121
caste system 53, 54, 215–16
catheters, urinary 55
Census 2001 120–1, 151
chaplains, hospital 47, 48, 213
charms 25–6
chi 22
child and family centred
        care 131–49
    carrying babies/children 135–6
    child-rearing practices 134,
        135–42
    children with learning difficulties
        104–5
    and children's perspectives on
        health 134
    culture and families 132–5
    development 140–1
    dressing children/babies 138–9
    emotional health needs 180–1
    emotional well-being 181–2
    feeding babies/children 137–8
    good practice 144–7
    hygiene practices 137
    illness/disease patterns 143–4

language and communication
142–3
'looked after' children 180
migrant children 177–82
name giving 139–40
play 140–1
problem behaviours 181
racism and 141–2
settling babies/children 135–6
unaccompanied minors 179–80
child protection issues 179–80
childbirth 110–13, 131–2, 177
and Hinduism 132, 216
and Islam 51–2, 106, 118, 131–2
men's role in 118–19
see also postnatal care
Children's Act 134, 180
chills 34
Chinese people/culture 23, 65–6, 68,
94, 125
naming system 65–6
see also traditional Chinese
medicine
Christianity 43
beliefs and practices 46–9, 213
Christian rites 47
denominations 213
holy days 46, 213
Orthodox 48–9
'Cinderella' services 151
circumcision 219
Civil Partnership Act 2004 117
clitoris, removal 109–10
clothing 75
children/babies 138–9
Hindu requirements 54, 216
Islamic requirements 139, 217
Sikh requirements 220
codes of conduct 1–2, 58–9, 75, 197
cold/heat polarity 22–3, 24, 65
colds 25, 34
collective cultures 93–4
colour symbolism 187
'colour-blind' services 93
communicable diseases 170
communication 7, 8, 69, 75
and child and family centred care
142–3
and mental health services 89–91,
92–6
see also interpreters; language;
language barriers
community psychiatric nurses 21
complementary therapies see
alternative and complementary
therapies
concept approach 207
confidentiality issues 7, 92, 179
conflict 38, 40
conformism 133

Confucianism 66, 94
contraception 49, 111, 119
control issues 34
counselling 93–4, 175
transcultural 93
course approach 207
cultural assessment 67–75
cultural awareness 63–4, 72
cultural beliefs 60
and child and family centred care
132
and male health/health care 123–4
and the needs of women 105–7
'cultural bereavement' 152
cultural care
accommodation 67, 68, 119
in context 1–3
developments promoting 61–3
knowledge required for 58–76
preservation 67, 68, 119
re-patterning 67, 68, 119
skills required for 58–76
cultural competence 68, 70–1, 72,
206–10
cultural difference/diversity 7
and professional practice 199–212
'cultural individuals' 61
cultural interactionist approach 191
cultural knowledge 58–76, 72
'knowing how' 65, 66
'knowing that' 65–6
cultural norms 5, 132
cultural safety model 59–60
cultural self-awareness 72
cultural sensitivity 72
cultural time 70
cultural values 2, 4, 5, 69, 132, 135
culture 12–14
changing nature 4
meaning of 1, 3, 4–9
of the nurse 5, 14
nursing 5, 6, 8–9, 17–18, 38, 188–91
organizational 5, 6, 7–8, 195–7
patient 5, 6, 9, 191–5
professional 5
culture conflict 87
culture shock 6, 72
culture-bound syndromes 82–3
curers 20–1
curses 82

death 48, 185–98, 216
biomedical death 186
clinical death 185
emotional labour of 189
euthanasia 46, 186
good practice 197
hidden nature 189–91
meaning of bereavement 186–8
meaning of death 185–6

nursing practice and care 188–97
phases of bereavement 187
point of death (time) 186
rites of passage 186
social death 185, 186
'Delivering Race Equality in Mental
Health Care' 86
demography 151
denial of health care 173
Department of Health 1, 2, 12, 43, 44,
60, 124, 200, 202
depression 32, 82, 87–8, 92, 109, 176
detention centres 173, 178
developing countries, asylum
seekers/refugees 167
diabetes 9, 48, 217
African-Caribbeans and 13–14,
37–8, 73, 159
men and 125, 126
older people and 159, 161–2
diet 75
African-Caribbean 37–8, 138
babies/children 137–8, 145–6
Hindu 54, 137–8, 216
Islamic 50, 137, 218
Jewish 137, 146, 219
Sikh 220
dignity 2, 58, 59, 60
in mental health care 85
women and 107–8
discrimination 2, 156–7
against migrants 173
double 85, 92
and mental health 81, 92, 96
racial 200–3, 209, 210, 211
see also anti-discriminative
practice; prejudice; racism
distortion 7
distress see emotional distress
'dividual', concept of 133
divination 28
domestic violence 100, 118
dosas (humours) 24
double discrimination 85, 92
'double life' 179
'drapetomania' 80

eating disorders 83
economic deprivation 84, 85
eczema 32
education 179, 180
multicultural 206–8
sex 119
Eid 51, 217
Eightfold Path 214
elimination 75
emotional distress 78, 88–9
displays of 143
working with 174–6, 182
emotional health needs, of young

migrants 180–1
emotional well-being 181–2
enculturation 69
English National Board 1
environmental control 70
equal opportunities 202–3, 205
erectile dysfunction 125
ethnic monitoring 12
ethnicity 11–14
    meaning of 1–4, 11–12
ethno-history 72
euthanasia 46, 186
'evil eye' 20, 82, 102
eye contact 89–90

families
    culture and 132–5
    decision-making 134
    extended 99–100, 104, 133–4
    nuclear 133
    shame, bring on 101
    see also child and family centred
        care
fasting 48, 51, 137
fatalism 33, 34
female genital mutilation (FGM)
    109–10, 179
fevers 35
financial difficulties 84, 85, 172
Finnish people 17
five elements 23–4
flower giving 70
folk health care sector 27–8, 73, 157
forgetting, active 175
Four Noble Truths 214

generalizations 18
genetics 84, 101
genital examinations 51
Giger and Davidhizar's model of
    transcultural nursing
    assessment and intervention
    69–70
glue ear 146
glycosuria 5–6, 9
God 19, 44, 213, 219
Gods 52, 214, 215
grief 187, 188
Gurdwara 219
Guyanan culture/people 154
Gypsy Travellers (Roma) 17, 24–5,
    28, 34
    child and family centred issues
        137, 139, 141–2
    dress 139
    marriage 134
    mental health 87
    washing 63–4
    women 101, 105, 106

hakims 24, 32–3, 157
happiness 17
harassment 202, 204
healers 20–1, 27–9, 39, 41, 82–3
health advocates 7, 8
health beliefs 16–24
    across the lifespan 16
    based on biomedicine 18–19, 21,
        29, 33–4
    based on naturalistic systems
        22–4, 29, 33–4
    based on personalistic systems
        19–21, 29, 37
    caring for people with different
        36–8
    change over time 17
    eliciting 38–41
    and older people 157–8
    of student nurses 26–7
    systems 18–24
    working with 32–41
    and world views 16
health care pluralism 32–41
health care sectors 24–9
    folk sector 27–8, 73, 157
    popular/lay sector 24–7, 34–5
    professional sector 29
health maintenance practices 17, 19
'health protectors' 25–6
health risk behaviours 127–8
heart attack 48, 126, 159
heart disease, ischaemic 126, 159
heat/cold polarity 22–3, 24, 65
help seeking behaviours 125–7
herbal remedies 28
Hinduism 21, 33, 37, 43, 127
    beliefs and practices 52–5, 215–17
    child and family centred care
        137–8, 140
    childbirth 132, 216
    clothing 54, 216
    and death and bereavement 187,
        216
    diet 54, 137–8, 216
    holy days 55
    naming system 54, 140, 217
    women 101–2, 103
HIV 176–7
holism 29–30, 41
    see also naturalistic systems
holy days 46, 51, 55, 60, 147, 213, 217,
    219
Hoodoo 20
Hopi Indians 28
hospital rules and regulations 29, 158
hseih ping (trancelike state) 83
hygiene practices 75, 137, 215, 216
    see also washing
hypertension 159
hysterectomy 107

icons 48–9
illness beliefs, working with 32–41
illness patterns
    childhood 143–4
    of older people 159–60
incontinence 112
independence 133
India 103, 109
individual, valuing of 133
individualism 87, 93, 133
inequality
    gender 99, 102, 103, 109, 111
    race 86, 93
    infibulation 109–10
'Inside Out' report 85
institutional racism 10, 199, 202, 206,
    209, 211
Integrated Care Pathways 67
Intensive Care Units (ICUs) 194–5
internationally recruited nurses
    (IRNs) 201–2
interpreters 7–8, 91–2
'intimate zone' 69
Iran 131–2, 136
Irish people 81, 84, 86–7, 151
Islam Foundation Muslim Guide 52
Islam and the Muslim Faith 5–9, 21,
    26, 43, 64
    beliefs and practices 49–52, 217–18
    child and family centred care
        131–2, 134, 137, 140
    childbirth 51–2, 106, 118, 131–2
    death and bereavement 187,
        194–5, 218
    diet 50, 137, 218
    dress 139, 217
    euthanasia 186
    five pillars of 217
    hakims 32–3, 157
    health risk behaviours 127–8
    and health care practice 49–52,
        217–18
    holy days 51, 217
    men 118, 127
    mental health issues 94–5
    naming system 140, 218
    and nursing as a career 205
    Shia Islam 49–50
    substance abuse 127
    Sunni Islam 49
    washing 50–1, 145, 217
    women 100–1, 103, 105–8, 111, 217
Israel 121–2

Japanese culture 63, 103, 104, 106,
    136
Jehovah Witness Hospital Liaison
    Committee 45
Jehovah's Witnesses 43, 45–6
Jesus 45, 48, 213, 218

Jewish refugees 168
Jinns 21
Judaism 105, 107, 209
  beliefs and practices summary
    218–19
  child and family centred practice
    146–7
  death 186, 192–3
  diet 137, 146, 219
  holy days 147, 219
  Orthodox 105, 107, 146–7, 192–3,
    218, 219
  Progressive 192, 193, 218

kapha 24
karma 215
kleptomania 83
knowledge see cultural knowledge
koro 83
kosher food 137, 146, 219

labelling, in mental health 79
language
  and child and family centred care
    142–3
  nursing 17–18, 38
  see also communication;
    interpreters
language barriers 7–8, 89–92, 143
  and children 179
  and older people 155, 156, 161–2
last offices 189
Lawrence, Stephen 199
learning difficulties, children with
    104–5
Leininger, Madeleine 61–2, 67–8, 72,
    206–8
  model of transcultural care
    diversity and universality
    67–8, 119
  levels of need analysis 68
life expectancy 123–4
life story-telling 182
link workers 7, 8
listening skills 175
Littlewood's anthropological nursing
    model within the nursing
    process framework 71–2
'living between two cultures' 179

Macpherson Inquiry 1999 199, 211
magico-religious systems see
    personalistic systems
Malawian culture/people 170
male health care issues 116–30
  and cultural beliefs 123–4
  genital examinations 51
  health risk behaviours 127–8
  help seeking behaviours 125–7
  male breadwinners 116

male carers 120–1
male child-rearing role 99, 119
male health service use 127–8
male life expectancy 123–4
role of men in society 116–20,
    123–4
male nurses 121–3
  caring for female patients 122–3
Maori people 59
marriage 100–2
  arranged 100–1
  first cousin 100, 101
masculinity 117
medical profession 29
medication 146, 157–8
men see male health care issues
Men's Health Forum 124, 128, 129
menstruation 107, 139
  as unclean 105, 106, 216
mental health 78–98
  assessments 94–6
  concepts of abnormality 78–80
  concepts of normality 78–80
  culture-bound syndromes 82–3
  gateways to services 85
  and intercultural communication
    89–91, 92–6
  interpreters 91–2
  issues in care and treatment 84–9
  and migrants, refugees and
    asylum seekers 172–6
  pseudopatient experiments 79
  and racism 81, 85, 92–6, 96
  services 84, 85, 86, 90–1
  transcultural psychiatry 80–2
Mental Health Act, sectioning under
    82, 84
mental health nurses 36
Mexican people/culture 26
midwifery 39
migrants 165–84
  children and young people's health
    177–82
  health 165–9, 176–82
  health care 169–76
  mental health 81–2, 86, 172–6, 179
  nurses 200–2
  women's health needs 176–7
migration
  and health 165–9, 176–7
  and older people 150–4
  periods of adjustment 166
  pull factors 153, 165
  push factors 153, 165
mind-body connection 88
modesty 51, 139, 146, 147, 195, 216
Mohammed 50, 217
mosques 50, 195
motherhood 100, 104–5
  see also child and family centred

care; childbirth; pregnancy
mourning 78, 187–8
multiculturalism 3, 61–3
  and death and bereavement 195,
    197
  male health care issues 116–30
  multicultural education 206–8
  and women's health care 99–115
multidisciplinary approach 207
Muslims see Islam and the Muslim
    Faith

Namibia 119
naming systems 54, 65–6, 139–40,
    217, 220–1
National Association of Health
    Authorities and Trusts
    (NAHAT) 43–4
National Health Service (NHS) 1
  black and ethnic minority nurses
    200–4, 211
  Trusts 1, 43–4, 195, 202
National Review of Nursing
    Education 3
naturalistic systems 22–4, 29, 41
Navaho Indians 28
needs
  emotional health 180–1
  levels of 68
  religious and cultural of staff 60
  women's 105–7, 176–7
Nepal 119
New Zealand Nursing Council 59
Nigeria 20
non-compliance 158
normality
  concepts of 78–80
  as value judgement 79
norms
  cultural 5, 132
  and health beliefs 18
  social 99
  traditional masculine 127
nudity 51, 139, 195
nursing culture 5, 6, 8–9, 38
  and death and bereavement
    188–91
  and health beliefs 17–18
nursing homes 209
nursing language 17–18, 38
Nursing and Midwifery Council
    (NMC), professional code 2,
    58–9, 75, 197
nursing practice
  death 188–97
  and health beliefs 17–18
  and superstition 35–6
  see also professional practice, and
    cultural diversity
Nursing Standard 202

obeah curse 82
obesity 126
older people 150–63, 209
    alternative explanations of
        behaviour 160
    demography 151
    health beliefs 157–8
    health and illness patterns 159–60
    marginalization 151
    migration 150–4
    myths and stereotypes 155–7
    service development 160–2
    treated as 'exotic' specimens 160
    triple jeopardy theory 155
organ donation/transplantation 186,
    193, 213
organizational culture 5, 6, 7–8,
    195–7
osteomalacia 159
'otherness' 208

pain management 193, 194
pain relief, refusal 66
Pakistani people/culture 50, 74, 100,
    107, 109, 120, 136
Papadopoulos, Tilki and Taylor's
    model of developing cultural
    competence 72
Paros 151
Pathans 135–6
Patients' Charter Standard 1, 55, 60
persecution 152
personal space 69
personalistic systems 19–21, 29, 35,
    41
pitta (dosa/humour) 24
play 140–1
pluralism, health care 32–41
police 84, 85, 199
Policy Studies Institute (PSI) 202
Polish people/culture 152, 156, 161–2
pollution taboos 55, 63–4, 215
popular/lay health sector 24–7, 34–5
post-mortem care 189–90, 192, 220
post-mortems 193, 213, 218
post-traumatic stress disorder
    (PTSD) 173–4
postnatal care 23, 25
poverty 159, 171, 173
power imbalances 90, 93
prayer 47, 50–1, 55, 195, 213, 217
    call to (adhan) 52
pregnancy 51, 106, 177, 178
    termination of 46, 49, 177
prejudice 90, 96, 142, 151, 154, 201,
    211
primary care 29
privacy issues 107–8
professional health care sector 29
    see also biomedicine

professional practice, and cultural
    diversity 199–212
    cultural competence 206–10
    equal opportunities 202–3
    history of black and ethnic
        minority nurses in the NHS
        200–2
    recruitment 203–5
    see also nursing practice
prostate cancer 125
prostatectomy 53–5, 65
psychiatric labels 174
psychiatry, transcultural 80–2
psychological distress 78
'public zone' 69
Punjabi culture 64
Purnell's model of cultural
    competence 70–1
Purves, Rosie 202

Qur'an 9, 26, 50, 51, 101, 106, 110, 139,
    195, 217, 218

race 12–14
    conflict theories 10
    consensus theories 10
    data 12
    meaning of 1, 3, 4, 9–11
    and mental health diagnosis 80, 81,
        84–5
race equality teachers 210
Race Relations (Amendment) Act
    2000 199
racial superiority 80–1, 93, 141
racism 10
    and child and family centred care
        141–2
    direct/overt 201, 211
    'I'm not racist but...' attitude 10–11
    indirect/covert 201, 202, 211
    individual 10
    institutional 10, 199, 202, 206, 209,
        211
    and mental health 81, 85, 92–6, 96
    and nurse education 209–10
    in nursing 199, 200–4, 206, 209–11
Ramadan 51, 137, 217
rape 177
rapport 40
rectal examinations 158
reductionism 29
refugee camps 169, 171, 178
Refugee Convention 1951 166–7
refugees 72, 82, 128, 152, 165, 166–84
    children and young people's health
        177–82
    death and bereavement 188
    health care 169–72
    image 167–8
    mental health issues 172–6, 179

mental/physical trauma 169, 170,
    171–6, 177, 179, 180
    numbers 167
    women's health 176–7
reincarnation 215
religious adornments 139
religious beliefs 43–56, 60, 213–21
    Buddhism 214–15
    Christianity 46–9, 213
    and death and bereavement 191–2
    and health care practice 45–55,
        213–21
    Hinduism 52–5, 215–17
    Islam 49–52, 217–18
    Jehovah's Witnesses 45–6
    Judaism 218–19
    Sikhism 219–21
    and spirituality 43–4
religious fundamentalism 94–5
respect 85
rickets 144
risk *see* health risk behaviours
rites of passage 186
rituals
    death 186–7, 189–90, 213, 215
    professional 5
road traffic accidents 45–6
Roman Catholicism 26, 46–9, 213
Roper, Logan and Tierney's model of
    nursing 73–5
Royal College of Nursing (RCN) 7,
    110, 201, 211
    annual conferences 199
Rwanda 166

same sex unions 117
saunas 17
schizophrenia 80, 81, 84–5, 86, 92
schooling 179
    exclusion from 180
Seacole, Mary 200
selection hypothesis 81
self-determination 34
self-harm 81, 86
self-help groups 27
sex education 119
sexual health
    female migrants 176–7
    male 125, 126
sexuality 75
shaman 20–1
shared care 144–5
shinkeishitsu 83
Shiva (Hindu God) 52, 215
sickle-cell anaemia 144
Sikhism 8, 64, 127
    beliefs and practices summary
        219–21
    child and family centred care
        138–40

and death and bereavement 193–4, 220
  five signs of 193–4, 219–20
  naming system 140, 220–1
Sitala Satam 102
skills, for cultural care 58–76
slavery 80
smoking 33, 126–7
social norms 99
social organization 69
social time 69–70
socialization 4
Somalian people/culture 110, 142
somatization 87–9, 175, 177
sorcery 20
South Asian people/culture
  death and bereavement 188
  diet 138
  dress 139
  mental health issues 90, 93–4
  and nursing as a career 205
  older people 159
  women 81, 86, 87–8, 100–1
space 69
spirit possession 83
spirituality 43–4
State Enrolled Nurses (SENs) 200, 204
State Registered Nurses (SRNs) 200
status
  of nursing 8–9, 103, 203, 204
  of women 103, 109
stereotypes 18
  of Asian women 110–11
  cultural 62, 64, 207
  of dangerousness 92
  of extended family support 100, 104
  gender 110–11, 121
  of 'normal families' 132
  of nursing 203–4
  of older people 155–7
  racial 85–8, 92–3, 211
sterilization 46, 49
stigma
  of mental health problems 174, 175, 181
  of sexual violence 177
stoicism 14stress hypothesis 81
stroke 126
student nurses 3, 100–1
  cultural competence 206–10
  and death and bereavement 188–9, 197
  and institutional racism 200–1
substance abuse 127
suffering 214
suicide 81, 86, 109, 124, 186
sun-tans 17
'Sunrise' model 67

supernatural forces, health beliefs based on 19–21, 28, 112
superstition 35–6, 41, 82–3
  regarding death 189, 190
susto 82–3
swaddling 136
Swedish people 125

taboos
  death 189
  mental health problems 174, 175
  pollution 55, 63–4, 215
  rectal examinations 158
Taoism 66
terminal illness 193–5
termination of pregnancy 46, 49, 177
testicular cancer 128
thalassaemia 144
'them and us' cultures 209
therapeutic relationship, power imbalances 90, 93
Tibetan refugees 73
time 69–70
torture 169, 171–2, 179, 180
traditional Chinese medicine 22–3, 33–4, 41, 66, 94
transcultural nursing care (TCN) 61–3, 67–9, 72–3, 96, 206–9
transcultural psychiatry 80–2
transcultural therapy and counselling 93
transformationist approach 208
transmissionist approach 208
triple jeopardy theory 155
Turkey 122

ulcer, leg 65–6
unaccompanied minors 179–80
undernutrition 178
unit approach 207
United Kingdom Central Council for Nursing, Midwifery and Health Visiting (UKCC), 1992 Code of Professional Practice 1–2, 58
Untouchables 53, 216
urinary catheters 55

Vaids 33
value judgements 79
values, cultural 2, 4, 5, 69, 132, 135
  regarding child-rearing practices 135
  respect for 2
vata 24
Vietnamese Americans 70
Vietnamese culture/people 112, 136
Vishnu 52, 215
visiting rules 158
vitamin D deficiency 144, 159
voluntary organizations 27

Voodoo 20

washing
  pollution taboos 63–4, 215
  ritual 50–1, 54, 63–4, 145, 215, 216, 217
weight loss 13–14
Western medicine see biomedicine
Westernization 133
white superiority 80–1, 93, 141
'wild man' syndrome 83
witchcraft 20
women
  as carers 102–5
  and cultural beliefs 109–13
  and the family 133–4
  and health care in a multicultural society 99–115
  migrants, refugees and asylum seekers 176–7
  needs of 105–7, 176–7
  nurses 8, 99, 102–3
  as primary breadwinners 99, 102
  and privacy and dignity 107–8
  role in society 99–102, 109–13
  working 99, 102–4
work, denial of the right to 173
working in partnership 144–5
World Health Organization (WHO) 110, 174
written information 7

yin and yang 22–3, 66, 94
Yoruba people 20
Yugoslavian migrants 37

zar 83